Victo...

Hy...

Mad in England - A memoir

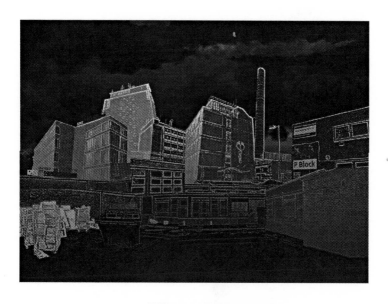

Victor J Kennedy

Over one million people each year commit suicide
- World Health organization

Mad in England - A memoir

Published by:
Chipmunkapublishing Ltd
PO Box 6872
Brentwood
Essex
CM13 1ZT
United Kingdom

http://www.chipmunkapublishing.com

Chipmunkapublishing is dedicated to raising awareness of all mental health issues and facts

Victor J Kennedy

Introduction

It's six months before my ten year anniversary and I'm just putting pen to paper now. I've waited until the time felt right to do it although I've had my chances to begin, like in 1997 when I designed all the covers while working as a junior designer for my old boss Reggie. It was going to be a best seller, I was going to be famed for such a groundbreaking book, not to mention its trendy jacket. But I never started writing because I wasn't well. I was Hypomanic.

What is Hypomanic? Well, for a start it's not a club night or a compilation album by The Ministry of Sound but it sounds pretty cool, if like me in 1997 you'd spent the first half of that decade experimenting with recreational drugs. Even without controlled substances, it's still possible to experience the state of Hypomania through stress.

Early Hypomania can be a pleasurable state of elevated mood, elation, optimism and confidence. Treatment at this stage is usually not desired or even necessary. For some, in early hypomania what they experience may be irritability, rapid thoughts which cause confusion and sudden angry outbursts. This state can cause problems in relationships, not only personal, but social and work-related relationships as well.

If undetected a Hypomanic episode will continue its increasing velocity into full blown Mania. More about that later.

One of the many reasons I wanted to write this book is because of my lack of understanding that at 23 led to my losing the second half of the nineties, not to mention my mind. If this book ever makes it onto a library shelf in a university campus and therefore by association into a student's hand, then they may avoid treading the same destructive path as I have since 1995.

If you have seen the film Back to the Future, in Doctor Emmett's 1955 Hill Valley garage, he draws Marty McFly a diagram on a chalk board. His theory was that if anything should be altered in 1955, an alternate reality would be waiting for Marty, should he return to 1985. Doctor Emmett drew a straight line, representing an unaltered timeline of Marty's life, his past, his present and his future. How it was meant to be. Then the Doc split a line off the original timeline, like a fork in the road at 1955 and drew a parallel line representing the new reality waiting in 1985. What on earth would Marty return to in that new reality?

In 1995 my old reality ended and I am now living in the new one with a new destination and an entirely different outcome. I often have mixed feelings about what happened in 1995 and in the paradigm I've just created, I wonder in hindsight at the grass back over on the other side of the fence, on that other reality which I split and broke away from on February 19th 1995. What did I lose, what have I gained? It's heartbreaking wasting time thinking about it but I can't help myself. Here I am, with this diagnosis, a label, in an alternate reality feeling always the defective human being but with a special power which cannot always be hidden or disguised but is forever mysterious to those who don't understand due to its volatility.

Being mysterious can be equally as threatening as it is attractive. When I was first introduced to the term by a psychiatric team who were assessing my state of mind, I interpreted their voices in the phonetic sense and my internal dictionary spelt Hyper Manic Episode. I'd been called 'hyper' before, obviously slang for hyperactive. I was a quiet child but I guess we've all been called 'hyper' at some point in our lives. In England it is a term of endearment. It can be delivered to a small child as an order to calm down. This of course after the child has been encouraged to eat sweets and fizzy drinks full of E numbers. That kind of discipline can confuse a young mind because the high, that accelerated state, is chased by all of us from the moment we're conscious of it. We call it happiness.

I think, I became conscious sometime in 1975. Of course this is some estimation based on my first memories, not necessarily which image first blessed my retina as a three-year-old kid from Bradford. I've always had a reputation for over articulation and description of dreams. I'd run down in the morning and choke on corn flakes getting it all out. I don't particularly have the subconscious mind traffic I had as a young boy growing, although I do still dream. What I'm getting at, is that around the time that ABBA's Dancing Queen was number one, I was being visited by some extraordinary visions in my bed when I was awake! I was so young I could only label them 'monsters' and run into my parents bedroom crying because I was so petrified. Whether I was seeing them or they were visiting me is an argument. However, at five years old, I saw things which were not of my perceived reality and moved out of the wallpaper towards me in my little bed until I could take no more and made a hurried dash for my loving parents.

Maybe this means I had all this in me back then, just waiting for the right conditions to blow up, like a time-bomb ticking towards 1995. The bottom line is, they come back. Whoever they are, be it death or some kind of demons, I have experimented in bed while everyone else is asleep, in darkness and I can access it on demand now. The thing is, when it comes it's always the same, it terrifies me. It's going to get me one day.

This is a true story. My truth. My point of view. If you talked to everyone else who was there in 1995, you would get many other truths but this one is mine. This is how I saw it.

Chapter 1 - Leaving Home

It was the end of a very long summer and I'd just got back from a 'mad one' in Benalmadena on the Costa Del Sol. All my long hair had been cut off during that intense week away with the lads. They told me I looked like a Bosnian refugee and I thought that was a great label, a good ice breaker, because deep down I knew I looked awful. What had they done? Not only was I devastated at my Samson like transformation but just before we'd flown out for a debauched, lager fuelled 'holiday' me and Faye had ended a two-and a half-year relationship. She was taking a year out in Paris after her A levels and I was going to university in London to study Graphic Information Design. To separate made sense but that didn't make it easy. She was my first love. The night we split up finished at 3am, after sitting on my single bed since the late afternoon, holding each other and crying. The next morning she was on a flight to France and a week later I joined my mates - the painters, carpet fitters and builders - on a last minute flight to Spain.
I now weighed about ten stone, give or take a few pounds. Seven days previously I was ten and a half but match fit. I'd done a full pre-season with Millhead Crusaders, my local football team, played in all the friendlies and the first couple of games of the north Lancashire league before this holiday came up as a drunken suggestion down the pub. I wished I'd never gone. That holiday went down in folklore and the stories that came back still do the rounds. "What goes on tour, stays on tour", but it didn't stay on tour. On the flight back to Manchester I'd got some weird bladder 'thing' hurting me at 35,000 feet and the morning after we got back I asked my mum to take me to casualty. My mum has worked most of her life in the X-Ray Department, starting in Bradford Royal Infirmary during the sixties before I was born. She knows everyone in the hospital so it was great if you ever got hurt at school or injured playing football. All the other people in the waiting room staring angrily as you

jumped the queue. The current staff knew me at the Westmorland General as well, not only from various accidents and scrapes I'd picked up since we moved to Millhead in '88 but also from hanging around waiting for my mum to finish work.

My mum got me straight through into a back room with Maureen, a large middle aged nurse who obviously had a son my age. She asked me loads of embarrassing questions while my mum waited outside. Turns out I'd 'acquired' non-specific urethritis, a sexually transmitted disease. Maureen was professional but I knew she'd tell my mum over a cup of tea or a fag break. Boys will be boys. However, the really dark bit hit me when Maureen said I had been really stupid putting my life at risk by not only behaving in such a hedonistic manner but also for not using any protection. I was told I would have to return in three months at Christmas for a HIV test. When I asked why three months and not now, she said it would take that long for the virus to grow and therefore appear in a test. Grow?

What sort of a freshers week was I going to have? Then I started to think wider and longer, making projections and scenarios. My life had only just begun. I wished I hadn't gone on that holiday.

All this was not particularly good preparation for moving 250 miles south of Cumbria, away from my family and new friends, not to mention my culture. My dad moved the family to Millhead in 1988 for his job in Kendal, I'd grown up in a city, back in Bradford stealing cars, robbing supermarkets and dossing around with my fellow Yorkshire urchins but after four years living out a Hucklebury Finn lifestyle in the Lake District with the builders and joiners, London was inevitably going to hurt. Especially as this was the start of something big. I was going to be successful now I'd finally been accepted on a university degree course. I was going to have B.A.(Hons) written after my name, you know. I'd been rejected from many universities in the past two years including Leeds, Edinburgh, Nottingham and my

Victor J Kennedy

beloved Manchester. I wanted to be in Manchester in 1989 because of The Stone Roses and The Happy Mondays. A stupid reason to choose a Graphic Design course but I wasn't interested in studying at 17 and I shouldn't have been applying anyway without a Foundation course behind me. The studying would be a side show to the main attraction, just being in 'MAD'chester amongst it, as it happened, as everything unfolded - history. I know now that's all perception and that particular desire was based on chasing and exploring drugs. I hadn't taken drugs at 17, the first time I took anything was after finally being accepted on my Foundation Course in Carlisle. I was 19 and it was winter time, very dark and very cold. The night was branded Phobia and Altern-8 were supposed to be playing but had not turned up, so the people organizing the 'legal' sports centre rave had drafted in The Prodigy. Me and my student friends scored from a dealer in Chapeltown, Leeds the previous week. He had a gun on the bar beside him while he counted the money before handing over about 50 ecstasy tablets, so I am told. Up and down the queue, everyone got one, "got sorted". I was frightened to death when I felt it pass through my throat and into my belly. I knew I could never go back, never be innocent and clean again. I was now a drug taker, no longer a sportsman. I could only ever be a reformed drug taker in the future, that's if that pill didn't kill me first.

I got in without a search, started dancing and sniffing Vicks and sticking my thumbs up at people, just because everyone else was doing it. After about 20 minutes, during something like Gat Decor's Passion, I came up. It was pretty cool. Bollocks, it was fucking amazing! I didn't need to be in Manchester. It was all in my head now. I was there, making history.

Obviously, as Pete Tong once told us, we continued. We continued taking ecstasy, speed, LSD and smoking spliffs right through Christmas into the new year until we finished the course in June. Then we went home, back to our loving parents for the longest ever summer break of our lives.

Mad in England - A memoir

I ended up in London by accident. The Graphic Information Design degree course in Harrow was my second choice. Nottingham was my preferred place as well as my preferred Graphic Design course. It had a very good reputation for producing talent. It became my preferred place after myself and three student friends had visited all the prospective courses and venues over two weeks in March to help us make a considered decision. It was a full-on tour. Nottingham was unbelievable. A clean city, everyone was friendly, especially the girls on the campus and 'there were five women to every man'. We went to London and visited all the 'trendy' places - like Central Saint Martins - which I thought were full of shit at the time but I think that was the WCN working class northerner in me. When we visited Harrow, everyone started laughing, me included. None of us could understand the course itself, Graphic Information Design? Apparently GID not only deals with the fashionable, decorative and pleasing aspect of Graphic Design but places emphasis on the importance of the user of the designed material and the information that person needs to decode. Phew! The campus was the funniest. As you got off the tube at Northwick Park Station you could see this monstrosity in front of you, which reminded me of my school teaching block. Buttershaw Upper Comprehensive in Bradford was portrayed as the school in the film Rita, Sue & Bob too. If you've seen the film you'll understand me when I say the words shit hole.

The University of Westminster had become the new name for The Polytechnic of Central London, which in turn had acquired Harrow Technical College and 'transformed' it into it's media campus. Anyway, it looked rubbish so I put it down for a laugh on my forms as my second choice because I was convinced I would be accepted at Nottingham. That one single decision of mine, changed the course of my life. Not only the course changed from design for print to design for screen (with the imminent commercial birth of the internet) but also the new friends I would be meeting when I got there. The people I would be thrown together with were not going to be in Nottingham, they were going to be in London and therefore they would be very different animals. That is, if you based your preconceptions similarly to Dick Whittington's reports that the streets were paved with gold. I was in London by accident, I didn't go after any golden streets. I was supposed to be in Nottingham.

My dad was helping my weak 10 stone frame pack up a Volkswagon Passat Estate throughout that Saturday morning in September. The day I left home.

It wasn't his car. He had borrowed it from his business partner's wife. It was her car, their second car and it was massive. I had my drawing board strapped to it's roof, which Reggie had very kindly donated as a thank you. Reggie was my boss, my father figure, apart from my dad of course. Reggie always sorted me out a job, always as a junior. He also thought I looked like a Bosnian refugee with my short hair. I had spent the most of that summer at Reggie's, spray mounting artwork for the Cumbria Tourist Board Guide and spending hours shooting it in a darkroom with a reprographic camera. It was very 'old school' graphics and very hard work.

My dad, my real father figure, was doing his usual stressed out dad thing. It was his idea for me to drive the Passat for the first initial 250 miles down the M6 and M1. We were coming off at Junction 5 and negotiating the last part through undiscovered country from Watford to Harrow on the A41, something he had never done. Then after his relaxing five hours in the passenger seat, we would unpack this lot into my £50 a week bedsit in Roxborough Road. He would then get straight back into the drivers seat for another five hours back north to junction 36 of the M6. It was all planned with military precision. That was my dad. It still is today, even in his sixties.

He'd set a deadline of 9am to get going and it was looking like we might miss it, only by five minutes or so but that was pissing him off no end. He had ten hours in a car ahead of

him and nothing was going to stop him making last orders at
the Cross Keys tonight when he got back for that satisfying
pint of bitter. I could feel his stress without him saying a
word. It's always been like that since I was a little boy. He
never hit me or my sister, well he did once or twice but it
was deserved. The point is, he never ruled with violence, just
the promise of it. Either in his voice or his eyes. That was
always much more frightening. My mum used to go out
every Thursday with the girls back in Bradford. When the
Panorama theme tune came on the telly he would click his
fingers and point to the ceiling and say "bed"!
Immediately me and my sister would get out of our seats,
without saying a word and go to bed, no questions.
Don't get me wrong my dad was a right laugh most of the
time but I was always scared of him, until I became as big as
him but we'll come back to that later.
The night before, I told my mum over a cup of tea and
biscuits that I'd been having dreams about dying. Probably
all the subconscious worry about the HIV test that was
before me at Christmas on my return. Lying on her lap while
she stroked my hair, I said I had a feeling I was going to die
and I couldn't explain it. She dismissed it and told me to stop
worrying, it'd all be okay. I never told her anything about the
hospital with her friend Maureen. My mum knew I was on
antibiotics but I presumed, no, actually I hoped she thought
it was just a bladder infection from drinking too much, or
whatever. I didn't like to think my mum thought of me as a
wrong 'un. I wanted to always be her little boy. The baby, as
she referred to me being two years younger than my sister.
Obviously I had not told her anything about the drugs in
Carlisle either. She would have been devastated. But that
was all to come out later.
I kissed her and gave her a massive hug, I got in the car
having previously tuned in Radio 1, which I thought was a
safe bet after packing all my C90 tapes in a box.
In reality, I had to settle for the odd decent track to emerge
from a deluge of Maria Carey, Right Said Fred, Boys II Men

and Technotronic. You know how it is, the one in Radio 1 stands for one decent record all day. The old man wanted sport on, or at least male voices talking bollocks and stating amazing facts or batting statistics from the end of the cricket season. The overhead signs flashed by; Preston, Manchester, Warrington, Knutsford until eventually the beast that is Birmingham loomed large with it's RAC centre. I did think to myself, how did they ever respond quickly from that base? Traffic crawled and progress was slow. On a good day, you could do the 250 miles from London to Millhead in four hours before speed cameras were invented. Our delay upset my dad. His estimations were out. How was he going to make up the lost time and get his pint? Not my problem. I put Radio 1 back on just to annoy him further.

Driving such mammoth distances mean invariably your passenger drops off with boredom. Not my dad. Mind you, he'd just go quiet and not say owt, which would make me nervous like a ten year old again. What is he thinking? Is my driving shite, am I too close to the driver in front, am I too fast? It's all bollocks because my old man taught me to drive anyway. He taught me everything. I AM my dad! He did a right job on me all my life. A good job. However, I didn't have that opinion in 1992 driving south that day. He was doing my head in and I couldn't wait to get there and get rid. Start my new life without the chains. Freedom! Do what I please. Harrow did not know what was going to hit it. And over the next three years, I didn't know what was going to hit me either.

After careful negotiation of the A41 we approached the built up areas of Wealdstone and yet more traffic. The weather down here was much warmer and the sunshine made us both pull down our visors to avoid getting blinded. This bit was the most excruciating part because we were so near, yet so far. Stuck in London traffic, crawling along at a snail's pace as the interior of the Passat became unbearably hot. We attempted to wind down the windows. It was the first time we had actually tried to do this in over six hours since leaving Cumbria but the winder mechanism turned out to be unconnected to the windows. They were both fucked! I could not believe it and my dad's eyes rolled back like a Great White as it sinks it's teeth in. We got the sun roof open and the genius that is my dad, kept opening his door when the vehicle stopped – which was quite often in London traffic. The engine was so hot the fan just blew warm air in. I couldn't afford to lose anymore weight at 10 stone but I'm sure the last two miles I dropped a further couple of pounds in sweat but we made it. I'd arrived!

We parked outside the bedsit and rang Katie's bell, number eleven. She was the scottish fashion student I studied with on foundation in Carlisle the previous year. Her aunt who lives nearby, sorted these two rooms for us both. I gave number nine (Ian Rush) a buzz too, that would be my room in about three minutes time. She came running down all excited screaming and kissing and hugging me and my dad, she was going right over the top and I was getting a bit nervous and apprehensive instantly. Had I made the right decision living here instead of the halls of residence? Only time would tell.

Victor J Kennedy

Chapter 2 - New Arrival

Because I was travelling from so far away and based on my old man's tiny income, plus the fact he already had to fork out for my sister at Newcastle Polytechnic, I got accepted into the halls of residence on Marylebone Road near Baker Street. I had decided to turn it down on the basis of Katie's financial advice, which turned out to be an influence I will always be grateful for, mainly because I avoided more hedonism. Halls are shocking and I consider myself fucking liberal.

Katie guaranteed I would save "soooo much money" by living in a £50 a week bedsit next door to her near Harrow-on-the-Hill, which her 'southern' based auntie knew all about. Harrow was a bit of a dive but Harrow-on-the-Hill was posh, they even have a boys public school, kind of like a poor man's Eton. David Ellery, the Premiership Referee, was a teacher there, I didn't give a shit or know about any other 'old boys' just that the grounds had graffiti chipped into the bricks dating back to the Nineteenth Century, unless some of the current crop of little bleeders were putting false "I woz ere" messages. My bedsit was on Roxborough Road, half way between Harrow and Harrow-on-the-Hill. The bedsit was not posh.

Katie was Scottish from just the wrong side of Carlisle and like myself did her Foundation Course at the Art & Design College. She used to go out with my mate Wes but he was now in Edinburgh. She was coming to London to be a famous fashion designer, at least that was the impression I got. She would be trained in the same stable as Vivien Westwood, Harrow Fashion BA (Hons). Katie wasn't concerned about the naff architecture of the campus. As long as she looked great nothing else mattered. I had never lived away from my parents and I certainly had never experienced living in such close quarters to a girl. My sister didn't count. She was never like this. What I mean is, Katie was away from home too. My view of my sister was always under my dad's roof so I never saw her misbehaviour. My sister was not a fashion student either so that was probably why living with Katie opened my eyes. I was seeing and learning all about the stuff you don't see behind closed doors. Pressure, expectation, aggression and insecurity.

Like I said before, I was in London by accident and therefore no thoughts of strategy on Harrow campus had occupied my head since I got accepted. My head was up my arse about the HIV and AIDS which I could have caught in Benalmadena but I didn't tell Katie that, I didn't tell anyone apart from Dean the surfer friend from Devon I was soon to meet.

After one of those uncomfortable father-son hugs my dad left for Cumbria in the Passat with no windows, Katie and I agreed to swap spare keys to each other's bedsits, just in case we lost our keys when we were pissed up or whatever. It seemed like a good idea until lectures started. About a week later Katie turned into my alarm clock. For five days a week, she would knock twice on my door at six a.m. and then let herself in. At first I was startled, almost intimidated but by October I got so used to it happening that Katie would have to physically shake me before starting her fashion show ritual, her strategy on Harrow campus. She only needed my male eyes and my male opinion but it was never about snaring a guy from college. She was there to study but she wanted to look fabulous, darling! I got the impression she was dressing more for the other girls on her course, even though about 35 per cent of her course were gay blokes. This is what I meant by the pressure, expectation, aggression and insecurity. I was dreading the tantrums and tears if all the other girls on Katie's course were adopting a similar fashion strategy to stand out and get noticed by peers and tutors. Not to mention the multiple outfit cat walk extravaganzas to their flat mate from six in the morning, three and a half hours before you even have to be at college. I'm not going into hair and make up too, there are too many combinations but yeah, you look good in that, can I go back to sleep now?

Victor J Kennedy

I devised a strategy to get through the Graphic Information Design course but it wasn't based around external appearance. I just knew I was going to be the best. Sounds arrogant but I had the dedication and the drive to work harder and unfortunately for me in the coming years, longer than anyone else. My Foundation course tutor told all of us before applying for uni that, you have to understand if you're in a pub or a club getting off your face, there is another student somewhere who is studying hard on their portfolio and they will take your place. I knew all those swatty, boring, spods were at Nottingham now, enjoying five women to every man. So I decided that kind of failure was not going to happen down here in London. Not on my course.

Katie and me went out round Harrow for the couple of nights before college and discovered Trinity. It was a gothic themed bar with over elaborated dripping candles, dark corners and a dodgy first floor that bowed when the place was full and the crowd were 'jumping around' to The House of Pain. The manager freaked out when the DJ played tracks like that probably because with a full house, the floor might give way. There was also some pikey bloke who looked like Swampy, the tunnel activist might have looked, had he ever come out of the ground for a Socialist Worker magazine shoot - a quintessential white rasta with dreadlocks and a beer belly who was ten years past it. He had a right cockney accent and used to shout at us after last orders, "Get 'em down your Gregory Pecks and get out!"

Trinity would turn out to be the 'cool' place to go after the student union bar was either drank dry or closed because of some sort of unsavory altercation involving drugs, sex or fighting.

First day at college was obviously bizarre and just full. It was the 28th September 1992, the first day of a twelve week term until we broke for Christmas on the 18th December. In the coming years we would go all American and three terms would be abolished in favour of two long semesters which broke in February. The first time this actually happened would turn out to be in my third and final year in 1995.

I remember on the Monday morning getting up and listening to Sting's 'If I Ever Lose My Faith In You'. Sounds shit I know but I liked the track and spray mounting for Reggie and his cronies over the summer had introduced me to much of Sting's solo back catalogue. However, this single was currently in the charts. I was listening to it on a Sony Walkman which my dad bought me as a birthday 'stroke christmas' present a couple of years back. The 'stroke christmas' present singular, is one of the draw backs of being born on the 13th January. To be fair, what he purchased was shit hot and I had full respect for my dad, although I know he just walked into Dixons and said in his best Brian Clough voice, "Young man, give me the best bloody Walkman you've got in the shop." and before the lad could reply, my dad would interrupt, "I don't care what it costs just get me the best one. Now!"

To get to college me and Katie had to walk across an open park area off the hill where people walked their dogs, a fucking mine field at night coming home, especially when you were blathered. She's got her hair in Princess Leia buns and I'm bopping along next to her with a Bosnian skinhead, my best jeans and trainers on and Sting in my ears doing his Stevie Wonder mouth organ tribute. What a strange couple we must have looked. She made me take off my headphones when we got to the traffic lights as there were other students appearing from alleyways and street corners the closer we got towards the front entrance. I naturally started sharking. I am a man after all. There were a few potentials but for one, I could have AIDS and for another, I could bet everyone assumed I was with Katie so I had no chance anyway. I was happy with the arrangement but only until the 18th December, then I was up to Lancaster hospital for a blood test in between playing the returning son.

We queued together to register and pick up the student union cards, then onto the Grants section for the bad news, which for me turned out to be good news. 'This award is based on accommodation in Hall/Lodging and will be paid in termly instalments of: £1,117.02.' Why bother putting 2p on the end of it?

I took my cheque and said "Ciao, darling!" to Katie with the proviso we meet back at the refectory before either of us went home. She went off to the Fashion and Illustration block and I in the opposite direction (and strutted like a cat) to the Graphic Information Design studio below the Library on the ground floor. When I slid through the door, cool as you like, I walked into a free for all. The tutors had not turned up yet but left a note on the door that we should choose a desk we would like to sit in and they'd be back a.s.a.p. Because I am cool, I chose the desk at the back of the class by the window so I could check the skirt making it's way to the library. I sat down next to Alan, the greatest comedy mind I've ever had the pleasure of working alongside but he looked like a Goth to me, all in black. I moved away nearer Carl. Carl had long blond hair and the total skater look off to a tee. Loved his BMX, loved his music and loved his dancing. I called himed Twinkle Toes because he could dance round defenders on a football pitch too. Me and him caned nearly every club in London in our first year, like a relentless project – one a week. I sat down right in the corner and opened the desk top to put my impressive collection of pens and pencils in but to my horror, someone else had dumped all their dirty, scummy belongings in there earlier and gone for a fag. As if he'd just read my last thought, this scarey looking bastard with a black goatee which the devil would've been proud of, comes back from his fag, or a fucking drug deal he'd just done, or perhaps a murder in the college bogs? I don't know and I don't care, I am just moving. Sorry for any inconvenience sir.

He was Rory. He was cool. Rory was the eldest in a very extraordinary family from Pinner. He was in his thirties. He was what is known as a mature student. He commuted to college every day on his £3,000 mountain bike until it got nicked. Not by me I might add.

I surveyed the room as I ran away from him, only joking, I walked away cool as you like. Everyone else on my course had either one eye, were over 40, looked like a murderer or had already become best mates and staring at me like I'd got one eye and had murdered someone. I got three quarters of the way across the room and looked at these two guys. I got an instant good feeling about them so I sat down and emptied my felt tips and protractors into the desk. These two were called Todd and Roy but before the first term had finished they had both left, which I took personally. Another guy sat down just after me. He must've had a good feeling about Bosian skinheaded-looking blokes. He was Jason, from Leicester a.k.a. Jase and he loved his Shamen so we really did get on, especially when they played Brixton Academy at the height of the Ebenezer Goode phenomenon but we liked the old stuff better. Jase always looked fucked. Knackered, bad skin, bloodshot eyes, the fucking lot! But I never saw him take any drugs and I'm not suggesting he did take any drugs, apart from Night Nurse and the occasional drop of Optrex for his gammy red eyes. I can only suggest this might have been something to do with the pressure from his Landlady in Wealdstone, who was a pensioner and lived on site, in the house with Jase! It's life Jase but not as we know it.

To my right was Dean and Diago being crazy surf dudes from Devon. I only thought they made custard in Devon but hey, there's only curry in Bradford, right? They already knew each other from Foundation course and were 'roomies' in halls in Baker Street but not for long. They were coming to Harrow.

I mentioned Dean earlier. I only confided in him about my pending HIV test because I needed the support and out of this lot, I only trusted him. The blonde surfer Dean Knight, to give him his full name, is one of the real gems you may meet in your life if you're lucky. He introduced me to spirituality, amongst many, many other positive mental attitudes and points of view about the world. I cannot speak highly enough of him, apart from his one claim of naming his first born daughter Summer. I guess it could've been worse, something like Frank Zappa's daughter's name Moon Unit doesn't fall off the tongue as easy as Summer Knight. To my left was Nath and Lewis. Nath Foreman was wearing a burgundy baseball cap and a mucky bomber jacket. He looked "Booley." "Booley" is short for Boulevarder, it means someone who lives on a council estate in Bradford. He smoked profusely, Lewis did too but only because Nath was plying him free 'baccy like a bear hunter setting traps. Lewis was so very cool looking but back then he wasn't cool at all, as it turned out.

I'm totally comfortable with my sexuality and I was back then but I kind of fancied Lewis. When I say kind of, I more like had an admiration for his most excellent appearance for the opposite sex to enjoy. If I could've instantly lost my Bosnian barnet and looked like anyone on that campus it would've been Lewis. I'm sure Nath was thinking the same, that's where the endless supply of ciggies came from. I would've easily destroyed over twenty women in the first term alone if I still had my long Jesus locks from before Benalmadena and that's exactly what Lewis did, while wearing Jesus beads round his neck and Jesus 501s, his Jesus goatee and the incredible Nike Hurache trainers to top the whole Jesus sandals thing off. The way he went about it was equally god like, he was so blessed by his looks it must've got boring for him. At some point throughout the first term I was getting extremely jealous as he was taking the girls I wanted, or maybe the girls were taking him. The handy thing about Lewis was he also came from Devon, over 200 miles away which automatically made him eligible for a place in halls of residence. The great thing about halls of residence was the distance of about ten miles from the Campus at Northwick Park Station to where they were near Baker Street on the Metropolitan line. Poor Lewis had to tube off

Mad in England - A memoir

home at the end of every day and leave me with all his
Harrow based ladies, who were now becoming great friends
with Katie, a social revenue stream Nath had also identified
and vocalised with me.

At the end of everyday Nath climbed into a metallic electric
blue Fiat Uno and drove back to "Watford, mate." which was
where Nath's Boulevard was and I was happy with that story.
Everything seemed to add up. Nothing awry there to report.
At the back of me and to my right was Jahan, Estella, Ravi,
and Jafit. In time they were to be known as "The Ethnics" a
name they adopted from Lewis and 'used' by everyone at our
end of the room who were included in the 'joke' which I
never understood. I'm born and bred in Bradford, I played
football at 10 years old with Hardeep Bhatt, the top scorer in
the Bradford Schools District League 1981/82 with over 100
goals. I played Basketball with Tayib, Ibrahim and Winston
in 1985 for Buttershaw Upper School. I was in the M.A.P.A.
boys Newby Celtic 5-a-side team which beat West Bowling
3-2 at Park Side Sports Centre in 1987 against Chris
Kiwomya, who ended up at Arsenal and QPR. I don't think
the politically correct term "Ethnic Minorities" existed until
the Nineties but either way, I felt that lot in the corner were
soft for putting up with that kind of reverse put down by a
middle class farm boy from Devon. If Lewis had labelled my
table "The Pigeon Fanciers" I would've punched his lights
out. As I got to know Jahan I found him to be a very
peaceful guy and I think that kind of edge is why that group
of three tables at the back adopted the name "The Ethnics"
because they could see Lewis differently to me at that time. I
know Jahan liked him and the three of us struck up quite a
heavy spliff habit later on outside the college bar. "Spliff"
was Lewis's nick-name, given to him by Nath. They called
me "Northern Exposure" after the Channel 4 Canadian cult
show. I thought I'd let them have that.

I cased the room when I'd sat down for some decent looking
women. Behind me, Jafit was always flashing a fantastic
smile but she had a boyfriend. Then there was Shumana, the

22

Victor J Kennedy

Liberian sex tease. She was so beautiful and innocent, which turned out to be a Venus fly trap thing and therefore she wasn't innocent at all, far from it. I had to try it on but she was having none of it. She didn't like me after that. Bizarrely enough she would comment on how dirty the insides of my ears were and would often bring in ear buds, inviting me, in front of everyone, onto her lap to rid her eyes of staring into my ears while a lecturer was in the room.

There were one or two other girls that fit within my 'Weird Science' erogenous mental setup at that time. Hermina was opposite me and struck up a girly friendship with Shumana instantly but unfortunately, left the course too early. She didn't like the lower classes though so I didn't stand a chance. Anthea, however, didn't mind, but she had a boyfriend too, which made sense because she had the most fantastic arse and regularly wore 501s for the lads.

At the other end of the class was Ruth McGregor. She was nice but very laddish, before the laddette was invented but she had that something you like in a potential girlfriend. She was very kind and struck up a huge friendship with Carl the skaterboy.

I have to mention Mauli at this point because he is intrinsic to this story, only because he was used and abused over the years by me and Nath like some kind of pawn. I have to take responsibility for my part in ruining some aspects of Mauli's degree and his three years in London before he went back to Malaysia for good. I've never heard from him since.

It was not coincidental, the diversity of that room's contents. There was a recruitment policy by Elena Fryer, the First Year Course Tutor. She was the daughter of the sweet giant Fryer's and she introduced me to and reminded me regularly of the importance of sexual equality. You should never refer to a ship as 'She!' It's just a ship. Not a woman!

As a group we had to lose all expectations of ability, sex, race and just get on with it. I hated that classroom at first. I wanted to go north to Manchester Metropolitan. London was great but I had my head on about being the best and these chumps were going to let me down. I also didn't get on with one of the other tutors, Eric Glaser, and he knew it. He wound me up about my 8pt text being illegible for pensioners. He gave me my worst mark of my degree by a country mile, with 57% for his Typolinguistics module. It still bugs me.

Each student had been given the first course brief by a University of Westminster letter during the summer, asking us to complete four pieces of work which represented our summer, or what the summer of '92 meant to us.

My traumas had turned into four detailed gouache paintings on different coloured A3 paper. The first titled 'Happy but Sad' was all about losing Faye and was cheese factor ten! It had images of me phoning her from a London phonebox and her reading my letters under the Eiffel Tower. I had no shame whatsoever.

Another had a headline of 'C is for Happy' with a brain amongst sums and mathematical symbols because that's what brains do, right? I'd retaken my GCSE Maths in Carlisle and got my result in August, hurrah! A deft and some what showy typographical trick on '2 Much to Drink' illustrated my crazy holiday in Benalmadena by showing my lost watch, broken sunglasses and drunken frolics at night, oh what fun. The last A3 was dark grey paper with black satanic scribblings of a guy in a hospital bed having his blood pressure checked. This was titled 'Afraid' and was a front for my current fears about HIV but I didn't tell my new classmates that. I made up a story about a bladder infection and that I'd spent some time in hospital over the summer having tests.

While we were putting this work up on the walls of the studio, it was evident that I had been very open about my feelings when others had just brought a few holiday snaps or evidence of a summer job in a factory.

After the first presentation, followed by a critique from the tutors, we had to encapsulate these pieces in some form of delivery mechanism which added another level of meaning

Victor J Kennedy

to an audience looking at it. Over the next few days I decided to recreate a Spray Mount bottle, which was the brand name for a glue used in paste up artwork, the verb of which is Spray Mounting and my summer working for Reggie was full of that. I used a three litre plastic Coke bottle, cut it open and sprayed it blue. Then I recreated the packaging look and feel but replaced the words Spray Mount with Summer Memories, do you see what I cleverly did there? After that, all four A3 posters were reduced down onto discs and were contained inside the two halves of the large plastic Spray Mount bottle ready for an audience. I even shot it with my SLR and tripod against an infinity background gradient to make it look even more handsome. Some of the other students made comments which could be taken either way, as a compliment or a slight against your attitude and dedication to perfection. This would become a recurring pattern throughout my degree. I'd gained an instant reputation and it stuck. I personally didn't think I'd "overdone it" in the slightest. The skills in Macintosh Software and hand finishing from practising professionals I had picked up at Goddard Murray Associates over the previous eighteen months before my Foundation Course were invaluable. It also meant I was eighteen months ahead of the people who took their A Levels instead of dropping out, like I did.

This created a problem for me in that the others, or at least ninety percent of the other students in my year could not compete with my standards. They didn't come up to scratch conceptually and their finishing skills were really poor, which was not their fault. At twenty years old I hadn't worked this out or even considered their point of view. None of these thoughts were vocalised although a natural hierarchy had established itself after the first brief.

We were told by Elena Fryer, to choose two student representatives for the first year who will sit in crisis meetings with the faculty staff every so often. It's an extra responsibility like being on the student union but without any tangible benefits. You basically represent your classmates' anger and disillusionment in the form of questions or requests to the powers that be. Then you bring the good or bad response back to your fellow students after the confrontation.

When Elena left the room we huddled together to decide first of all, who can be bothered to do it and secondly, if no one volunteers then who would we like to do it? Ok, no one stepped forward so a few names were thrown around and instantly the nominees stepped away from the plate until Jafit said yes, which everyone agreed was cool because she had so far come across as responsible. Then my name came up, which was flattering considering I had only just met them all so I said yes. Nobody objected, I checked their faces for twitching or grimacing, I couldn't see any and I became the second rep.

When Elena returned to find out who we had chosen I don't think she was very impressed due to the fact I winked at her, which is a social faux pas in her feminist world and she let me know that straight away in front of the whole class. It was really embarrassing and demeaning because my whole upbringing in Yorkshire taught me that a wink was affectionate and hardly offensive. After she had put me in my place Elena told us all to pack our pencil cases and go home.

My first day was over in the blink of an eye and we didn't do much else apart from sign things and queue up to sign more things. My bag was full of crappy forms and handouts with the lovely new University of Westminster logo emblazoned across everything. One of the handouts said there was a sports fayre coming up on Friday the 2nd October which I was looking forward to because there was of course a University football team to join.

I made it back to Katie on time, she was kissing and hugging lots of equally strangely dressed girls along with a few dodgy looking blokes who referred to everyone as 'sweetie'. They looked like they'd been mates forever. I looked like a

Victor J Kennedy

plank until she introduced me to them all. I had no chance of remembering their names but they all kissed and hugged me too so that was nice, well, apart from the men. This crowd were to become my social salvation and if it was not for living with Katie I would not have been accepted as quickly, if at all.

Once we had been introduced and said our goodbyes, me and Katie headed north, back to Roxborough Park and our fifty pound a week bedsits for a Pot Noodle and Eastenders.

Mad in England - A memoir

Chapter 3 - Settling In

A lot of my time in the bedsit was spent sat on this quite uncomfortable white high chair I bought from Argos. It was so cheap even the upholstery was in white PVC which made my arse sweat in those long hours perfecting my work for college on the large drawing board. It had a cracked parallel motion that Reggie had donated to me before I left his employment. The large open space of the drawing board was ideal for me, I could even balance the phone on it next to the single armchair which had been left by a previous tenant. Katie convinced me to open the phone line, which we would share but was in my name and of course British Telecom would come after me if it wasn't paid. I wasn't really keen on that idea but I wanted my mum to be able to ring me every Sunday as she had done in Carlisle the previous year. Apart from the armchair there were three other pieces of furniture; a tiny wardrobe with drawers inside, a sideboard from 1950 and of course, my single bed. With the drawing board taking up most of the floor space and the fact the door opened inwards created a problem. I wisely solved my space issue by putting my bed up against the kitchenette installed next to the window at the far side of the room, the sideboard became my bedside table and the wardrobe, with my portable TV on top welcomed you by the door, perfect! Obviously all the tenants in the building had to share the bathrooms on each floor, which I found horrendous so washed myself in my kitchen sink every morning to avoid the queues and embarrassing conversation on the stairs with a towel over my arm. They also didn't have a shower fitted which meant I would have to submerge myself in a bath shared by about fifteen other people who were bound to be hairy and probably masturbated in there anyway. I decided once I had joined the college football team most of my personal hygiene would get sorted in the showers after training or games. There was no washing machine in the whole building, which pissed me off even more when I took my

Victor J Kennedy

first black bin liner of washing to the 'local' launderette one
Sunday. It was so far away my shoulder nearly came out of
the socket. I would read the papers or write letters to friends
at better universities dotted around the country while I
serviced washed, tumble dried and then shrunk my clothes,
which were now pink or grey. The Gateway supermarket
was nearer than the launderette but only marginally, so I
tried to spread my shopping throughout the week to save my
arms. I developed an addiction to their frozen mincemeat
which was based on the fact that the packet fit neatly in the
freezer section of my dwarfed fridge which lived under the
kitchenette work surface back at my bedsit. This meant that I
could make the same 'Italian' dish everyday of the working
week using the five onions, five peppers, five sauces and the
huge packet of dried pasta. The one flaw in relying on frozen
mincemeat was the electricity meter, next to the wardrobe,
which was powered by fifty pence pieces. It seemed to last
three hours before my TV, fridge plus lights went off and
left me in darkness. Before salmonella could grip the
defrosting meat I would get down on my hands and knees,
fumbling around in the dark for the emergency spare fifty
pence coin I kept under the meter. If that failed I would have
to put on my jacket and pop down the petrol station at
midnight to buy something I didn't want just to get fifty
pence change.

While the lights were on and I wasn't cooking, sleeping or
working I would organise all the things I wanted to do now I
had moved to London. The first was to watch England play a
competitive match at Wembley, well I say competitive but
this was 1992 and Graham Taylor was the manager of
England – enough said. It was a shame that England were so
rubbish at that time because I definitely would've followed
them to USA'94 had we qualified. My first ever game as a
fan in the old stadium was witnessing a 1-1 draw with
Norway on Wednesday the 14th October. David Platt scored
for England and Rekdal, totally unmarked, replied for the
visitors. It was disappointing firstly, because we drew and

secondly, Paul Gascoigne wasn't playing due to injury and thirdly, because Wembley looked tiny to my naked eye. The TV pictures always made it look massive in all the FA Cup Finals, where some players got cramp due to the size of the pitch and the heat of course.

Wembley Park tube station was only three stops from Harrow-on-the-Hill on the Metropolitan line so I could also set off late to international games, arriving just as it kicked off, in time to pick up cheap tickets from the touts who had over subscribed and now needed to get rid sharpish.

Also being a northerner in London, another hallowed venue I wanted to put in my 'been there done that' portfolio was Top of the Pops. Well, not on it but in the crowd so I sent a polite letter to the BBC for instructions on how I would get tickets. They sent one back telling me the waiting list was now closed, please apply again in six months.

I wrote a lot of letters in the first few months just because, selfishly, I thought it would feel good getting replies. I had friends from Foundation course all over the country, plus my old mates from Bradford and the friends I'd made in South Lakeland. I had a pretty standardised approach but would personalise some with flyers I'd picked up in clothes shops to make it look like I was having a whale of a time. Most people sent letters back taking the piss out of my letter, some would even return the favour and send me flyers from their towns or cities. However, one mate who hadn't made it through clearing and was stuck at home with his mum for another year used to send me his replies inside sandwiches. Yes, posted through the front door and sitting on the mat, a battered and bruised homemade ham salad sarnie wrapped in cling film with a stamp on. Inside it a folded A4 rant about students not eating properly. Brilliant!

I made sure I got 'cool' now I lived in London after I found a discount offer for a twelve month subscription to ID magazine. It was a stupid idea as money was tight but I managed to rip off one or two outfits from it by using the excellent Flip in Covent Garden to mimic the look I saw in the magazine.

In my other spare moments inside the fifteen square feet of my bedsit I would meticulously plan my twenty first birthday which was arriving in January at a rate of knots. I contacted Maestros on Manningham Lane in Bradford, a club where I had breakdanced as a twelve year old nearly ten years before. I got about a hundred free tickets and a buy one get one free voucher for some cheap bubbly. I got in touch with Shaw Hadwin Transport to book a fiftytwo seater coach to integrate the friends from Millhead with the Bradford ones via the A65. I even started designing a flyer of my own with the headline "21. He's Made It! Now You Should Too." Another task in my initial weeks was to make sure I was registered with a doctor and dentist. The dentist was hassle-free but the doctor did a basic health check on me. I handed him a warm plastic jar of piss, he proceeded to dip litmus paper into, while he stared at it and sucked through his teeth. Not piss, air! He sucked air through his teeth like a builder or a mechanic does before he tells you it's gonna cost ya! He told me there were high levels of yeast in it and sent me down the GUM clinic (Genito-urinary medicine) for a test. The 'clinic' turned out to be next to college in Northwick Park Hospital which I found highly embarrassing when a guy called Gavin from my course was sitting in the waiting room and acknowledged me with a knowing Jedi nod of his head! Anyway, they did some horrible things to me involving Petri dishes and steel rods. Then took the piss (again). Within thirty minutes of the test a nurse took me into a private room and informed me I had NSU Non-specific urethritis, which is 'sort of' a sexually transmitted infection and could be cleared up with antibiotics, which they gave me as I left. The whole experience shit me up badly because I knew I'd picked that NSU up in Benalmadena which heightened my sensitivity to what I had to confront at Christmas when the three months incubation period was up. It made my mind up to stay away from any girls until the year passes and I got tested for HIV.

. . . but I could still go out.

After lots of promotion and posters around the campus, everyone from Katie's fashion crew and of course me, were ready to party at the freshers ball on Wednesday 7th October at The Ministry of Sound. The University of Westminster is huge and Harrow was just one campus The School of Design and Media but there were many others dotted around central London who would all be attending the ball. We had the choice of a long tube journey to Elephant & Castle with the mother of all taxi fares on the way home, that's if we even found a cab at 4am on a Thursday morning around the arse-end of Southwark east. Somebody didn't fancy it and had organized a lift in a dodgy builder's transit van which was filthy inside but about twenty five of us squeezed in, slammed the doors and sat in darkness while drinking cans or passing round spliffs until we arrived. I was well excited in the queue, this was it. I was living the life I imagined while listening to Pete Tong on my radio in Cumbria, it's not where you're from it's where you're at and I was here. When I got through the entrance, I was frisked then started queuing again to drop off my jacket. I could hear Jamiroquai's 'When You Gonna Learn' twelve inch intro with the didgeridoo funky riff. I had never heard it before but I loved it. It felt appropriate and very cool. I waltzed in and mingled while checking everyone out in the surroundings of this monster venue. I clocked a few people from my course including Lewis who already looked off his face. We waved at each other like we'd been mates for years. I got a drink from the bar, which was subsidized by the N.U.S. but I was anxious for a buzz and began to inquire/socialise with various freaky looking individuals who I thought might be able to 'sort me out.' This approach was futile and got in the way of meeting real people who had accepted it was a booze oriented evening as the bar hadn't accommodated the ecstasy contingent by forgetting to stock bottles of water. I moved around the club from floor to floor, dancing for a bit, staring at faces for a bit, asking myself big questions like 'what on earth am I doing here?' which I wouldn't be asking if I was having MDMA rushes from the ecstasy. Eventually I was pissed which helped a bit but I still felt isolated even though I spent most of the later part of the night sat crossed legged in a cinema room with Katie and the fashion lot. Don't get me wrong, the evening was far from a disaster but it was 'empty' for me. The same judgement applied for The Ministry of Sound as it had for Wembley, it was just not as great as I'd expected and I felt like a fraud when I wrote letters to friends telling them about the 'amazing' freshers ball and therefore my association with it but I wanted everything to be perfect. To be the highest experience. To really live.

At the Sports Fayre held in the gym the previous Friday to the freshers ball, I put my name down to trial for the university football team but one of the other vendors by the exit called to me as I was leaving the gym so I had a look at what they were offering. It was an opportunity to do a solo static line parachute jump from 2,500 feet for charity. There would be full training over a period of weeks at the Bolsover Street campus in central London and then a weekend staying over at Peterborough airfield with more training before doing the jump early on the Sunday morning which turned out to be Halloween.

Like I said before, I wanted everything to be perfect. To be the highest experience. To really live and this was an opportunity to do all three, plus I wanted to confront the feelings I'd had at the end of the summer about dying. I signed up and that night rang my mum to tell her I was going to face those fears I'd been having before I left for London. She told me I was stupid. Firstly for thinking like that and secondly, for putting my life at risk by doing a parachute jump.

The parachute people sent me all this stuff about the importance of raising enough money to cover the costs for your jump. The charity was Radio Lollipop - a childrens hospital radio station who had enclosed sponsorship forms with an ID badge to attach a photo and wear round my neck when I was canvassing. I needed to raise £180, half of which was to cover my jump costs. I decided to take a stroll up Harrow-on-the-Hill as it was guaranteed to be a minted area so I thought I might do well. What I didn't anticipate was that everyone wanted to pay up front so I wouldn't have to knock on their doors ever again. I was getting fivers and tenners stuffed in my hand, some of whom didn't give me their name, they just slammed the door. I found it bizarre but I raised the sum plus the cash in one visit. The training was pretty straightforward. Lots of star jumps and counting to three 'thousands' before checking canopy. Things got difficult at the airbase. We started doing jumps from a huge platform with a large fan attached to slow the person's speed to exactly that of a real jump. We were landing on a crash mat from about thirty feet high which hurt if you got it wrong. The instructor talked alot about broken ankles which contributed to my nerves. I got worse after we had kitted up with chute, reserve and bright orange crash helmet on. We all sat outside on wooden benches waiting to be taken up by this dodgy looking red Cessna light aircraft which was well past it's sell by date. I was three benches back so had to wait till mid afternoon before my moment arrived. This gave me severe squeaky bum syndrome because I was thinking about things too much and the first lot had returned to tell us all how much they had shit themselves. They were not wrong. By the time my legs were hanging out of an aircraft at 2,500 feet with a fucking noisy propeller engine just next to my face and a red-faced instructor bellowing at me to jump I was not keen, I can tell you! I jumped and couldn't even shout the countdown because my larynx was in my undercrackers. I remember the instructor telling me to look up at the plane disappearing and that would give me better shape in the freefall before the chute opened but I sort of blacked out in all the assaults on my senses and luckily my chute opened to complete silence. I say silence, it's quiet compared to the massive engine noise you just left behind plus you are too high to hear any ground noise like traffic but what you can hear are the whoops of delight from the other people from your group floating down around you. That's when I got my desired rush, a feeling of elation and survival which no drug had ever given me before. The landing was a bit rough but I got through it, gathered up the chute and ran for the mini bus taking us back to the airfield. There was alot of talking and excitement on that bus, I could even suggest we nearly bonded until the others wanted another go - like it was a fucking fairground ride! I'd just worked out that for the first time in my life I had let go of a machine which pretty much guaranteed my safety and fallen towards the earth in charge of my own well-being if anything went wrong. That is not a fairground ride. Anyway, apparently you could pay another twenty quid and go up again. I couldn't look chicken could I? So I agreed to join them although I felt one parachute jump was enough to test my theory about dying.

When we got back to the airfield they made us pack our chutes on these long tables for the next person to use, which shit me up that some other amateur thrill-seeker had packed mine. We put a fresh chute on and paid up at this burger van then sat back down on the benches. The nearer we got to the front the more petrified I would get until an instructor came back from the landing area telling us a girl had broken her ankle due to bad light so we should stop now. All jumps were off. Inside I was cheering because I'd managed to body swerve it with my coolness intact. I never disclosed any of these details in my letters back home. Super Vic and all that.

Back at college due to our course becoming modular based, along with many others in 1992 we had the opportunity to take what they called a PolyLang module which is basically a language on top of your studies just in case you failed a core module in Graphic Information Design. I didn't really plan on failing anything but I did have ambitions to go to

Italy in my second year on the Professional Practice module. You had to sort out a work placement anywhere you felt like going for about eight weeks plus the Easter holidays if you wanted. I had ambitions to work at Memphis with Ettore Sottsass in Milan. The work placement thing would be the excuse and justification to lecturers as well as myself and I ended up studying Italian for a year as a consequence.

I love Italian food but I'm not a huge fan of pizza, not since myself, Dean and Diago, the surf dudes from Devon began a Wednesday night habit of visiting Pizzaland on Baker Street near halls of residence. We would go there before making our way to the Bolsover Student Bar to meet the drunken Rugby boys and Hockey Girls, none of which we even knew. Pizzaland offered a basic menu of Pizza, lots of it, in many different ways but always on a thick doughy base which was in fact Pizzaland's marketing trick. Their offer of £3.99 to 'Eat as much as you like' was like a red rag to a bull when you consider what the average income of a student living in London was. The problem being that after about four slices you were pretty much satisfied but being pikey students, myself, Dean and Diago decided to sit there for hours force feeding each other to see how many we could actually eat. I folded at nine, Dean dropped out after eleven but Diago went out on a limb and scoffed fourteen! It wasn't a pretty sight.

It got worse when they invited me back to halls for a rest before pouring lager down our throats at Bolsover. It was my first visit to halls of residence and I was looking forward to seeing what I was missing. They lived on the tenth floor out of about fifteen I think. When the lift doors opened I walked into chaos. We went straight into the kitchen for a glass of water where a massive argument was going on about bread, jam, fish fingers and Frosties. Who had eaten who's and not replaced them. From which cupboard and what part of the fridge against how many fags ponced plus bottles of wine drank. In the middle of this a girl walks in and tells Dean that Lewis had shagged 'what's her name with the big tits' on

Victor J Kennedy

the fifth floor behind her back and she'd just overheard someone talking about it on the seventh floor staircase.
I asked what floor Lewis was on and popped down to visit. He was dancing outside his room with a spliff in his hand and a smile on his face. I asked him where he'd got it from and he explained to me how brilliant it was. He told me that there were two dealers in the building one of which Lewis had befriended. Turned out Lewis's dealer mate had a Ford Fiesta which his mum gave him so he decided to make some extra income by taking orders from inside the halls of things like skunk, resin, even Nepalese palm balls, if you so desired. He would then drive to Amsterdam at the weekend, pick it all up from a cafe, stick it in the glove compartment and drive back through customs looking cool as you like but with a squeaky bum – nice! I peered in Lewis's tiny smoke-filled room and two chicks were huddled up on his single bed. He was blasting out some nondescript reggae, probably to go with the beads round his neck I guess. An angry geek burst out of a room down the corridor shouting at 'whoever' was playing that racket to turn it down because he was trying to study. Study? In this place? In the middle of the commotion there was a massive bang on the window. We all turned round to see solidifying fat on the outside of the windows. I asked what had just happened and someone said it was probably another chip pan fire on twelve, they regularly dealt with it by throwing the whole pan out of the window. I looked out the window to see if it had hit anyone below but there was a flat pebble roof full of fag butts and chip pans. As I looked up to the skyline I was taken aback by it's beauty and sat down in the darkened lounge to drink my water while enjoying the very still and silent dark sky of London. I'd been in the Lake District where I'd witnessed some breathtaking scenery but I was a city boy and this made as big an impression on me as anything up north. This view turned out to be the only decent thing going for the filthy, decrepit halls of residence and I was thankful to Katie for my own fridge and cupboards full of my own food under

my own lock and key. The glass of water didn't help, it inflated the nine slices of dough in my stomach and I had to go home on the tube in severe discomfort with my belt and top button undone.

At college we had entered our first module Visual Representation, introduced to us by the third year lecturer, seventy-year-old, head of course and Scottish genius of Raymond Beattie. So what is Visual Representation? Visual Representation describes the way in which we, as human communicators represent information. Whether it be visual, sound, touch, smell or taste the idea or information from sender to interpreter should be coherent and enjoyable. As a designer you must look hard at represented information and ask yourself, is there another way that might give greater understanding of the message being sent. The brief explained the task ahead:

You are asked to explore the representation of the human face, examining some of the ideas reviewed in the lectures and new ones. Also, you are asked to use different media - Drawing, Photography, Montage, Words, Numbers, etc. You are asked to select one face; (it may be your own) and to represent it and information about it. You may examine: 1. Key elements that define a face 2. Proportion 3. Topography 4. Character 5. Colour 6. Light and shade 7. Economy of description 8. Denotational techniques and systems 9. Descriptions in 3-D space and 2-D space 10. Symmetry, asymmetry 11. Time and age 12. Topology 13. Culture 14. Context 15. Perceptual Considerations etc. You will be asked to verbally present and explain your representations and the informational descriptive content of each.

Raymond sure wrote a mean brief, I mean the amount of syllables check on their own deserved an award. I noticed he had a habit of saying 'reciprocal' and 'neural networks' a lot, both of which I had no idea what they meant but by the end of the three years he would make sure we all understood. If any of us put on a crap Scottish accent and said either 'reciprocal' or 'neural networks' then the rest of the class knew who was being taken the piss out of. Thing is, Raymond was cool. He was the best thing about that course but you only found that out in the third year when you got him full time.

After a few weeks of taking photos, drawing, cutting pieces of wood and folding card our work was coming together. There were huge pixellated murals of Asian children's faces, coat hanger wire framed skulls, whole heads photo montaged in single dimensional planes, blurred faces, stretched faces and loads of indepth study on basic face recognition. I got personal again by opening up my whole head, taking the skin off and peering into the inside of my brain which displayed the basic setup of values I'd established at that time of my life. It was all created using a box inside a box coated in photography and illustration. My rationale read, 'I decided to represent not only the face but the whole head and it's contents, right down to what's inside my head. There are six planes - top to bottom, side to side and back to front. A box format is perfect because it has six sides. The outside layer is obviously the outside of the head. But open the box and it reveals the next layers of muscle, bone and then brain. Look further into the head and find my inner thoughts, the type size represents a hierarchy.' The hierarchy was printed white text out of black and it went in this order, most important first: Serenity, Love, Faith, Fulfilment, Health, Survive, Joy, Excitement, Security, Happiness, Fitness, Knowledge, Success, Respect, Sex, Power, Protection, Money.

This was not self-awareness it was an advert saying 'Buy into Vic's way of life!' By challenging the rest of my class when I presented this 'naked' response to Raymond's brief brought me no real introspection or insight about my state of mind at that time. The whole piece reminded me of a similar thing I produced about three years before while I was doing an art and design BTEC First Award in Kendal. The brief was moods, the media was clay and I made a pyramid with one side white and smooth, one side black and unevenly textured, one side had a door to get inside and the last side had a person coming out of the pyramid as if to escape. I told the tutor it was all about my different moods from dark and irregular to light and effortless. Both pieces were about showing on the outside what's going on inside. Looking at them now makes me sad because they were a subconscious cry for help but the context of the work and my desire to succeed masked the real issue.

A few people on the course didn't quite take the visual representation brief as seriously as me, some hardly turned up and others blatantly paid it no respect whatsoever. After photocopying four photos of his face onto different coloured fluorescent paper, spray mounting over them with text printed on tracing paper, cutting it all out and then attaching the four faces to a rusty metal plate with string Nath wrote, 'It came to me one afternoon in bed, how I should tackle this challenging brief but I ignored it. Then it came to me later that morning and prompted me to snap into action and play with some layouts. Minutes passed like hours, days like decades and then one day I thought how nice it would be if I could integrate my face somewhere in my design unit. The brain wave paid off, within moments I had completed a four levelled visual representation on separate cards. Find out next week how Nath's visual representation challenge ends.' He used this approach for a different brief on black and white photography by doing absolutely nothing throughout and then bringing in some colour holiday snaps of him and his girlfriend in the South of France. He mounted them on the wall next to everyone else's black and white work then with massive balls, stood up and presented to us in front of the tutors. His confidence and patter was unbelievable but he convinced the tutors that although they were colour photographs there was an essence of black and white about them. He passed the module. When the rest of us found out pretty much everybody slagged him off good and proper. The tutors got a mauling too and in my head the episode totally ridiculed the course.

Victor J Kennedy

November brought the death of my grandfather Keith from a massive stroke. When I say grandfather I mean step-grandfather as my nan, Lesley had divorced and remarried Keith long before I was born, hence I'd grown up calling and treating him as my grandfather. A plumber by trade, he was very active and was always fixing things. Before I left for London he had fixed a lamp shade for me which was now in the bedsit next to the phone through which I heard the news. I stared at the lamp and thought to myself, that's the last thing he ever touched in my life. My mum didn't think I should go to the funeral up in Bradford and interrupt my studies so I agreed not to. After I put the phone down I wrote my nan a letter to try and cheer her up but I bet it only made her cry. This was the first death of any immediate family for me even though he was not blood it affected me and made me think about death again, something I thought I'd left behind on that airfield near Peterborough.

There was a midweek night out organised to something called 'Seduction'. The flyers had images of naked models who'd been body painted as gangsters. It was at The Milk Bar which at the time was a 'must go' because Björk had allegedly just recorded 'There's More To Life Than This' while she moved through the club into the toilets and back again. A few of us from GID arranged to go together in Carl-the-skater dude's car which turned out to be a bit of a shock when he came to pick me up. It was a Triumph 2.5PI circa 1969 just like the one my grandfather Keith had when I grew up. I'd had a death wish between leaving college picking up eight cans of Carlsberg Special Brew on the way home and Carl arriving. There were two left which I had in my hands as I walked out the front door. Carl asked me to finish them on the spot before I got in his motor and slid around the cherry leather upholstery. So I obliged. Down in one! We picked up Dean and Diago who by now had moved out of halls and had a place above a chip shop in Harrow. They'd had a few cheap ones too. It was a pretty raucous journey and Carl was blatantly regretting ever offering the lift, especially when we demanded a piss stop in Wembley. When we arrived on Charing Cross Road I was totally off my face and behaving like an animal. We queued, we got rid of our jackets, we took another piss and then entered the arena. It was full of familiar faces from my course and Katie's friends too. I saw that the sweet and innocent Shumana was dancing on the edge of the dance floor so I steamed in. I grabbed her, put my arms around her and told her she was 'fookin' sexy' or something. She smelled my breath and turned her head away so in my drunken state I read that as a sign that she wanted a snog. When I tried to do that she pushed me away and I staggered backwards turning to my left to see half the campus looking towards the dance floor. I stuck two fingers up at them all and barged my way through to the stage, climbed up and started doing my Happy Monday's Bez freaky dancing impression. Things were getting pretty blurred and I couldn't really see the crowd but I could hear the music which sounded great so I really started raving. After five minutes or so other people had joined me on stage and I had really started moving around showing off. I moved to my right hand side to execute some fantastic move and I just completely fell off the side of the stage into a sticky, dusty corner with fag ends and broken glass everywhere. Nobody came to my aid because nobody saw me and if they did they probably thought I was cock who didn't deserve help anyway. I picked myself up and went to the bogs where I realised things were going down hill fast. I had to get out before I spun out so I went up the stairs to the exit without my jacket and sat down where everyone has a piss from The Astoria but I didn't know that because I was new to London. You know the feeling, just before you spew, it's like everything else is moving but you're not. I was semi-conscious from all the 9% ABV Lager inside me ticking like a timebomb until my body emptied itself, again and again. At one point a girl sat next to me and put my jacket over my shoulders but I couldn't say who it was. I was in a dark place until I blacked out and woke up in bed the next day without a clue of how I got there.

This attitude towards excess was another problem I saw as a solution to my state and my experience. I wasn't a risk-taker apart from jumping out of planes but I felt free to try anything for a high at this point. I was in the country's capital city so everything was there to be experienced. One thing I regularly experienced throughout my first term was Whirl Y Gig in Shoreditch Town Hall on a Saturday night. The posters read Music & People of All Ages & Places with DJ Monkey Pilot & The Dance Trance Sound System and you could take your own booze in a plastic bag, perfect for students. Every surface except the floor of The Town Hall was draped and wrapped in psychedelic style with a huge canopy rising high above the dance-floor. There were huge balloons constantly being released from above the DJ booth which the hippies' kids would play with. The parachute dance, the climax to the evening, had to be seen to be believed. To the sound of dreamy music, the new-age bald blokes who'd earlier been playing the bongos by the side of the dance floor, now held and flapped a circular parachute over the sitting audience as circus lights played across its rippling surface. It was amazing whether you'd taken a pill or not but the feeling of unity when the entire dance floor sat down, cross legged, passing free spliffs around was the whole point of going. The only downside was a midnight finish due to the residential area. This meant the Harrow contingent who left five minutes early (usually me, Dean, Diago and Katie) had to run from the venue all the way back to Liverpool Street Tube to catch the last train home. Not great when you'd just spent the last thirty minutes smoking dope.

Since Dean and Diago moved to Harrow we had become good friends. We spent alot of time hanging out together at their flat, where Dean would teach me guitar and all about surfing. We had all decided to start working out together at lunchtimes in the college gym 'for the chicks' but as an excuse we'd say it was for football and surfing. In December armed with free tickets from Katie, myself and Dean went to The Clothes Show Live event in Earls Court. We looked around everything but all we could afford were these multicoloured Lycra tops just launched by a new designer with a bargain bin full of seconds. These tops were like skin-tight cycling shirts but with short sleeves. In fact, they hardly had sleeves at all. They were really gay but I'd seen a straight bloke on Blind Date wearing one so we thought, seen as we'd got in such good shape at the gym, these tops would be perfect to show our muscles off to the 'chicks' in nightclubs. We knew what we were doing but we just couldn't give a fuck, it was going to be a laugh and with Dean it always was.

Christmas came and it was time to go home for three weeks of mum's cooking, beers with the lads and of course my HIV test at Royal Lancaster Infirmary.

The day of the test I borrowed my mum's car with an excuse that I was going shopping in Lancaster on my own, which I never did. In fact, I never went shopping full stop so it was a shit story but she never pulled me up for it. I arrived at the hospital and made my way to the GUM clinic and told the girl at reception I had an appointment under the name V J Kennedy. She checked her computer for a moment, which felt like ages until she said "yes, number L92/623. Could you please fill in this form and bring it back to me when you're finished, just take a seat." I was just a number now. I looked around for a seat, there were alot of glum faces who probably were numbers too so I made sure there were at least two seats between me and them. The form seemed really intrusive and thorough but I gave them everything they needed to know. When I handed it back to the receptionist she thanked me while handing me a leaflet to read as I waited. It was basic propaganda about preparing for the worst case scenario, HIV positive. It left me cold but it wasn't supposed to. My name was called. I got up and walked towards the sound of the soft female voice. It was an older woman in plain clothes. She smiled at me and offered her hand towards a private room. I followed her in and sat down opposite her. She wasn't a nurse and this in fact wasn't the test yet, she was a counsellor. We talked for ten minutes about what I knew about HIV and AIDS, what I thought my risk of being infected was, what impact I thought a positive, indeterminate or negative result would have on my life and how I thought I would react to receiving them, what kind of support system I had including who I would tell if I tested HIV antibody positive and how I have coped with problems in the past. She was really nice but that ten minutes had increased my heart rate dramatically because I hardly thought about any of the things she brought up. To be honest, I was arguably the most frightened I had ever been in my life up to that point. Serious contemplation about the concept of mortality had not entered my head until I was sat back in that waiting room for another long, agonizing five minutes before they took my blood. That part was easy, a needle in and out of my arm then leave, only I had to go to a post-test consultation with some sadistic doctor who, after asking me for my preferred method of notification, offered me condoms and another leaflet on safe sex, which to be honest was the last thing on my mind. I chose to be notified by telephone but they would not ring me. I had to ring them using a password I agreed with sado-doctor. So notification would be the 11th January, exactly two days before my twentyfirst birthday, my coming of age. If it came back positive I gave myself seven years to my twentyeighth birthday before I died a horrible death, a figure I'd read somewhere or heard in a pub.

As I left the hospital and walked towards the car park I noticed a church on the opposite side of the road and immediately ran across to find salvation. When I was a kid my mum sent me to Sunday school and I believed, even to the point of praying before I went to sleep at night to make me a better pupil at school. I wouldn't say that recently I'd practised the best relationship with God but I felt I'd given him enough attention over the years to deserve a some help now when I really felt I needed it.

I walked into the church and it was totally empty and very, very dark. As I approached the alter, I called out to see if the vicar was in the vestry but there was no reply. I looked around at the various stained glass windows and iconography before kneeling on the three concrete steps at the front of the church in prayer. I assumed the classic position then opened up like never before. The emotions ran through me until I began to empty all the anxiety, which had grown over the last three months, through my tear ducts.

I cried through fear, self-pity, desperation and guilt in the search for forgiveness, to be let off this one misdemeanor so I could continue on my current path. So I could stay alive.

I was all over the place, totally alone in a building suffering what some people might say was a religious experience. I would disagree. One of the effects of fear is to disturb the senses and distort the mind to the point where things appear different to what they are. I'd just had a particular reaction to a highly stressful situation. That was how I coped with stress.

After five minutes I wiped my eyes, left the church looking cool and ran back across the road to the hospital car park to finish my 'shopping' and get the car home.

Victor J Kennedy

Chapter 4 - Getting Confident

Friday 8th January 1993, my twentyfirst birthday party.
Organised with military precision, flyers and free entry to a
discotheque. In fact, I was probably going to make a few
quid on the coach fares because I upped the price on each
seat thinking I wouldn't fill fifty two seats but everyone
came back to me saying "yes". A few years back when
everyone turned eighteen, we always seemed to go to
Blackburn, Blackpool or Charnock Richard services on the
M6 to this wierd nightclub round the back of the petrol
station. That was all inside Lancashire and tonight was going
to be their first Yorkshire experience, a magical mystery tour
down the winding A65 to Bradford's premier nightclub
Maestro's. Known in the eighties as Dollars and Dimes, it
was the place I first learned to breakdance, just down from
Valley Parade, the home of the mighty Bantams - Bradford
City FC. Everyone from Millhead seemed to be on the
coach, it was strange seeing all these faces getting on and
handing me a card or a token prezzie. Even my best mates
from Carlisle had turned up but it was odd seeing them
acknowledge Maestro's dress policy in their suits and shiny
shoes rather than tie-dyed t-shirts and baggy jeans.
The journey was a raucous one with singing and comedy
routines. But the combination of booze and the unforgiving
corners of the A65 was having an unwelcome effect on most
of the group so that by the time we reached the club,
everyone made straight for the toilets, an experience not to
be forgotten.
Fountain and fish pond in the middle of the room, free hand
cream, aftershave (top brands of course) and a free shoe-
shine machine dispensing black polish. In the nineties,
brown shoes were the go but it didn't matter. The attitude
was one of "I'm a northern bloke, away from home and I
don't give a shit!" There were a lot of two-tone shoes to be
seen on the dance floor that night.

Mad in England - A memoir

After an hour or so, my Bradford schoolmates arrived so that a section of the huge nightclub was occupied by almost 100 people with me at its fulcrum. It felt surreal watching three disparate groups socialising and I knew it would never happen again - unless, of course, I had a traditional English wedding and actually gave a shit about inviting them. But at twenty one I cared about these people, the community and history, the importance of keeping in touch. If I'd had reverted to type I would have drunk every one of the pints lined up for me on 'my' table, next to 'my' cards and presents but I didn't. I actually stayed sober because I spent time talking to them all, even my first love Jodi Brown took fifteen difficult minutes explaining that by looking at her figure I wouldn't believe she'd given birth to two kids since I left Bradford. To be honest, I couldn't see her waist or her arse in the darkness of the nightclub but her face was still as beautiful as it was in 1988.

I made sure that as I walked around I took photos of all my mates for posterity while at the same time, striking poses in theirs. It was the last dance, everyone paired up for a cuddle and a smooch. That was when it hit me, I was single. I'd sent an invite to Paris in the hope that Faye would make it but her parents had moved to Wales so she wouldn't even be coming back to the Lake District again. I was still in love with her and all the letter writing and phone calls were just breaking my heart. She'd found a French bloke, a twat, in his thirties with a wife and kid but a taste for attractive, young Scottish girls. He even installed her, rent free in his 'special' flat. A place where he could conduct his dual life. She was being used and I was helpless. I looked at the dance floor and knew I was better off on the sidelines, a spectator for this bit. My birthday did not include love. Infact, since Benalmadena, and my arrival in London, I'd been loveless and depressed. The classic line 'he threw himself into his work' comes to mind but I'd been wrestling with change for nearly four months and I'd not even enjoyed being single. I needed a bird. A solid girlfriend, not a shag. A companion.

Victor J Kennedy

But to do that I had to be free of AIDS or at least the threat of it, the obstruction had to be removed or I could not progress.

Monday 11th January 1993, first day back at college after Christmas, everyone is mingling and chatting around the studio waiting for a tutor to arrive. I was anxious, almost sweating and I had more front than Blackpool. All pleasant and nice, asking a few questions about presents and mistletoe, "where were you for New Year?" that type of thing. I had no idea what their responses were, in fact, they all sounded like Charlie Brown's teacher – that trombone sound. I was trying to waste time until I saw Dean was free. I couldn't speak to him in front of people because he knew my results were in today. We'd had a heart-to-heart round his flat before Christmas and I blobbed the lot. He was really understanding and said he would be there for me. What he didn't know at this point was that the clinic had agreed a password with me so I could ring up from a phonebox and get the result verbally, I was paranoid about a letter or anything that could be stolen or duplicated. I still felt ashamed of having it. I saw Diago hop down from the table they were both sitting on and move towards the back of the classroom. I saw my opportunity, ended my chat with Jason and jumped up alongside Dean by the window. "Alright bro?"

"Dude, how the hell are you? You look well, in fact you look mighty fine sir!" Dean often spoke in an American west coast surfer drawl, crossed with his Devon twang. Sometimes he even sounded Aussie but it all lightened things up.

"I'm good man, feeling better than I did before Chrimbo."
"Ahh, yeah mate. How did everything go at the hospital?"
"It was really scarey, they gave me counselling and everything! About every scenario. Every fucking outcome."
"What, like good as well as bad?"
"Dude, you get a good result – why do you need counselling?"

"Jees, sorry man. I'm not thinking straight this morning. So what's the current state of affairs? Do you know anything yet?"

"Nope, I've got this telephone number to ring today with a password we both agreed on. Then they tell me over the phone."

"The whole deal? Wow! That's one heavy phone call. When you gotta do this by?"

"Any time after 9:30am."

"Man, it's practically 10 o'clock. What are we waiting for? I don't think I've got any change but let's go to the refectory and catch some brain food, then do the deed!"

"What's brain food?"

"Carton of milk and a Flapjack. Come on my friend."

I instantly felt better. Even before the brain food. Dean was very matter of fact, that's what I liked about him. He would never make things complicated and if they already were he had a calming effect on everyone. He had loads of emotional intelligence and his viewpoint on the world was always open. I'd never met someone like that when I was growing up.

He walked me into the main entrance area and asked me to put out my hand so I did. He placed five twenty pence pieces in my hand and said, "Go forth my brave friend, get the answer you so require." I felt self conscious doing it in college so we bailed out onto Watford Road and walked until we found a public phonebox. It smelled of cigarettes inside and I could see Northwick Park Hospital through the trees, which was an omen I didn't like. The telephone would keep me remote from Lancashire hospitals but my eyes could still see one.

I dialled the number, Dean right by my side, the receptionist answered and I popped in a twenty pence. "Er, hi. I'm er, ringing to pick up my er, results."

"What's your name?"

"Victor Kennedy."

"Date of birth?"

Victor J Kennedy

"Thirteenth of the first, nineteen seventy two."

"What is your agreed password?"

"Briarwood. It's Briarwood. Can you hold?" Then the pips started going and I started freaking out, trying to find another twenty pence piece. It seemed like an eternity. Dean quickly put another in and the girl's voice came back.

"Your test results have returned negative."

"Negative!?"

"Yes luv, they're negative. All of them."

"Thanks, thanks a lot, that's great news. Great to hear that."

"Is there anything else you need Mr. Kennedy?"

"No. That's everything thanks. Oh, actually, can you say thank you to all the people who dealt with me?"

"I'll pass that message on Mr. Kennedy."

"Thanks very much!"

"Goodbye Mr. Kennedy."

"Thanks a lot, see you later."

I slammed the phone down and we both screamed. He hugged me and picked me up, then squeezed so hard it was like Chewbacca was hugging me. It felt great, like the weight of the world had been lifted. I felt like a new man in that stinky phonebox and Dean was there, making me feel like I'd won a gold medal. He didn't have to do that. I don't think I'd have had the same empathy if the roles were reversed. I couldn't think of anyone else other than myself. If it didn't happen to me I couldn't imagine how it might feel, that I might need to play a supporting role.

That day changed a lot of things. We instantly decided that I should have some sex. That I should organise my 'London' 21st Birthday Party. I also decided that Dean deserved to be paid back for what he'd just done for me. I would be a loyal friend to him if anything else and if he ever needed my help, he got it.

Back at the classroom nobody was any wiser that I had just gone through a life-changing moment, for a start we were both finishing off the arse end of a flapjack with big smiling

51

milk moustaches. The tutors were back and we were late.
But not by much.

We were all briefed by Eric and Elena on Typolinguistics. It
was all about analysing the font Baskerville and creating two
posters; one about italic swooshes and the other was
redesigning an information sheet on Glandular fever. The
text was given to us on an A4 sheet, we just had to make it
easy for students to understand. I thought it must have been
one of Elena's tricks, to teach us to look after ourselves and
recognise when we are at risk from something that often
happens to students. So I ignored it and ended up getting
61% for that module. In that particular briefing Elena also
tried to pre-empt students failing their first year by pushing
us all to learn a language. This is how it all worked. You
needed over 100 credits to qualify for the second year. There
were 8 modules, 15 credits each, representing 120 credits. If
you failed one single module you could still pass with 105
credits. Elena obviously knew that, based on previous
experience, if she assembled a class of equal opportunities
and kids from minorities who had some talent but lacked an
abundance of it, then they (the tutor who gambled/wished on
them in the first place) were likely to lose a few of them at
the end of year one, due to them not being too bright. This is
where the module Polylang came in. Polylang, I can only
guess, is probably a term from Polytechnic. The University
of Westminster was previously The Polytechnic of Central
London. Polytechnic Language Labs all shrunk down into a
new and easy to remember descriptor – the Polylang
module. Now for a start, I wasn't going to fail anything. No
way! No fucking way! So I didn't need Polylang to bail me
out but Elena got on my case. She suggested a module in the
second year called Professional Practice was an opportunity
to work in some swanky design agency in a far away place
and that got me thinking. I was still in the throws of a World
Cup hangover after Gazza's heroics in Italia '90 and he was
now starring for Lazio on Channel 4's Football Italia. After
some thought I decided to take Italian on the Polylang

Victor J Kennedy

module because I wanted to do my Professional Practice module in Milan at the product design studio Memphis, working for Ettori Sottsass and watching Gazza destroy AC or Inter in the San Sero at the weekends. That was my plan and before long, I had a bedsit full of stickers. Everything was labelled in Italian, from the pots and pans to the television remote control. But it all turned out to be futile in the end because I only just passed with 53% and struggled to remember anything once the stickers were taken down. One sentence I do remember from my aural exam, the section where I was booking a room in a hotel whilst complaining and it is the only thing to this day that I can say to any Italians I meet, often in their restaurant whilst I am drunk. "Il palazzo i puistosto brutto!" Which apparently means, "This building is very ugly!"

So the word was put out by Dean and Diago that my birthday was to be on Wednesday night in the central London student union bar, the Bolsover Bar. They both organised a meal for me and a select group of friends beforehand at our favourite place; Pizzaland on Baker Street. I turned up in my brand spanking new Levi 501s in white. I also had my Grandad's nylon t-shirt from 1952, yeah I was looking hot, slightly self-conscious but I looked like I'd been shopping frantically at Flip in Covent Garden, currently the coolest second-hand shop in town. Poor old Oxfam.

Once the meal was out of the way and the comedy cards were exchanged, including Dean and Diago's homemade stuck-on condom 'Always wear a wetsuit' ensemble, Katie very kindly popped the cards into her tiny gold handbag for safe-keeping and we were on to the main event. As we walked down Marylebone Road, past halls of residence, she began explaining what I could only perceive as her birthday present to me. Her latest 'best friend' Tanya Baker, from the fashion course was already being groomed as perfect girlfriend material. According to Katie, the gorgeous Tanya from Essex recently split up with her boyfriend Mike, who himself was a second year Graphics student at St. Martins.

Mad in England - A memoir

She had allegedly told Tanya all about me and how
vulnerable and kind I had been over the last few months in
London. Maybe Katie also informed Tanya about how many
women I was alledged to have slept with during that crazy
year I was in Carlisle? Not to mention the fact I still had a
girlfriend back in Millhead while I was at it. Yeah, typical
bastard male but Faye did the dirty on me first, at a party in
the second May bank holiday of 1991 and it broke my heart.
I reacted the way only a 19 year-old-male could react and
got revenge with my penis. But I couldn't leave the scores at
1-1 could I? Now she had created the monster, I had to finish
on top – literally. That was my problem, I always had to win
but I'd not yet discovered that personal insight. Hopefully
Katie didn't mention that bit and I would have the chance to
woo Tanya on my own terms that night.
We all bailed into the lower ground floor bar, littered with
various sports bags piled up from the Rugby boys and
Hockey girls who'd caught the coaches back through rush
hour from the playing fields of Chiswick at 6pm.That was
almost four hours ago now and everyone was jumping
around and going mad to ABBA or House of Pain or some
obscure shit the DJ felt we should all be exposed to. People
were snogging in seedy dark corners, while others shouted
conversations in each other's ears from point blank range.
Somebody ran off to get a round of watered down NUS
Carlsberg and I made my way around to the sweaty speakers
to check faces and empty seats. They were all there, the
fashion lot, funky dancing and smiling ear to ear. Everyone
seemed to be smoking, it could've been the dry ice but
through it all I could see this girl in dungarees, those
tradesman overalls with multiple pockets to carry every tool
imaginable. She had a vest on underneath and no bra,
difficult to detect because her long mousey blonde hair was
covering everything. It looked like she had hobnail boots on
too but as much as she covered herself up, it seemed to do
the opposite in my imagination. I totally wanted to see what
was underneath. I wouldn't call it love or lust at first sight

Victor J Kennedy

but I was hooked and I wanted to know more. Dean passed a pint into my hand and then whacked his pint against it, wished me Happy Birthday and went into the crowd. Katie was now talking to the girl in the Dungarees and Katie was now waving me over. I was so glad I knew Katie. She introduced us, it was in fact Tanya, how lovely! We had a shit conversation, shouting at each other in front of the speakers. She seemed to laugh at my gags and smiled a lot but I couldn't work out what was wrong until this skinny 6ft guy turns up with two drinks and holds one out to her. She nervously introduced him as Mike and he said some bollocks in my ear which I didn't hear clearly so I nodded, smiled and legged it. What a shocker! That must've been miles more embarrassing for her than it was for me. I think it was a car crash of promises and expectation with a few misunderstandings and a lack of communication thrown in for good measure.

The best 21st birthday present I got was inside January's issue of Creative Review. I'd subscribed to Creative Review Magazine since I worked at Reggie's in 1989 so I'd got about 36 issues sitting in a cupboard at home and decided they were full of shit. Most of the content came from the same people/agencies/colleges and I was fed up with it. It's not like the coffee-table-tat is exactly cheap, is it? Financially, I mean. Anyway, in November I decided to tell them what a 20-year-old's eyes were seeing in a nicely written letter, bearing in mind 1992 was before email became widespread. Once the January edition came out, I had instant popularity! The rest of my classmates were celebrating with me when they saw my letter was published on page 7. Kind of like the brightest stars, it fell into the stratosphere like this:

College bias claim
It was interesting to read your article, "D&AD Redesign" (November issue). So interesting that it caused me to finally put pen to paper. It is reassuring to know that D&AD is prepared to make changes. It is also welcome news that

Mad in England - A memoir

Neville Brody is in support of the small designer and his or her concerns.

Would I be right saying the art directors have, in the past, had tunnel vision towards a certain section of the design community, thus giving young designers from less established design groups an even harder time getting noticed?

We could call this a monopoly (from the large companies' point of view), but we won't!

This brings me nicely to my point and my aim to relieve mounting stress.

Would I also be correct in saying the new generation of designers are the most important to promote? Now I do not have any prejudice against Central St. Martin's (it's work is always excellent), but a majority of the student work featured in Creative Review is from there or other 'established' colleges. If the Art Directors' Association does change for the better by not alienating the small designer then could Creative Review echo it's progression forwards by widening its own vision towards less established colleges.

A time for change? Or does St Martin's have hotels on Mayfair and Park Lane?

P.S. I hope this letter does not prejudice my work from future inclusions in your magazine!

Victor Kennedy
Graphic Information Design Student at
University of Westminster
Roxborough Park
Harrow
Middx

Editor's note: We do not have any bias towards Central St Martin's, or indeed any other so-called 'established' institution. The fact is these colleges seem to place far more emphasis than their country cousins on sending in examples of interesting work.

Victor J Kennedy

A public spanking from the Editor of Creative Review for talking bollocks from the back of the class. Seems that will be my only ever contribution to the content of that institution. Unless I change my name to Neville Brody and start producing some 'examples of interesting work'. Editor's discretion of course.

I seemed to develop a copywriter's taste for writing letters to creative people in high places and swiftly followed one rant with another to Kriss Potter, Head of Graphic Design on the campus of Design for Communications Media at Manchester Metropolitan University, my beloved Manchester. I'd had a couple of bad weeks doing the module Diagram Design for Megan, a tutor I really respected not only because she interviewed me, thus offering me the place but because she talked so much sense. More than Eric and Elena put together. Megan once coined the infamous phrase "GID is fun" to counteract students on the Graphic Information Design course complaining at how boring it is. During the module I'd successfully presented a representation of an Egyptian sunset and sunrise, using only a circle, a square and a triangle. However, my evaporation cycle diagram was heavily criticised, in front of the class in a public critique by Megan, due to a thumbs-up icon I had invented to represent good or bad. The diagram was a nod to the colour coding of traffic lights. Red meaning bad or a thumbs-down, amber was a sideways undecided thumb and green was a big thumbs-up! She didn't like my icon, she said it didn't look like a thumb. In fact she said the hand didn't even look human. Probably because the three different hands were painted red, orange and green. They didn't look very healthy hands but hands, or at least fists with extended thumbs all the same. I hated that comment, I couldn't take feeling like being ridiculed in front of my peers. It felt like I was being treated unfairly when I had tried so hard. I was up really late for days making it. Some of the other work I'd seen that afternoon on that wall was poor in comparison and I could only question their conviction towards this degree and the quality of the creative work coming out of it. Those type of thought processes would lead me to the conclusion that Harrow or rather those people, that group of students and tutors were not good enough for me to learn new things. I felt like I was teaching them! I imagined that I would be given 'new things' if I moved to a 'better' course, which in my mind, at that point was Manchester. I was clearly a hypocrite if I was planning to leave but I'd pre-empted the failure.

Dear Mr Price,
Further to my letters and informal interview earlier in the year regarding a place on the Graphic Design section of BA (Hons) Design for Communications Media, I would like to thank you again for your time but with regret let you know that Harrow College offered me a place after 2nd choice interviews and I have accepted.
I still believe Manchester and it's course were right for me, especially as you gave me a chance even though my luck was down and out.
The reason I am writing this letter is if, in the unlikely event, things do not work out in London and I find I don't enjoy it then would I possibly be able to transfer to your second year at the start of next year's intake and if so how could I do it?
I know you are very busy so if it is too much time and trouble to inform me then it doesn't matter now, I will contact you at the time if I want to do it.
Many thanks again for seeing me. All the best with the new students.
Yours sincerely,
Victor Kennedy

He held me to my word and never replied to my letter so I soldiered on. Of course, there were certain people on my course I respected as competition. One of those was Nathan Foreman. I hadn't spoke that much to him, mainly because he dived into his blue Fiat Uno and zoomed off back to Watford as soon as the bell went. However, the last couple of weeks we'd worked together making a Diagram Design presentation to Megan and the rest of the group as a pair of TV presenters. It was sort of a pastiche on Channel 4's The Word but with cows. We both did a great job and there was an obvious chemistry between us, especially on the improvisation where we were laughing at each other and the audience joined in. It felt very comfortable and I think Nath felt the same way. Over time our rapport turned into trust and we began to swap information. This culminated on a particular evening after I'd spent days convincing Ruth McGregor, the cool chick who sat beind Nathan, to let me borrow her brother's Nintendo Entertainment System. She told me he had a Duck Shooting game and we couldn't work out how the technology could match a pixel on a TV screen with the plastic rifle controller attached to the NES. She eventually brought it in for me to try out. Nath had noticed this conversation going on and joined in. Before long he had my bedsit address and we made a date for later on. That very night, just as I'd finished my Italian pasta wok extravaganza, the buzzer went off and it was Nath! I let him in, he squeezed through the door and had a quick look round the room and paid it a few compliments, "Not bad, not bad at all. Is that your drawing board?"

"Yeah, the only things in the room were the bed, that armchair, the wardrobe, that lovely seventies sideboard and obviously the kitchen."

"What about the batphone?" he joked, after seeing the classic eighties British Telecom telephone sitting on the corner of the drawing board.

"Oh yeah, she's a beauty isn't she? That's mine and Katie's umbilical chord back to our mum's."

"Katie from fashion?"

"Yeah she lives here too. In fact, she sorted me out with this bedsit when we got accepted. Didn't fancy halls. But I was accepted."

"What, the ones in town that Lewis, Dean and Diago are in?"
"Yep, Marylebone Road." And then it hit me. Nath hadn't been involved with any of the social stuff whatsoever. He didn't know about all the fun we were having outside of the course. All the parties, that sort of stuff. He didn't even know Dean and Diago were out of halls and above the chippy in Harrow.
"So where does Katie live?"
"Just down the corridor. She got first dibs because her Aunt lives down here and sorted these bedsits out for us."
"She order two? One for you?"
"Yeah, I didn't get to see it till the day I actually moved in. Her flat is a bit nicer and I bet she swapped a bit of furniture as well. I would've done the same!"
"I thought you were together, the way you always seemed to be chatting at college?"
"Oh no, it's not like that. She was on the same Foundation Course as me."
"In Bradford?"
"No, no. My parents... well, actually the family moved from Bradford in 1998 to Kendal in Cumbria. You know, Kendal mint cake and all that."
"Yeah, yeah. The Lake District."
"Well, not quite. It's a little village near junction 36 of the M6 called Millhead. But it does fall just inside Cumbria, where it meets Lancashire and North Yorkshire. That's how I ended up in Carlisle. I wanted to go to Bradford, that's where all my mates were but I was no longer inside that Education Authority, couldn't get a grant unless I stayed in Cumbria."
"So did anything happen between you and Katie at Carlisle?"
"Do you fancy her or something?"
"No Vic, I've got a girlfriend."
"What, from college?"
"No, from back home. Don't change the subject, tell me about you and Katie."

Victor J Kennedy

"Nothing happened. She went out with one of my best mates. They were a couple for quite a while but it fizzled out at the end. He's in Edinburgh now so don't worry, he's too far away." I gave him a wink.

"But you two are good friends, right? You wouldn't have ended up living together if you weren"t."

"We were accepted onto the same campus in the same city, near her auntie who very kindly sorted my room for my first year at university. Maybe Katie needed someone she trusted to be nearby. First time London? Think of me as her muscle. Especially if you ever come back late on a Friday night and upset her."

"I don't fancy her. She's not my type."

"So who is?"

"What, at college?"

"Yes, at college. Who've you got your eye on?"

"No-one."

"Ah, come on. There must be someone?"

"Let's get the Nintendo working and if I beat you at Duck Shooting, I'll tell you." He grabbed a few wires and a started plugging the console into my portable telly. Then he grabbed the rifle, pointing it right at me while I made two coffees. He was joking, of course.

Between us we got it working and I quickly learned how competitive Nath was. I learned a lot of things about Nath that night, as he did about me but in hindsight I think that was the whole point of his 'popping in.' He left my flat safe in the knowledge that I'd invited him to join the Friday night fashion girl drinking posse. He had successfully infiltrated the Harrow social network and he never told me which girl he fancied either. I lost at duck shooting but he did say he had a girlfriend. . .

In early February all GID students were given free tickets to the annual Icograda student design seminar in the Odeon Cinema Marble Arch. No, we would not be watching a film. We would be listening to 'giants' from the industry lecturing us about the 'magic' they do within their specialism. Turns

out my mate Nev was gonna be there. Yeah, Neville Brody.
I wondered if he'd seen my fabulous article quoting his name
in Creative Review in last month's issue. Various other
speakers came on and I cannot remember their names
because they were so boring I have forgotten all about them,
never mind what they said. One bloke was called Alan who
did typography in bright colours and loved serifs but that is
about it. The other students felt so bored they began abusing
them in the Q&A at the end. These spods in Icograda polo
shirts hold microphones around the theatre audience and you
hold your hand up. When the presenter sees you, the
microphone is thrust in front of your face and your voice
booms over the speakers, superb! There had been some
funny questions earlier but once Neville had finished rattling
on about various software programs like Photoshop, it's
filters and nice effects using the blur tool, this Geordie lad
down the front puts his hand up. Neville points at him and in
goes the mic, "I have these pens like. They're brilliant pens
mind, but they keep drying up if I don't use them often
enough. It's indian ink and the label of the pen is called
Rotring. I just wondered how you manage to keep all your
pens so clean and if you've got any tips you could give us?"
The audience was split. Half were trying not to piss
themselves and the other half were mumbling noises of
dissatisfaction at the heretic from the north east. My mind
was racing at this point, what question could I give him to
make him think? To make him realise the point about hand
skills the Geordie bloke was making. Maybe he wasn't being
that clever, maybe he was just doing a 'Vic Reeves' and
asking a bizarre one to get a laugh? Neville answered with
something to the effect of, "Wow, Rotring pens! I haven't
used one of those for years. Probably since I started using
the mac. But if I remember, you put the tip in boiling water
and add a little vinegar until the blockage clears."
I thought that was a rubbish answer and he wound me up
even more for copping out. He might have been a brilliant
Graphic Designer but he was a shit public speaker and he

would never make it in stand up. His brain didn't think quick enough. Or he was the opposite and wanted to keep it real and say nothing controversial. So I stuck my hand up high, he pointed at me, in comes the microphone and over the loud speakers booms, "Don't you feel a bit of a fraud standing up there, presenting Photoshop effects to the Photoshop generation? I mean, the machine i.e. the macintosh computer and it's software supply all those effects and we all know the right buttons to press to get the same end result as you've got up there on the screen. Haven't you been deskilled by a computer?"

"Good question. But I have to ask, haven't we all been deskilled by a computer? There is a fundamental shift in the way we, as human beings compose and deliver commercial artwork. This has been brought about with the invention of the desktop computer. It is not the be all and end all of mark making. Graphite was not the end of charcoal and Indian ink was not the end of graphite. The Macintosh is a tool. Photoshop is a tool, nothing more. If you are already aware of the different effects available then I suggest you experiment while you have the time because when you leave college you will struggle to find that time. Establish a good repetoire to avoid being deskilled. Next question."

So that was me completely ended. Maybe the spikier the question the spikier his response? I guess I asked for it, over loud speaker as well! At the end as we all bailed out a few mates from the course patted me on the back and told me it was a good question but I thought it was all bollocks. The world still seemed to be set up the same way as it was before I asked the question. Keeping the status quo. We got back to the Harrow campus and spent the rest of the day with the fashion lot and some of the boys from illustraion, getting pissed in the bar, skiving lectures and talking rubbish.

Noel Palmer from Wigan, one of the younger and more interesting tutors, in a mate kind of way, spoke good Spanish. In fact he knew a lot about Spain because he had lived there in the past. He took it upon himself to organise a sabbatical in the cultural city of Barcelona, one year after the Olympics had finished. It felt like a school trip in one sense and a holiday away with your mates in another. We would get a break from dossing around the Harrow campus to dossing around the centre of Barcelona instead.

After being waltzed around like sheep, through passport control and boy-girl, boy-girl seating arrangements on aircraft and trains, we arrived on Las Ramblas. We were down an alleyway, right next to the prostitute area in a hotel with a big tree growing in reception. I say tree, it was like a grape vine that had got out of control. It was at this point when many future relationships were decided – who shares with whom? It was a scramble and natural selection took over. It split the group in many ways and decided who would hang around Barcelona together. Sort of like a gang mentality. Not me though, I spent alot of the time on my own. Didn't want anyone slowing me down while I ticked all the boxes; Olympic Stadium, Science Museum, Gaude Park and Sagrada Familia. When I was part of a gang, I chose to be with Rory, Alan, Salim, Jase, Twinkle and of course Dean and Diago. If we weren't all together then there would be smaller gang variations checking out Salvador Dali's Museum on the train up to Figueres or watching Barcelona hammer Athletico Madrid 5-1 at the Nou Camp in front of 55,000 fans who sounded like 100,000. We sunbathed on the beach and swam in the cool February sea, while surviving the whole week on visits to Pans & Company for a bocadillo. Basically, it's a white breadstick and a filling of cheese and ham. It was very easy to order when you spoke no Spanish whatsoever. There is a major flaw to this food strategy and you don't find out until the end of the week when you finally realise you haven't 'been' for five days. The other core 'gang' consisted of a few hangers-on but a fairly basic foursome of Nath, Lewis, Shumana and Hermina. Basically, over the past couple of months, Shumana had been coerced by Lewis to publicly give personal information about herself and her sexual

Victor J Kennedy

preferences. It was difficult to work out if Shumana was advertising herself or whether Lewis was being intrusive because all of it was done in the classroom in a casual way. He was sort of wooing her for the crowd. Flirting for the audience. He could be heard chatting her up, probing and seeing how far he could take it. He didn't seem to be hurting her or damaging her psychologically but I assumed he wasn't partcularly interested in her wellbeing or respecting another person being who may not be as sexually experienced as he was. As soon as she confessed, under duress that she was in fact a virgin, every guy in the room was alerted to her attention. This is where I question Shumana's motives for releasing that information. Whether it was true or not, it represented a power shift where Lewis (or Lewis's brain to be more specific) was no longer in control of that relationship. His penis was not in control either, Shumana was now firmly in control (of him) and before long the innocent Liberian-sex-child had Lewis snared as her boyfriend. She would do things like making him hold hands with her, as your mum did when you were crossing the road as a kid and he had to comply.

It may have looked like "Lewis pulled Shumana in Barcelona" but in actual fact Shumana didn't 'pull' anyone, she pushed them around by using her pretty face, fantastic figure and the 'promise' of an untouched vagina. And I'll admit, I wanted it (excitement, passion, desire) too but that 'promise' didn't force me towards hanging out with the other 'gang' in the social frameworking of that five day Catalan Fiesta because I didn't go to Barcelona for sex with a classmate. In fact, I didn't go to Barcelona for sex full stop. I went to become a better designer.

We met Mariscal, the guy who designed 'Cobi' the '92 Olympic mascot. Noel took us to his studio where Mariscal did a presentation and showed us around the building. Then he signed autographs. It was that type of thing I was hungry for and I have to thank Noel for sorting it all out. I had a very close relationship with Noel after that trip. He was a fellow northerner on a campus with very few other familiar accents and that gave me comfort.

On return it wasn't that long before Lewis and Shumana split up. I can't comment on why they split up because I don't know. What I do know is that Lewis told me he never made it all the way around the baseball field. Boys will be boys and all that.

After we returned it was heads down again, picking up the course work where we'd left off and a new module added for good measure. Design in Society was an ongoing Wednesday morning lecture series which we'd been doing since the start of the year. It was great because I had permission to leave early from Bobby at the gym, who was my football manager on Wednesday afternoons. If we had an away match I would only have to sit through an hour or so of semiotics and the history of the printing press before sloping off out the back door. At this point of the year I was more into my football than my degree and having to write a Communications Revolutions essay of 25,000 words was not an attractive prospect and I received my second worst mark of 59% for the beautifully bound document I had decorated with Palatino at 10pt. It had to be the early exits for football and another 'life lesson' by another frustrated female lecturer, unable to 'engage' me with her prose that helped attain that mark. This was a combination of factors I would start to recognise. It was called politics and I hadn't been aware of any in Bradford or The Lake District or even Carlisle before now. It was there, of course, but let's just say the veil had recently been lifted. The end of ignorance and innocence. And authentic communication? Apparently, Oscar Wilde said of London, that it was the most powerful society in the world. I used to take the piss out of people on the tube because I couldn't believe strangers never talked to each other. I would swing down the hand rails as the Metropolitain train headed for Baker Street and shout, "Gladiators ready! Contenders ready!" but no one laughed or raised an eyebrow. In fact, they looked afraid of me and I

Victor J Kennedy

suddenly felt self-conscious. You do that on a bus in
Bradford and someone else will either take the piss out of
you or join in the irony and have a laugh. Same in the chippy
or down the market, it's just banter. Uncomplicated giggles.
But you cannot do that in London and the combination of
that with the crap tutors made me hit the fountain pen to
Manchester Metropolitain University once again.

Dear Mr Davies,
I am writing to back up my phone message to request advice
or any help you could offer me on the subject of transferring
to a second year Graphic Design course.
I am not sure of your knowledge of my contact with Mr.
Kriss Potter as I wrote to him last September after my
interview but I have enclosed a copy of the letter returned to
me last year as I began here in Harrow.
Everything surrounding my student life here is excellent. I
am perfectly happy with the place I am living in and the
people I am with. It is just that I am beginning to think that
as the course progresses, I find Graphic Information Design
is not what I expected. This is not a snap decision but an aim
to pre-empt any move in the wrong direction for myself.
I would be eternally grateful of a chance to interview for
second year on BA(Hons) Design for Communication Media
– Graphic Design or any sound piece of advice of what to do
next.
Please use the enclosed SAE and I look forward to your
swift reply. Many Thanks.
Yours sincerely,

Victor Kennedy

24 March 1993
Dear Mr Kennedy
Further to your request for entry onto the second year of the
Communications Media, option Graphic Design, I regret to
inform you that the course is full.

Mad in England - A memoir

Should a place become available again over the summer
period I will contact you again.

Yours sincerely,

Veronica Long (Ms)
Assistant Administration Officer. Department of
Communication Media

I was lying a bit when I said I was very happy there in
Harrow living in a £50 a week bedsit while socially, being
surrounded by gay men who love sewing machines. I was an
alien. A fish out of water. In fact, unconsciously I think I
was homesick for the north and still grieving over the end of
my two and a half years with Faye. Whether or not it was
subconscious, I was getting out of my head more frequently.
Me and Twinkle went to see D:Ream at the Reach for the
Sky night in the Limelight on Charing Cross Road. There
was also a regular trippy visit to Whrlygig in Shoreditch
every Saturday night. There was a midweek Seduction down
the Milk Bar, not to mention Cafe de Paris with Judge Jules
and Carl Phillips. Then there was The Dome at Tuffnell Park
for Listen with Mother. Not forgetting Somethin' Else at
Subterrania in Ladbroke Grove. There was Jeremy Healy in
Club Med at the Gardening Club, Covent Garden and Leave
My Wife Alone at Ormonds in Mayfair. If I wasn't pissed up
at these things then I'd be on some horrible speed or a crappy
E I'd paid peanuts for midweek at college from a druggie
bloke called Jeremy, who couldn't have been a dealer
because he took so much of it all himself. Twinkle never
took anything and I never asked him or told him I was doing
what I was doing either, which was abnormal. Not abnormal
to take drugs in 1993 but abnormal because half the point of
taking drugs is to come up at the same time as your mates
and experience it all together. My experience of all this was
solo, it was private up to now because I hadn't met anyone I
trusted. It was my little habit and as long as it didn't disrupt

my football or my work or anything else then everything would carry on the same and nobody would know.

Just before Easter, the phone rang and it was Faye from Paris. She asked if she could stay at mine overnight as she had an interview for a summer job with a travel company based in Southampton the following week. Of course, I agreed and duly prepared for her arrival. She landed at Heathrow from Charles De Gaulle and I met her off the platform at Harrow-on-the-Hill station. All the way back we talked the same way as we did before we split and although she was telling me all about her current squeeze from Paris, the 30-year-old serial adulterer with the shagging pad for his bits on the side, I still thought it was fair game for me to sleep with her that night. She didn't know that yet. When Faye got in the bedsit, it was evident to her that a single bed was going to be difficult. She needed her sleep and all that, big important interview in the morning. I changed the subject and got out the wine, put some old tunes on that would stoke up the memories and we chatted away till midnight. Then all of a sudden she grabbed her toothbrush and said, "Ok, it's time for bed for me. Can you show me where your bathroom is?" I took her down the corridor and when she got back she was wearing just a black lace teddy. My eyes were popping out.

"Don't get any ideas Mr. Ok?"

"Honestly. Never crossed my mind." She walked over to the bed, turned around to pull the duvet back and on close inspection through the lace I saw this red mark above her coccyx, "What's the mark on your arse?"

"What mark?" she said, as she twisted around on the bed trying to see it.

"That mark. Just there." I sat down next to her and touched it. There was broken skin but it was healing.

"Ah yes, that mark. Erm, it's a friction burn."

"A friction burn? From what?"

"Use your imagination Vic." she rolled over and I picked up my toothbrush.

Mad in England - A memoir

"He must've been going ten to the dozen to make a mark like that!" I contested as I began brushing my teeth in the kitchen sink.

"Look, let's not start an argument because it's bedtime. I've got a new boyfriend and I know this isn't the ideal situation to be in but I need you to just get into bed and sleep. It's a big day for me tomorrow." In my head I was screaming, while at the same time another voice was shouting out the fact she just invited me into bed. I still had a chance so although my heart was getting ripped in two and I was in bed, lights off, with someone else's girlfriend who used to be mine. I still kept putting my hand between her legs and accidently feeling her tits. It felt horrible and yet horny in a revengeful way. When the lights were off, she was just another sex object. She was no longer my first love from 1990. After fifteen minutes of apologies and warnings she snapped, "Get out. Get off me and get out of the bed! Do you have another quilt?"

"What? What did I do? I thought we could do it one last time. For old times-sake and no-one will ever know. Come on... just one more."

"No, I'm sorry. You have to sleep on the floor."

"This is totally not fair." I was like a little kid. I lifted up the matress and pulled out a blow up matress and started to inflate it with the light on. By the time I'd finished she was lying down again and I pulled the bed to one side, waking her up before pulling out my old sleeping bag from 1977, complete with Star Wars characters printed on it. I scowled at her and turned the light off, jumped into the bag making the usual squeeky li-lo noises and then silently cried myself to sleep. In the morning, she simply ate breakfast got changed and left for Southampton having saved about £16 on a B&B.

My head was totally fucked for a week after that visit and it represented a turning point in my life because the following Friday after the bar had closed, Katie brought Tanya back to our bedsits in a very drunken and giddy state. Also slightly

Victor J Kennedy

randy, on a bit of a promise but not from me – from Katie on
behalf but unbeknownst by me until they burst through my
door using the spare key. Turns out Tanya was finally single
and had jettisoned ex-boyfriend Mike from St. Martins.
Katie giggled and talked drunken-ladette-small-talk for a
while and then left Tanya with me and the spare key. We
had an incredible night, which over the following five weeks
turned into a whirlwind romance. On the sixth week Tanya
moved out of her parent's in Buckhurst Hill into a house in
Kenton, about a mile from my bedsit. Within weeks Katie
moved out of the bedsit and joined Tanya with another girl
called Sara from the fashion course.

Once installed they had a seventies house warming party,
complete with a seventies DJ. It was a fancy dress theme
called Charlies Angels. You get it? The three girls living in
the house were the Angels and of course there would be
loads of 'Charlie' (and the rest) being distributed to guests. It
was around this time I was touted around as Tanya's
boyfriend, mainly because we were always together in the
bar and the relationship had lasted longer than just a drunken
shag but it was still in that blurred part.

Clad in smelly old leather jackets from the Charity shop, me
and Twinkle pulled up to the 'two up, two down, typical
rented student house' in his seventies white Triumph, after
it's mileometer had just reset. It was a bizarre coincidence to
be in the car making up the three extra miles around the
streets of Kenton and Wembley at 999997 just to make sure
we could watch the historic moment as the numbers all
rotated back to 000000. It was something 'cool' to show the
girls at the party. Twinkle's car was the same make and
model as my grandad's car during the eighties. It was the
first fuel injection car ever made, according to Keith, who
had aquired it from a dead friend's widow. I remember as a
ten year old, burning my shin on the exhaust pipe as I helped
my mum, nan and sister push it down a hill while he tried to
jump-start it. This minor childhood trauma happened
somewhere between Morecambe and Skipton on the A65. It

left a perfect circle of burnt skin on my leg and etched the Triumph 2000 PI on my brain forever.

Me and Twinkle arrived in Kenton like Starsky & Hutch to a lot of over-the-top screaming, by a very drunk and relieved Katie at the front door, I could tell she was anxious about the turn out. Tanya came out and we had a snog, I asked her if many were inside and she took my hand and dragged me in. It was packed. All the fashion lot, some of the Illustration boys and Dean and Diago dressed as Thunderbirds Scott and Virgil Tracey! It seems the Covent Garden second hand shop Flip had a deal on band stand outfits that afternoon.

The party took it's normal course with copious amounts of alcohol leading to different rooms doing different drugs. Coke or speed in the bathroom, spliff and reggae in a low-lit bedroom, Bongs, munchies and giggles in the kitchen and full-on ecstasy fuelled bouncing in the lounge next to the speakers. Eventually this party model usually leads to an incident, often a fight between the people at the party and some uninvited locals who are drunk combined with a hatred for students but this party did not follow that route. As people began to disperse around 3 or 4am and the chemicals inside made it tougher to recollected faces or time, I got talking to some bloke dressed in a Prodigy t-shirt on the couch who I assumed was one of us. We talked bollocks for ages while he built a spliff. Other people around us were crashed out, the music was now a compilation mix tape, the decks were still switched on but unmanned. This guy finished making the spliff and then lit up. It smelled different, not that usual sweet smell of resin burning and it crackled as he pulled on it. He took a big one back and all this brown smoke came out. He inhaled deeply. His eyes closed and then he sat back on the couch saying nothing. I thought to myself, fuck me that must be good stuff, I've got to try some. So just as the ash was about to fall out of his relaxed hand onto the sofa, I asked him for a go. He passed it lazily but by then it had gone out. I got on my hands and knees to pick up a lighter I spotted on the floor. After a few sparks it lit and I put the roll up to my lips and connected to the fire. My lungs expanded, the brown smoke appeared and then my body melted from my chest outwards. I coughed a bit but felt thoroughly 'monged' and joined him on the couch to enjoy it together with my new found compadre.

"Nice....man. What is that stuff?"

"Heroin."

"Heroin! You're fucking joking?"

"Nah man, don't do this now. I'm a bit.."

"Why didn't you tell me before I smoked it?"

"Mmmmnnnppphh..."

"Who've you come with? What course are you on?"

"I don't know what you mean, I'm on my own."

"Who invited you?

"No one, the door was open and I heard the music."

"So you live next door?"

"Nah, I was walking past."

"You just walked in off the street?"

"Yeah."

"Are you on your own?"

"Yeah."

"Can you leave please?"

"If you want?"

"Yeah, I think it's best." So we got up like two old men with arthiritis and shuffled our way to the front door and I 'kicked him out' or at least that was my story in the morning. To be honest, I was mortified with myself more than him. The thing is, I still didn't get it. I wasn't scared by that incident and I should have been. It should have shocked me into stopping or at least being more careful about what I put in my body but it only made me angry. I was still taking risks because I wanted excitement. I still felt I should supplement my evenings to help me experience 'everything' that little bit more. I continued my nightclub tours with Twinkle, I took a pill at Kentish Town Forum watching Arrested Development without Dean and Diago knowing a thing about it. At that time I would have taken drugs eating Sunday lunch in a pub.

Mad in England - A memoir

To make things worse, my letter writing to all and sundry
describing my antics in London, had attracted Peter Duffy to
come to stay. On the last day of school in 1988 we had
signed goodbyes, on each others shirts and all bought
address books to keep in touch. I had raided mine before
Christmas when I was lonely and looking for attention. One
of those letters went to Paul's old address and the diligent
pensioner living there in the nineties had forwarded it to
Paul's mum in Blackburn. She in turn sent it to Paul in
Falmouth, where he was completing his BTEC National in
Graphic Design. It arrived with perfect timing, just before he
started a work placement in London as part of the final
stages of the diploma. So it was my fault that he ended up
sleeping on my floor, eating all my food, moving my bedsit
around when I was away on holiday and shagging his
girlfriend in the communal bathroom whilst making loads of
noise in a Yorkshire accent. Everybody in the building
thought it was me in there and I got letters telling me I was
out of order for having sex in the bath from the other tenants
that had to use it. I only found out about all this after I'd
returned from a fabulous holiday in Tiverton with Dean.
He'd kindly invited me to stay with his mum and sister in
between spending seven hours a day in the water off Croyd
learning to surf. He let me borrow a board, a wetsuit and he
drove me to the beach everyday in a red mini which acted as
a makeshift shelter. We would stop off at a supermarket to
buy cheese and French bread to feast on inside the 1960's
Cooper after a day in the cold Easter waters. He talked to me
about the spirit of the sea and advised me to take a shell to
wear around my neck to remind me of my first time, to keep
the sea near me forever. His mum would play whale music
to us back in the house, while we drank wine, chilled out and
talked about their family's outlook on life. It was a million
miles from my upbringing and I was deeply affected by
where they were coming from. I now knew why I liked
Dean. It wasn't a coincidence. Something underneath was
alike. Once back in London with my crisp shaped shell, I

bought a piece of thin leather and drilled a hole in the top to thread it through. Dean helped tie it round my neck, like a ceremony. I felt like I had a new power, something extra to give me strength – a symbol of my new spiritual side.

Before I had chance to find out what Peter Duffy had done while I was in Devon, I dropped my bags off, did a full wash at the laundrette and then left for Edinburgh. Tanya came to Kings Cross to see me off, which I thought was really nice until she started crying on the platform and told me she loved me. It freaked me out all the way to the first stop Doncaster before I rid myself of any responsibility because I didn't feel the same way. I just wanted to focus on to squeezing the last of my Easter holidays out visiting my old mate Wes from Foundation course, who used to go out with Katie. I could also squeeze in a visit to Faye's best friend Julie Fitzsimmons, who was at Heriot-Watt Uni and had become my pen pal shoulder to cry on.

After the long train journey up I spent three days getting off my head with Wes and his new mates in his halls of residence by the Grass Market. At one particular party, a quiet lad called Daniel who was with us (quiet when sober but mental after a few sherbets) had been abusing a couple of black gay men, who were kissing in the kitchen. He was dishing out proper verbals to both of them in front of everyone else about how disgusting he thought they were. As the evening progressed Daniel passed out on the couch and another lad from halls called a few of us over to grab an arm and a leg. We put him down next to the pantry door under the stairs and this bloke grabs a broom, opens a condom, spits in it and stretches it over the end of the broom handle. We all stared at each other and he says, "Go on, then. Turn him over and pull his kegs down". So we did, then he poked the condom up his bum hole, fiddled around a bit and then removed the broom. "Tidy him up then!" So we pulled his pants and trousers back up leaving the condom attached, tucked his shirt in and fastened his belt. The guy then tells us to help him carry his victim outside to some alleyway full of rubbish bins by the Grass Market. Me and another bloke dropped out at this point but they found others to help. When they got back everyone was saying how out of order it was to do that, but the party was split by Daniel's earlier abuse of the two guys in the kitchen. Either way this bloke defended his actions by declaring himself as part of the 'gay liberation front'. I'm sure he was straight. We returned to halls, fell asleep on Wes's floor and woke up with Daniel returning and asking everyone what happened. Before anyone could speak, the bloke from 'the gay liberation front' opened his mouth, "You left the party with those two black lads you were shouting at earlier." To which Daniel said, "Oh, really?" and went solemnly back to his room.

I left Wes after that and went to see Julie who introduced me to all her friends who seemed to know every detail about me and in some cases had obviously read my letters to her, in which I bleated about my broken heart and that Faye should quit Paris and that 30-year-old married dickhead. We had a night out at Carbolic Frolic at the end of Princes Street. Sitting on double beds in the middle of a nightclub is very odd. Maybe the club owner wanted everyone to shag but they just got in the way and as a bloke, if you sat down next to a girl she had every excuse to call you a filthy letch even before you opened your mouth and delivered your first chat up line. Putting beds in nightclubs is a shit idea. On the second night we got really drunk in a communal area on the Heriot-Watt campus. A real 'preppy-rugga shirt hockey' night in with drinking games and snogging. I hated it. I hated academics studying traditional courses with exams at the end of them. There is no creativity and no skills to bring to the party apart from how much you can drink and whether you can still have sex after all that alcohol. We ended up having a water fight, which moved into the girls showers and it was at that point, fully clothed when Julie kissed me. I say 'kissed me' because we were wrestling under a shower head, which was switched on while I held her in there. As soon as it started, I thought to myself – this is a set-up, dried myself and went to bed. Five hours later I was on the train heading south, trying desperately to catch up on my sleep and totally denying anything had happened with Julie in that shower! I felt a total idiot because I only ever thought of her as a mate who offered me strength and advice through her kind letters. On return to the bedsit in Harrow, it was an absolute rubbish tip. Actually, it was a shit hole and Peter was lying on my bed with his shoes on and his arms behind his head watching TV.

"What the fuck's going on here?"

"What? Nothing. Just watching Italian football."

"Bollocks to that. Why is my bedsit all moved round?"

"Because I thought it worked better this way. My neck started to ache when the TV was on top of the wardrobe. You can see it better from here."

"So you could move it all round but you couldn't clean up? Look at the fucking state of the kitchen!"

"Look mate, I'll sort it all now." He got up and moved towards the kitchen, picking up some paper from the sideboard, "Here, you got some post and someone shoved this stupid complaint under the door."

"Complaint about what?" He passed everything to me.

"Well, when you were in Devon, I invited my girlfriend Susan down for the weekend. One thing led to another and after a few drinks on Saturday night we had sex in the bath and some people upstairs could hear us. I don't think we were being that loud. It's just nosey neighbours and they should keep their mouths shut."

I read the note, "Hold on a minute, they think it was me. Have you been upstairs to apologise?"

"No, I thought it was best to keep a low profile, seen as you're subletting the place anyway. I didn't want you to get in trouble."

"Subletting? Fuck off! You haven't paid me a penny since you arrived, you cunt. You hardly even contributed to my weekly shop either."

"Oh, come on mate. I've done the best I can. As soon as I get paid I'll give you some money."

"When will that be?"

"Before May bank holiday."

"Well it better fucking had be. End of this month I want you out. You're pissing me off now and this bedsit is too small to cope with annoying, lazy, tight Yorkshire flat mates. And once you've cleaned that mess up you can go upstairs and downstairs, knock on every fucker's door and apologise for shagging in their bath. Make sure you tell them it was not me and then go and clean the fucking bathroom top-to-toe. I'm off out you cunt." I slammed the door and walked down to Kenton to slag him off to Tanya and get a cuddle at the same time, obviously making sure I didn't mention that stupid snog in Edinburgh.

As the end of the month approached, after I failed to get an official ticket to watch England take on Holland in a World Cup '94 qualifier at Wembley, I jumped on the tube at Harrow with only two £10 notes in my pocket at 7:45 for an 8 o'clock kick off. As I left Wembley Park station at 8:05pm I was practically mobbed by touts left with too many tickets. I put on my best puppy dog eyes and opened my wallet. "I'm a student and I've only got twenty quid." It worked and I picked up a £22.00 ticket. It may not sound great to you but when I took my seat amongst all the boos for John Barnes, which I found bizarre, a couple of scousers asked me how much I paid for it and then laughed when I told them. It turns out the tout had bought it from them for £45, which made me feel good and lucky that I lived next door to the stadium. Barnes shoved it back down the boo boys throats with a brilliant free kick but the game ended 2-2. Three points dropped at home. When I got back to the house I felt bullish enough to kick Peter out of my bedsit. Not literally, but we did agree he had to go that weekend as it was the end of the month and he could settle up. The little shit left me £30 short and nicked one of my favourite tapes, which I managed to get back in the post by chasing his girlfriend

Susan. He left me no forwarding address and I never saw him again.

Nath had pissed me off as well, after making fun of the fact I was working out regularly with Dean and Diago. We knew we were doing it for show, for the 'chicks' but we also knew it would help Dan's surfing, my football and Diago's body building. Diago was well up for getting big. He lifted well above what me and Dean were doing. He also started taking that protein powder stuff in giant tubs. We all had a healthy routine on Monday, Wednesday and Friday lunchtimes, doing measured reps and helping each other through the workout. It was getting sunny and warmer now so we began to wear less and the six months of training was beginning to show. Nath knew I had been surfing in Devon over Easter and that I was close to Dean. One morning break myself and Nath were sitting outside the Alhambra video block on the grass talking about the following year. Discussing things like where and with whom we were going to live. It's etched in my mind because Nath 'turned up' at my bedsit again out of the blue to see how I was and he had mentioned a few possibilities, including how we could convince Mauli, the rich kid from Malaysia, to move in with us purely because he had a Macintosh Computer and "we could use it." Both myself and Nath conspired to get the 'uncool' Mauli in with us, even though he didn't fit our demographic. Nath knew I got on with Twinkle and suggested that foursome would be a great fix, if we got 'gay Seth' from fashion to let us have the house he was leaving when he graduated in a month's time. 'Gay Seth' was another mate of mine we used to quiz at the bar about what it felt like to have gay sex. Seth was someone who had something that Nath could use as a second hand contact through me. As far as I was concerned it all seemed logical and I was willing to broker everything if we could convince Twinkle and Mauls. After all, every one of us needed somewhere sorting out for next year. It was a scheme and it felt good to have a plan. We paused on the Alhambra's grassy knoll for a second after the agreement was made, I laid back on the grass and looked at the fluffy clouds travelling slowly across the Middlesex sky. Then Nath spouts out, "Are you going for your work out with Cheech and Cheong, then?" The words hit home like poisioned vocal daggers. I felt embarrassed, angry and a whole host of emotions but most of all I questioned myself for hanging out with Dean and Diago. That's what the comments were designed to do. All of a sudden, they were both complete losers in an instant. In one sentence Nath had managed to put them down to size by tagging them as fools and seed a thought that would motivate me to realign myself with my future housemate Nath. I sat up and looked at the scaffolding which had started to appear with the redevelopment of the campus and said, "Dan & Diago are alright you know. They're a good laugh."

"They're hilarious Vic." He stood up, dusted the grass off his denim jacket and walked off.

The building work continued into June and as Student Rep I was getting ear ache off people who thought it was going to get in the way of their studies. With all the meetings I was going to I was wondering about it myself. The works were due for completion in 1996, a full year after graduation and there was talk the Queen would be opening it as the 'largest media lab in Europe'. All very exciting for new entrants in 1996 but for us, the football pitches were already being cut up for the diggers to start the foundations of the new halls of residence. There was a lot of mud everywhere.

The grafitti on the mens toilets in the GID block were causing emotions to run high. The third years had decided to call their degree 'Infonauts' and someone scrawled 'Info nots' on the back of a toilet door. One of them saw it and reported back to the others and then all three classrooms who shared the bogs, fell out after some finger pointing went on. Nobody was found guilty but we all thought it was amusing. I went and had a look for myself. The handwriting looked liked Nath's but he denied it with a smile. That was the type of thing he'd do.

Victor J Kennedy

The end of the first year was not going well for me. In the last module Client Based Project, I was in a group that patently wanted the course to end and summer to start. We bummed around Harrow's town library trying to work out how to successfully label and signpost sections whilst the general public stared at us in disbelief. We were headless and rudderless too and the mark of 63% reflected that. For the Design in Society module marks came in, which had evolved from Wednesday morning lectures. The tutor had scribbled all over it.

You have produced a thoughtful essay and have made use of difficult texts such as Mcluhan. These have been handled well. Overall I feel it is sometimes difficult to know exactly what you are trying to say and as far as the reader is concerned there does not seem to be a structured way of answering the question.
B-/C+

I didn't think her response was clear because the mark was okay but her comments sounded bad. Elena also put the boot in on a triplicate form I got back from my 'informal chat' towards my Tutorial Record for level one.

Topics Covered: Liked the whole idea of exploring and pushing ideas around. Learning skills – really valuable experience from the design studio – management and organisational skills – useful for working in groups. Had to work hard to get where he is – flunked school. Poly Italian – 9th Module – wants to take it next year. Wants to be really good – being in London is really useful – meets designers etc. Has already been in Art and Design since 17 – learnt to be quite skillful at dealing with people. Realises that he can't lean back and be lazy because the competition is getting tougher.
Recommendations: *Will try to be more respectful to the idea of 'lectures.' Megans project – excellent – so much to

look into and explore – enjoyed client-based project – was unsure of the course when he started – got depressed – then it picked up but in March thought about transferring – now is okay and he really needs to push it hard – explore, fail and then find out through doing it. Proud of the fact that he tries hard on every project.

The Graphic Experience 60% B
The Graphic Language 85% A
Information Carriers 73% A
Visual Representation 71% A

Ok, I know they were top marks but the comments came out of my mouth and once written down I felt they were a punishment, only because of their honesty. Maybe Elena was just honest. I mean, she had already fixed me and others up for a chat with Abram Games for tea under a blossom tree in his back garden. She also took me to a Paul Rand lecture at the RSA in Savoy Place. I'd got to speak to these great men and learn from them just before they died and I guess I should have thanked her but I felt like we'd got off to such a bad start that she was against me.

As our course petered out and the Infonauts fell from the sky, Tanya invited me to the fashion course degree show at the Business Design Centre in Islington. It was unbelieveably bigger and better than our third years' degree show in Regent Street. Even famous fashion designer Jeff Banks from the Clothes Show was in the audience. 'Gay Seth' had asked me to go down the cat walk in rubber on all fours, attached to a lead which he would carry at the finale but I let him down gently with a "fuck off" and a "no chance!" But he did it anyway with one of the other lads from fashion in tow. There was a big roar from the crowd and I was a bit jealous and regretted being a chicken at the thought of an association of his message. After the show we got pissed in a local pub and then made our way down to Brixton Academy to watch Jamiroquai. Whilst in the queue, Tanya, Katie and some girl called Alma had to crouch down

Victor J Kennedy

between two cars to take a piss. Everyone in the queue from
Harrow was screaming and causing a fuss to create attention
and eventually there was a crowd watching them pissing.
That was actually more entertaining than the gig.

For a couple of weeks I'd been collecting boxes and packing
my things up from the bedsit. Diago had taped me Bob
Marley & The Wailers album Legend and I was listening to
No Woman No Cry when the buzzer went. It was Tanya and
Cathy with Nath. Back in the spring when Catherine moved
in with Dean and Diago above the chip shop, Nath had
become single. They both started dating after Easter and we
had all become really close. In fact we were the 'perfect
foursome' because by now Katie and Tanya were not as
close. Cathy was on the same Fashion course and Tanya
really liked her. They had organised to live together next
year with two blokes from GID. The very quiet Ross Deng
from Devon and the infamous Lewis, of all people!

I let Tanya in and she came up to my room, leaving those
two waiting in Cathy's Land Rover. I'd invited them to the
Lake District to stay at my parent's for a few days on the
proviso I got my gear transported back in that Land Rover.
On entering the room, Tanya burst into tears because the
room was stripped of any evidence that I'd been there and
that we'd had so many good times there since we got
together in January. It made me feel sorry for her and has
emotionally tainted that Bob Marley song everytime I hear
it. I told her I wasn't going away. She was coming with me
and that I would be back in September but she just tried to
hold it in and kept forcing a smile for the remainder of the
time we packed the vehicle with my stuff. Her eyes were
pink and she kept hiding them behind this cute mushroom
hat, which from that day forward became my pet name for
her; my 'Shroom.'

I shut the door, posted the key through the letter box which
I'd got so many wonderful letters through and jumped in the
back of the Land Rover. Cathy slammed the door and off we
went. It took hours and we had a ball when we got to

Millhead. We visited all the tourist bits like Hawkshead and Windermere. Back at my parents' I even showed those three things from my past, like my Star Wars figures which I'd kept from my childhood. Nath took particular interest in those and that fact I had hoarded them. They all found out much more about me, yet I knew little about them. Cathy had taken us back to her father's place in Aylesbury for one night of booze riddled partying but all I knew was that we had to vacate the cottage before her dad got back, which didn't sound good especially after I'd been spooked by photos of him on the fireplace. I'd obviously been to Tanya's parents in Buckhurst Hill for Sunday lunch now and again but I had no idea about Nath and in less then three months I was going to move in with him.

After another tear fuelled goodbye, my 'Shroom', Cathy and Nath set off back to London and I started unpacking my things to begin storing them in my parents garage. The first box I opened had a note from Dean in the top. I remembered he'd been round a couple of nights before to help me sort things out and he must have sneakily written it on a piece of card and slipped it in the box before sealing it with brown tape.

It read; Vic, The optimism of the action is better than the pessimism of the thought. Dean

Victor J Kennedy

Chapter 5 - Coming Together

I was home. Back up north with the whole summer ahead of me. I wanted to make it a good summer so I borrowed my mum's car and drove the seven miles into Kendal town centre to visit Reggie and everyone at Goddard Murray Design. I'd already written him a letter asking about the possibility of carrying on where I left off as the office junior. I needed the money and it was much more beneficial than working in a supermarket or a factory. Let's just say it was more relevant to my career path to be in a design studio as long as I could put up with the piss taking, which basically meant fulfilling the 'court jester' role and 'making 'em laugh.' I only had to take a few student quips from Sally and Sasha on reception and the job was mine. I started the next morning on £120 a week organising the transparency filing cabinet and making cups of tea. Every day I'd buy my lunch from Marks & Sparks and then either sit in the bandstand at Stromongate or in the park if it was sunny. And I bought The Sun so I could keep up with the London gossip, celebs flashing their knickers and the football. If I took my lunch back to work, Sally and Sasha would comment or tease me about the high calorie content. They weren't that much older than me, a few years, but flirting with them, especially Sally with her fantastic breasts, fired a young lad's imagination.

20/7/93
Dear Victor,
Hiya luv, how's it going? I hope you're having loads of fun up there and that work's going well. I start work tomorrow at Fairlop Waters, although I don't want to go at all, I've been trying to fool my mum all day that I'm not feeling too well, like when I was 12 and didn't want to go to school, she's not falling for it though!
Anyway, I thought I'd send these photos up for you to have a butchers at, also I've enclosed the picture from Chris's car,

although it's not very clear. Katie put it in my room for you before she left.

It seems so strange living back at home, I can't believe how quickly I've sunk back into it, all my friends seem to be doing exactly the same as when I moved away (sad but true). It was really nice to hear from you on Sunday, I've really missed talking to you since I got home.

I'm really looking forward to my Birthday, I wish it was in term time so you were around, Cathy, Alma and Seth etc. are coming down so it should be a laugh, Alf who is the manager of The Colorado – where I used to work has sorted it all out and let me hire the top half of the restaurant for nothing and then go into the club. The table's booked for 'around' 30 people so it should be really good.

Anyway enough about that! How are you? I hope everything's going well and that you're enjoying being home. I'm really sorry I got so upset when I left + the night before, I was being a twat - but what's new?!

Well that's about all I've got to waffle on about for now, please write or call soon. I'm missing you loads! Take care + have fun. Love Tanya xxxx

22/7/93

I've just finished my first shift at work + thought I'd add to this letter before I send it, Victor you wouldn't believe what this job's like. I've never seen so many 'fruity women' in all my life!

Everyone in the whole place has a brilliant suntan and perfect body!! What can you do!!?

I worked behind the bar with two blokes, one from here and one from Newcastle so it was quite a laugh, also I made £16 tips on top of my wages, so I didn't do too bad. Also after the bar shuts at 12 they give you something to eat and a pint, so it's okay really.

Anyway I'll shut up now and go to bed! Hope to hear from you soon. All my thoughts. Tanya xxxx

Victor J Kennedy

I got through my first week at Goddard Murray Associates and then received a phone call which freaked me out a bit. I was caught totally off guard by Tanya's mum, Carolyn one Sunday night. She basically asked me to go down to Essex in July for Tanya's 21st birthday as her surprise present. Everything would be paid for and supplied by Tanya's parents including my train fare if I could just 'turn up out of the blue' at the venue, The Colorado Exchange on Epping New Road at 8pm when everyone starts singing happy birthday. Straight away I said yes and put the phone down. First of all I thought, oh my god Tanya's been telling her mum about me and now they think I'm serious about her. The classic response of a frightened manchild by commitment. But then after a while I thought her mum was very kind for doing that for her daughter. The thing is, I felt more like the present than a participant on the long journey down there. It was like being Jeremy Beadle when her dad picked me up outside Woodford tube station and briefed me on the ensuing situation at the restaurant. We pulled up outside, Elvis was about to enter the building. Her dad got his camera ready as I straightened my top and tidied my hair. As soon as her mum saw me she started singing happy birthday, everyone joined in and I marched round the back of her seat. All her cousins and friends from uni were there, many faces I didn't know and a few I did. Nath was there, still pretending he liked Catherine. Cathy was next to him, unable to sing but laughing her head off at me standing behind Tanya. Eventually they got to the last line and that's when I tapped her on the shoulder. She screamed, then jumped up and hugged me really tightly. It felt like a release of anxiety and made me think back to my 21st birthday in January. You just want your 21st to go really well, especially when someone is there who you love. I could empathise with Tanya at that moment and I played my part but that was the whole point. I was a passenger, a puppet even! And deep down my heart wasn't in it. I wasn't in love with Tanya like she was in love with me.

Mad in England - A memoir

After an intense weekend of meet and greet from grandparents Edna and Cyril to cousin Sophie and sister Jen's famous model friends, I got myself back up north, a good two hundred and fifty miles away to my other life. My other life now seemed even more attractive than the one back in London. It wasn't necessarily my stirling work with a can of Spray Mount and a scalpel at Reggie's but my improved relationship with the rest of the old sixth form lot at Dermont School, who by now had finished a first year experimenting with drugs at various universities around the country. Twelve months before I only confided in a few of them who I knew would try it. This eventually included Faye, who was my obvious link to these school friends but she was no longer here. I was two years older than them and I guess the receptive ones had looked up to me on the regular 18th Birthday Party coach journeys to Blackburn's nightclubs. Twelve months later and this minority was now the majority. In fact not even just ex-Dermont School but all the locals around South Lakeland seemed to be getting 'sorted.' This is the thing really, by watching the media you would think that drugs were an inner city problem but rurally it was an epidemic. The cities are just a magnet. All that summer of 1993 I was off in a car, down the A65 every Saturday night to places like Up Your Ronson, KAOS and Orbit in Leeds. In fact, that summer I was in Leeds with more regularity than when I lived nine miles away in Bradford. We got skanked a few times with things like Anadins instead of Es which on one occasion I couldn't undo because the dealer was an uncompromising scarey Jamaican bloke. Once he had our £75 in his hand, he raged at my suggestion that I could feel a groove down the centre of all five pills after we'd exchanged hands under a table in the middle of the Rhythm Factory. I guess he could've been bluffing but he made me believe I would get shot if I continued my line of questioning. One night we also nearly had an accident on the way home. Just coming through Ilkley main crossroads, my mate Alvin who was driving, at some speed with a loud disco going on inside the car went through a red. A farmer who was on green and trying to transport some of his sheep at 4:30am just missed us by inches.

Julie returned from Edinburgh after experimenting with only alcohol and snogging blokes in the showers after a water fight, had her usual 'big' birthday party in August. We were off to Peppermint Place in Blackburn again, only instead of a fiftytwo seater coach there was an exclusive and intimate twentyone seater bus and my name was on the list. This was after an extremely difficult time back at her parent's lovely house in Silverdale for pre-party drinks. The main issue for me was, for a start I'd taken a 'Strawberry' LSD tab about thirty minutes before I arrived, I had not spoken to Julie since our snog in Edinburgh at Easter and secondly, I had 'come up' and had uncontrollable giggles at every single thing anyone said to me. I'm sure they knew. They knew alright! Her little brother Don definitely knew. He played for Warton with Scottish Ray and was in his first year at Dermont sixth form. Scottish Ray didn't suspect me but he stayed up the front of the bus with Julie. They looked to be getting on really well and by the end of the night they were snogging and dancing together which freaked everyone out who knew them at sixth form, when they were with other partners. Scott and Jacky were there too, of course. To all who didn't know the truth that I knew, Scott and Jacky were turning into the golden couple from that sixth form generation. Twelve months away at university and everyone had split up apart from them. Jacky was down in Acton staying with her brother for a 'year out.' A year out just means a year going out and getting pissed. She had a job but was studying for something and nobody knew but me (and Scott probably had a different version) that she had asked me over from Harrow to stay at her brothers and watch a video together. At the time I was naive and still grieving over Faye and my impending HIV but Jacky was not to know that and I think that night she pulled out all the tricks,

the alcohol, the confusion about which bedroom I was
staying in, walking into the bathroom in a neglige while I
was brushing my teeth. That type of thing. I asked her if she
had been with anyone while Scott was up in Leeds doing his
geography degree and she said yes! Like it was to be
expected. Like I was supposed to throw abandon to the wind
and have a go with a mates girlfriend. Well, I would've but
for the HIV test and she caught me off guard because I had
my 'friend' head on and not my 'unscrupulous sexual deviant'
one. This was now about ten months later and being free of
HIV but paying for LSD I took a bit of a shine to the idea of
Jacky having a filthy, soft spot for me. By the time we got
back from Blackburn, swerved Julie's parents and got back
to Scott's mum's in Leighton village, I was in a poor state.
Jacky however, was still sober because she left her car at
Scott's before we set off. She had to work in the morning
back in Yealand and had to go home. Yealand is situated
back through Millhead and Carnforth on the A6 towards
Kendal and Jacky, who knew my parents lived in Millhead,
offered me the 'ride home' with a cheeky little wink. Of
course I accepted and she obliged by taking a detour through
Dermont Park and pulling the car over. I didn't think of
Tanya or Scott or in fact anyone other than my groin area. It
was very lusty. It was outside. It was over very quickly.
I woke the next day feeling pretty crap with myself. The
feeling was not guilt because I pushed it into denial. I just
kept quiet and got drunk again at the nearest opportunity.
Work was fine. Work was a piece of piss really. I was doing
pre-season training with Crusaders and playing five-a-side at
Dermont School on Thursdays with Smudge and all the lads.
One of them, Jamo, a joiner from the village had finished
building his own house and was having a party. All of us
were invited but it was a boozy do rather than anything I was
doing with the students. So like a good chameleon I went
along, drank beer from a keg in his kitchen and socialised
with these pro-family oriented manual workers and their
wives or girlfriends. Lucy, the daughter of Andy, a painter

and decorator in the village had been making comments about how nice my backside looked in the 501 jeans I was wearing. I'd fancied her back in '88 when I first arrived in Millhead because she was so well developed compared to other 16 year old girls. She didn't like guys her own age, which was normal. She wanted older blokes with cars and moustaches. I never even bothered making a move because I knew the result. I was a skinny kid, no car or facial hair yet. By 1993 I knew she'd tried out a few of the Crusaders squad but with no real marriage results. I knew it was difficult for them too because her dad Andy used to play for Crusaders in the 60s and 70s. He was noteably a great player. In fact he was legendary round these parts. He still went for a drink down the clubhouse too so he would find out if you were treating his daughter badly. At Jamo's party she was on at me all night. There was not yet furniture in his house so it was packed with drunken people just like a pub. If I moved rooms she would come and find me and pat me on the bum and smile suggestively. Northern birds. Not backward at coming forward. She drank pints too. Kept up with me all the way until it came to crunch time, that is. We left together after midnight and staggered down the road to her parent's house. I knew Andy had a poker table in the cellar because a mate of mine called Phil had been their apprentice and told me they stack the paint down there. We snogged on the doorstep. The lights were off so dad was in bed. She unlocked the door and we quietly sneaked downstairs to the poker room. We faced each other next to the table and then we just went for it. All the cards and chips got pushed to one end, she quickly derobed and jumped on the green surface while I tried to pull my jeans down. It was a complete drunken mess and half way into my repetoire I realised she was asleep! What else can you do but pull your pants back up and leave in humiliation. I hope her dad didn't come down for a late night game of poker and find her spread-eagled.

Mad in England - A memoir

I didn't have time to worry about what I'd done (again) or how much of a crap boyfriend I was to Tanya but it was starting to creep into my head quite often, it slowly increased over a period of weeks after that. I would ask myself how I kept getting into these situations. I just loved the thrill of sex. Risky sex.

After his party I became closer to Jamo and at the U2 Zoo TV concert in Roundhay Park in Leeds we stood together right at the front. What I liked about Jamo was he was in his forties but he acted like he was my age. I aspired to be like that when I got to his age. The rest of the lads sat together on a grass hill at the back and away from the mayhem. They were all twats that day. Especially Graham Ince who was driving the mini bus. Everything by his rules and his timetable, even his jokes had to be the most funny and they were usually at my expense. We drank so much on the way to Leeds that when we got to Roundhay Park there were massive queues for the toilets so he suggested we all stand round in a circle and piss into a plastic carrier bag. That way any girls nearby would not see our cocks and get offended. All twelve lads agreed but once it got full, the tiny air holes started leaking piss so Graham stood back because he'd finished. Then he started pointing and shouting very loudly that, "Those blokes are pissing in a carrier bag!" and everyone turns around. After all the lads had walked away there was just me standing there pissing into a leaking carrier bag with four hundred women watching me and some were even pointing. This was the same group of lads who shaved my hair off in Benalmadena on that mad 'HIV' holiday the year before. I wouldn't call them friends. It was up for debate whether I was going to go with them this year or not. Nath had sent me a jokey postcard from the South of France asking me if I wanted to fly out there and spend some time at his parent's villa with him during late August and early September. I honestly thought he was taking the piss, especially about it being his parent's villa. That proposition seemed a million miles away on every level from where I currently was. The job with Reggie didn't pay enough and I was addicted to my working class Canary Island jaunts so I arranged a 'cheapie' with Julie and Scottish Ray, who I would've put money on to become an item after a sweaty holiday romance. It was a fairly risky venture due to my Edinburgh snog but I really wanted those two to have a some fun and see what comes out of it. Ray was depressed from being single and not at university, Julie was depressed from not finding a fella in Scotland. I told Tanya about the holiday over the phone and she tried her best to come along but couldn't get time off work at such short notice. She was perplexed about not being invited in the first place but then again I wasn't thinking that my two lives were joined up. I was living the one up north at the moment and the London one was not starting again for a good few weeks yet. She sent a letter which freaked me out a bit because I wasn't expecting it.

Dear Victor,
Alright treacle? Hows it hanging? I thought I'd write you a short note to see how you are and if you're having fun up there in Cumbria?
I've been missing you loads since you left and have taken to using my spare time by getting fit, so far this week I've been swimming every other day and have been to keep-fit twice, I'm also using my birthday present from you to tone those areas not exercised by either of these two sports! (say no more luv ha-ha!)
Anyway enough of that, I want to thank you so much for coming down for my 21st, it was brilliant to see you, I've never been so surprised to see anyone! I thought as a thank you I'd send you these extra things to fill your scrap book! [balloons and ticket to Thorpe Park]
(only joking!)
Anyway – not that much has been happening around here, I've had to work loads of shifts and from Wednesday will be working the days as well as the evenings! However, I've still

managed to fit in the odd drinking session, one large one on Friday when I went up to town with Sophie for a Party at David's work. There was loads of free drink and food which both Sophie and I obviously took full advantage of!

Well that's about all I've got to waffle on about for now. Dad, Luke etc. are coming up on the 26th August for a couple of days so I hope it'll be okay to come and see you then, please get in touch and say if this isn't possible so I can change the dates etc.

Hope to hear from you soon, take care and have fun. All my love Tanya xx

Myself, Julie and Ray ended up after suffering the menu on a cheap flight with a tent under our arm in Puerto Del Carmen, Lanzarote but dumped it as soon as Julie worked her magic with the guy at The Apartment Aquarius and got all three skint students into a self-catering place for seven days, costing us merely peanuts. Obviously the rest of the spending money saved was spent on booze and frequenting the local tacky nightclubs such as the Hippodrome, Paradise, Long Play, Dreams and Joker Discoteca. We survived on Calamari which I mistook for a large bag of Onion Rings in the deep freezer at the supermarcado. We had a great time, if you call reading books, listening to the walkman and sunbathing a great time but sadly those two didn't get together. No matter how drunk I got them both. I think there was too much history between them. They ended up like brother and sister.

My endeavours for Goddard Murray Associates over the summer and a cheap holiday in Lanzarote had left me some pocket money so I decided on my return to university I would have my very first CD player. I'd never been able to afford one before and it felt like I was the last person to own one so I shelled out for a portable Panasonic XBS and got Prince's Greatest Hits triple CD. I needed something to play in my new home; number 34 Crofts Road, Harrow. The Panasonic was placed into a rented blue Transit Van that my dad had organised. It fit neatly next to all the rest of my belongings. The old man was getting good at this journey now and we shared the driving so he could 'get used to its handling' on the motorway before the busy roads of Wealdstone set upon him. And set upon him they did! There was sweat dropping off his nose from the stress at other people, or "fucking London drivers!" as he referred to them. A lot of people up north refer to "that there London" and the fact they "couldn't live down there" or travel to work everyday on "that bloody tube, it's like a cattle lorry" but they never do. They just visit and say how shit they think it is and then leave. There's no answer to it. It's what maintains the divide. The thing is, London driving is a multicultural make up of international techniques of forcing your way around a giant metropolis as fast as you possibly can without dying in the process. It doesn't seem unreasonable to me. It's called a rat race.

We got to the house first and that meant I got the best room. We carried all my stuff up to the front bedroom and then locked the bedroom door before taking the van down to Mauli's first year digs to pick him and his belongings up as a favour. After a cup of tea and a good hour of packing the van was completely full. My stuff had only filled the van halfway. My dad was amazed at how much crap Mauli had managed to collect in twelve months living in a new country. We even had to leave some of it behind! By the time the van wobbled it's way across Harrow both Carl and Nath had arrived and were installed. Carl upstairs at the back and Nath in the front room below me. That left Mauli with the crappiest room in the house, right next to the kitchen with an oven that didn't work. The gas however, did work so we ate fried food for most of the first term. Our new landlord, Darren Fenchurch, was nowhere to be found unless it was rent pay day. He always turned up on time then but if we mentioned the cooker or anything else that didn't work he would tell a fib or make an excuse to do something about it later. It was great having Mauli with respect to eating fried food all the time but Malaysian food does lend itself to that mode of cooking and I loved it when it was Mauli's turn to cook. Twinkle just cooked sautied potatoes. I was the token Italian pasta mess and Nath would mix it up with steaks and French stuff he'd picked up from his mum, who was allegedly French. We had a good system for food shopping once a week, where three people go shopping to Tescos in Nath's car while the other person stays home and cooks. Whatever made it's way into the trolley was divided four equal ways financially. The three people return, unpack it and then everyone sits down upstairs in the smallest bedroom on duvets to eat the meal, watch TV and then play Mario Karts before doing some homework or mucking about. This room was a ridiculous choice of living room because everyone all wanted a large bedroom. The smallest bedroom then became the most popular room in the house. We were all squashed when we were in there and nobody cleaned up the plates or spilled food. It was disgusting because Nath smoked and everything stank. It was like hanging out in a wheelie bin. The Super Nintendo brought a lot of arguments and fall-outs between competitive Nath and strong-minded Mauli. Nath thought Mauli was weak and in a way Mauli appeared to be an easy target. Mauli though, would not stand for it and would fight Nath until either myself or Carl would step in to end the slaughter. It was a relationship that was soured right from the off and the whole situation was horrendous for everyone involved in the household, not just Mauli.

Using double standards, Nath treated Mauli with upmost respect when he needed to use his Apple Macintosh to get homework done. Then me and Carl started sneaking on it. Then Nath introduced a cruel homework rota, in Mauli's best interests of course. Everyone else got one hour on Mauli's computer to complete their project and when everyone else was finished, Mauli could have his computer back somewhere around midnight to finish his own homework. Obviously his work suffered in the long term because he was still awake in the early hours. The rota existed simply because the computer was in Mauli's bedroom and he "obviously needed to sleep, which would be difficult if someone else was still sat there working." During this second year at uni, Mauli did not get as much sleep as the other three leeches he had agreed to live with.

Our first outing as housemates was the Freshers' Ball on the campus at Red Lion Square, Holborn. The student union must have radically changed hands over the summer because Bad Manners and The Urban Cookie Collective were booked to perform. It was good to see Busta Bloodvessel in the flesh and what flesh it was but The Urban Cookie Collective mimed to that one song they got in the charts about the key and the secret. The whole thing was a cost cutting exercise, even the toilets were in a portakabin because the campus was being shut down soon. It was like having a disco on a building site and the whole thing probably cost about two hundred quid. "Not like last year, eh? Ministry of Sound was our Freshers' Ball last year. Absolutely brilliant!" That was the type of thing coming out of Nath's mouth to all the impressionable new first years, which was a lie. I never saw Nath at last years Freshers' Ball. Last year, I never focused on anything else other than finding some drugs but this year I made sure I'd brought a few wraps of speed back down from my trips to Leeds. We bumped into Lewis, Ross, Cathy and Tanya so I collared Lewis and Tanya, dived into a portakabin toliet and opened my wallet. Lewis got excited straight away, Tanya looked at me slightly surprised, "Where did you get that from?"
"Oh, it's from a mate back home."
"Is it Coke?"
"No, no. I can't afford that shit on northern wages. It's speedy gonzalez baby! Do you want some?"
"Yeah, why not?"
We all emerged grinning from the portakabin, collectively rubbing our forefinger over our gums while Twinkle, Nath, Cathy, Mauli and Rich stared back at us with no expressions

on their faces whatsoever. I thought they all looked square,
really boring and with no life inside them. I grabbed Tanya
and found a dancefloor with a DJ who was playing the
soundtrack to my state of mind and we just went for it. The
shivers, the rushes and the elation. Up and down for hours
until the place started to empty. Everybody got back together
for a pow wow about transport and I decided to seperate
from Twinkle, Mauls and Nath to go back for some sex at
Tanya's. Cathy disappeared but we assumed she was with
Nath so it was up to myself, Tanya, Lewis and Rich to get
back to Kenton station on the Bakerloo line. This was from
Holborn at about 5am. We decided to get a bus to Queen's
Park station and catch the first tube north somewhere
between 5:30 and 6am. Once we were on the over-ground
platform we all huddled together in a glass waiting room and
watched optimistically as goods trains flew past but no tubes
arrived. I got the bellyaches as I came down from the speed,
which was probably cut with Vim and I got most of it
because Tanya and Lewis were fine. As the minutes passed I
got worse, until once the busy tube had arrived I was lying
down on Tanya's lap in complete agony squeeling in pain. It
felt like my lower abdomen and bowels were about to turn
inside out. I remember looking up at her worried face. She
asked me to hold on. Lewis was on the sidelines giving crap
advice about how to put up with the come down but he knew
I was in a bad way. He'd seen things like this in halls in the
first year. Ross was silent but then Ross never said anything
to anyone anyway. They all helped me off the tube at
Kenton and once back in the house I was administered an
Alka Seltzer then put into bed by Tanya. She laid down
bedside me and said, "Let's not do speed anymore." Then her
alarm clock went off and the Steve Wright Breakfast Show
on Radio 1 started blaring out. She quickly turned it off and
soon we fell sound asleep.
Still feeling peeky, I staggered into the campus mid
afternoon to show my face to Eric Glaser, my
Typolinguistics 2 module tutor for that day. I'd impressed

him in the first couple of weeks of the new term with a cleverly folding card which looked like the Catalan cityscape and said "Gracias" when folded but announced "Barcelona!" once it had unfolded and revealed the hidden letters. He'd now given us a tougher task to redesign the Monotype Directory. Basically he wanted to see the cover, the contents, a sample spread and an index page. I'd got it all sorted and had begun knocking it out in the desktop publishing software Quark Express, using all the tips and tricks given to me by the Goddard Murray typesetters Kevin and Paul over the summer. They even showed me a bit of the software called Illustrator, a drawing program which was pretty much the same thing as Freehand, the software of choice at my university. I'd also been using Photoshop, a piece of software that lets you edit photographs and put wierd & wonderful effects on them. I was mucking about with my printouts on the photocopier that afternoon, resizing and cutting out the trace, then running back up the stairs to the library to photocopy it again. There was a queue due to the new card system introduced to further milk students of cash when they needed to print out or photocopy. If you ran out of credit you had to put your card into this box by the librarian and stick a pound coin in, then stick your card back in the box situated on top of the photocopier. A nice bit of red tape to get the stress levels up. I wasn't bothered because a) I didn't have a deadline and b) I had a bad come down from the night before. The queue got down to two people, me and a black girl who was in front of me. She was slightly taller than me and had a really short haircut. It wasn't until she got stuck with the photocopier that she turned around to ask me for help. She was absolutely stunning! Totally out of my league but she needed my help so I used my opportunity to check her out. My heart was going.
"What's happened to it now?"
"It's jammed I think?"
"Let's have a look at it. They're on their last legs these ones up here. You should go to the ones in the Alhambra at the

bottom of the teaching block. They're brilliant and the uni hasn't put these stupid card meters on them yet."

"I had a lesson down there this morning on the AV slide shows."

"So you're on GID?"

"What's GID?"

"Graphic Information Design, with Elena and Eric?"

"Ah yeah, that's me. Are you a third year then?"

"No, I'm a second year. Just across the corridor from you. If you need anything, I'm Victor."

"I'm Siobhan. Nice to meet you."

"Did you go to the Freshers' Ball last night?"

"No. I'm not really a fan of Bad Manners and I don't live in Harrow so it would've been difficult getting home on my own."

"Where do you live then?"

"Finsbury Park on the Victoria Line. It takes me quite a while to get home from Northwick Park."

"I bet it does! Anyway, that paper's unblocked now. Give it another try."

"Thanks a lot Victor."

"Call me Vic. Everyone else does."

"Ok Vic. See you later." Then she walked away with a really sexy strut but even though she smiled alot and lived alone, she must have loads of blokes chasing after her. All with much more about them than a second year Graphic Information Design student who happens to already have a long-term girlfriend.

When I got back downstairs we were briefed on another module called Visual Representation of Information, which was to choose an object and tell a story of how it became the object in the first place. I chose a piece of popcorn sitting on a dark red carpet. The carpet was in a cinema. The film was Terminator. The journey of the popcorn went in reverse from the moment Schwarzenegger scared the audience and the popcorn ended up on the carpet. It was a bit of borrowed interest on my part because I used the Terminator's view of the world to represent the information visually. I shot the popcorn with Jase in a Harrow cinema, I took screencrabs of the film Terminator and I found images of tractors, cornfields and farms to take the story backwards. Then using Photoshop, I made a storyboard that looked like the Terminator witnessed everything through its own eyes. I turned it into a flick book but my tutor Noel took me to one side and introduced me to a piece of software that would change the direction of my career and my life. Noel thought the piece of work would lend itself to interactivity rather than a sequence in a flick book. He took me to the third floor in the teaching block and sat me down amongst all the CMP students. That's Contemporary Media Practice to you and me. They were all coding and animating things on screen, even adding music to it. It was all very exciting and before the afternoon was out I knew the basics of Director, a piece of software that creates interactive projects onscreen. I was in awe. It felt like going back in time to 1986 when I first got hooked on my Commodore 64 computer. Maybe this time around I was hooked by the science fiction element in my answer to the brief. I just went for it and worked really hard to squeeze out 75% for that module. Nath went for it too by producing a beautiful and inspiring piece of work involving a cube spinning to the beats of Cypress Hill. Me and Nath paired up for the next module; Designer In Context and created an interactive educational lab called KIDS for parents who assess their children's ability to read and identify differences between represented words.

Working with Nath was great because we lived together and could take our time brainstorming till late at night. We knew we had loads of respect for each other's work and approach so when we joined forces we were frightening. The one thing I'd noticed on that KIDS project was that he led everything. Every idea, every string of thought was led by him, supplemented by me. Recently he'd joined Monday night football in the gym with the boys from illustration, the skilful Twinkle (where he got his nickname from) and me.

Mad in England - A memoir

Nath was not a football player, he was a hockey player but he ran around the indoor football court like his life depended on it. Amongst the boys there was no malice or competition up to the point of him joining the proceedings. It was just a kickabout and a chance to relax after college and run around, get in some exercise and then have a drink afterwards. Nath was bashing people around and diving into tackles, constantly trying to mimick things I did. He even started shouting "Vic's ball!" before I did. The fucker used to shout it at home when he passed me the steak for dinner. There was one night I found out how stupid, stubborn and competitive we both were. We turned up to the gym for football and it was called off so everyone left apart from me and Nath. There was a solitary basketball in there and he said,"Let's have a little one on one." He quickly got changed, right there in the gym and started bouncing the ball. "Come on softy." His goading paid off and I got changed. I walked towards him for some one-on-one. I played basketball at school so I felt confident. He dropped the ball to the floor and trapped it under his right foot. "You go over there in that goal and I'll stand in this one. First person to score ten goals from across the gym wins. You have to stand off your line though!" This was stupid and could break your foot but I wasn't going to lose. Not at football, even though he was trying to even up the score with a heavy ball. We were there for well over an hour of stress and competition, he was ruling out goals left, right and centre. All his meddling just stretched out the punishment to both our ankle ligaments, shot after shot until I won 10-8. He couldn't argue with that and I think his feet hurt as bad as mine did. It actually felt like he was trying to bully me. To try and break my sporting spirit to become more powerful than me but I maintained my position. I couldn't work out if I was disturbed by his behaviour or whether I found him funny in a sad way. In my life up to that point, in Bradford or The Lake District, I'd never come across an intense personality like Nath's before.

Victor J Kennedy

He was really complex underneath but appeared to be simple on top. Psychologists call it Machiavellian.

The remaining fashion girls Sera, Katie, Sam and Sonya had grouped together for the second year in a huge house in the middle of Harrow. They decided to have a 'huge' house warming party for the 'huge' house and gave it a theme. "It Came From Outerspace" invited revellers to turn up in some kind of get up related to science fiction or fact. Because it was fashion students who now had sewing machines in their bedrooms, the outfit stakes were high and inside 34 Crofts Road we had a major brainstorm to make sure we didn't let ourselves down. After less than thirty minutes of suggestions and wardrobe searches we came to the idea of Star Trek, the original series from the sixties with Mauli of course as Sulu and Carl in red as one of those token guards that always gets killed. Me and Nath squabbled for James T Kirk's identity but I argued Nath would make a great Spock because of his short black hair and my lighter colouring suited that of the Captain. Getting ready to go out, I couldn't help but think of all three of them as geeks. I even questioned what I was doing living with them and those thoughts spiralled me towards the last remaining wrap of speed sitting on my drawing board. They were so boring, they would never take drugs. I couldn't even tell them about it or include them because they were on a different planet. No pun intended. I took the whole lot in my James T Kirk outfit, cleaned off my nose and then went downstairs to join my crew on the long and cold November walk to the party. We needed an entrance for the gag to work, then I could ditch the losers and get off my face. Mauli got the biggest laugh and I guess that meant the rest of us were there to support and contextualise the Sulu thing going on. Mauli came of age that night but sadly he still didn't get a shag. I went straight upstairs to wash my face because I was freaking out due to taking too much speed at once. I had come up before everyone else had arrived but I bumped into Jeremy the drug dealer, on the first landing outside the toilet.

Mad in England - A memoir

"Are you alright Vic?"

"Yeah man, just done a bit too much, too early. You know what I mean?"

"It's a long night boyo. You want some smoke upstairs to calm down?"

"Yeah. Yeah I do. As long as it's not Heroin Jeremy. I've had a bad experience with that shit."

"No, don't worry. It's just bog standard resin. No monkey business."

"Lead the way sir." I followed him up to what I understood to be Sera's room, all gothic and a bit S&M. Lewis had shagged her recently and then told everyone all about it. Sera was fit but she was allegedly one of those girls who are paid by a club to accompany any old rich businessmen who visit London alone. It's a cliche that every girl who chooses that kind of income always says, "There's no sex involved. We just keep them company and look beautiful. And they are prepared to pay lots of money for it." I always reply to that kind of bullshit like this, "Shhheeeyyyeeeaaah right!" Anyway, lying down on her deep blue velvet bedspread, me and Jeremy spent a good couple of hours smoking and talking bollocks. I would have said, 'getting to know each other better' but that is never the case. The only thing I can remember him saying is, "Fancy some coke?" and me saying, "Yeah, why not?" We then proceeded to stay for a further few hours because I felt it was rude to snort his free coke and then walk away but in the end Sera came upstairs with a guy. Not a punter, just a guy. She asked us both to leave her boudior. That meant going downstairs and having to be sociable. There were not many left when I did get downstairs. All my crew members had beamed back aboard and most of the others I didn't recognise. Somebody was holding Katie's head over a bucket and gently stroking her hair. Other people were asleep. Tanya came waltzing out of the kitchen, "Where the fuck have you been? I've been on my own all night!"

"Just up stairs with Jeremy."

Victor J Kennedy

"All fucking night with a gay Welshman?"

"He's not gay is he?"

"Oh god. You are so naive."

"What?"

"Did he give you free drugs again? Don't answer that! Your eyes are practically all black anyway, you look a fucking state Vic."

"Do you wanna go home?"

"Not to my place, it's too far to walk to Kenton from here."

I took her back to mine and we squeezed into my single bed next to the bay window. She was asleep almost instantly. I couldn't sleep at all and just lay there listening to her breath while a whole onslaught of shitty paranoid thoughts went flushing through my brain like a turd through a toilet. It must've been good coke though because at least I never got any bellyaches.

I tried to keep my head down for a bit after that party. Just concentrate on my work, my football and my bird in that order. My coursework was easy while working with Nath. I was now a fully fledged first teamer on Wednesdays at Chiswick because Bobby Jindal had taken over as coach from the captain Alex and the rest of the old first team clique who picked themselves. Bobby knew me from last season up in the Sunday league around Middlesex so it turns out playing Sunday's can have its bonuses.

I took Tanya out to see Paul Weller at The Royal Albert Hall which was alright but my cheap tickets meant we would be in the heavens and could hardly see him. We definitely heard him though. My parents also came down in November to stay at The Ritz on some posh insurance jolly paid for by my dad's work. I had a day to spend with them and took a Time Out magazine to the hotel reception. We hugged each other and chatted over a coffee. After deliberation my mum decided to Christmas shop and the only thing worth watching turned out to be Wimbledon versus Everton at Crystal Palace's stadium. The crazy gang were ground sharing. So I had a day with my dad at the football. It wasn't

Mad in England - A memoir

that long before I saw my parents again only this year I
wouldn't be visiting Lancaster General for anything.
Christmas was a blur. I couldn't afford presents for my
family but my mum said being home and well was the
biggest present of all. My sister made a few quips about
being 'skivvy' over Christmas dinner and I defended myself
by explaining that while she was at Polytechnic with a grant
plus my dad's money, I got only a grant. I also had an
overdraft limit of £800 and I was well over that already. In
fact, so much so that Lloyds were harassing me with letters
to sort it or take out a fucking loan. My dad diffused the
situation by further taking the piss out of me. The Christmas
drinks at lunchtime in the village pub wearing our new
sweaters, he told everyone the story. I got really pissed on
Christmas Eve and returned from the pub after midnight,
raided the fridge. I took what I thought was a soup in
Tupperware and Microwaved it. Then I consumed it straight
from the plastic jug it was in. It turns out in the morning my
mum asks my dad where the Turkey Giblets are so she can
make a stock. He did his detective work and then had a
giggle all day making sure the whole world knew what I had
done. The rest of the Christmas and New Year break went
the same way. In the village of Millhead and the surrounding
areas I'd managed to become friends with the biggest
drinkers around. We even went to a local knockout pool
competition held in Flookborough at 11am on Boxing Day
and we were still drinking at 3am the next morning while
watching the final being contested by two drunks. It was the
first time I had ever drank myself sober. I even got punched
by a farmers wife while I was asleep on New Years Eve
after her drunken daughter Megan and boyfriend Mike had
crawled into the same bed I had collapsed into. The old dear
nearly bust my nose thinking we were having a threesome.
By the time I had to return to London I needed a holiday.
I returned to London after the Christmas holidays. I hooked
up with Tanya immediately so we went home for some rabid
unprotected sex. The kind of sex you have after being apart

106

for three weeks. Afterwards Tanya leant over from the bed and pulled an envelope from her jacket. "What's this?" I asked.

"Open it." she said. I ripped open the envelope and low and behold it was an early birthday card. As I opened it to read her greeting, a piece of paper fell out. I picked it up and unfolded it. It was a travel itinerary for two people to take a train from Waterloo to the Ferry port of Harwich, then two tickets to Hook and finally the train from Hook to Amsterdam. "Flipping heck! How much did that cost?"

"Shouldn't you say thank you first?"

"Shroom, it's obvious I'm grateful but bloody hell, nobody has ever spent this much money on my birthday present."

"It's not just for your birthday, it's for Christmas too and anyway I'll be coming as well so it's a bit of a holiday just in time for the semester break."

"Ah, that's very sneaky of you. An expensive weekend of debauchery just when all the hard work is finished."

"It won't be expensive."

"How can it not be expensive, you've already booked the travel!"

"We can claim it back when we return. Have you got any receipts for anything expensive that would fit in a suitcase?"

"You what?"

"Insurance! Me and Mike did it once and got the price of the whole holiday back."

"I'm still not with you luv?"

"When we get to Amsterdam we go straight to the Police station and report a stolen suitcase. Then they give us a copy of the report and the travel insurance company pay up. All we have to do is show the receipts to prove the value of the items that were stolen."

"Young lady, that is fraud and my father is an insurance broker. He would send me to my room should I get caught for doing such a crime."

"Don't worry, I'll do all the talking."

"To whom?"

Mad in England - A memoir

"To the loss adjuster who comes round to interview us to check our story. I'll do that bit. I did it for Mike last time and it worked."

"Please don't tell me this is something you do regularly."

"Oh no babe. I'm not a criminal but we're students and we cannot afford things like this but we still need to relax. We shouldn't have to work every bit of spare time away from college. And anyway, I didn't get to go to Lanzarote so this will make up for it."

She was a right one our Tanya was. It made me think her dad must've been an East End bank robber who retired to Essex and she had his criminal blood running through her pretty little veins. She had a heart of gold though and made a right effort to get everyone along for my 22nd birthday party at The Thai Cafe in Wealdstone. You could take your own booze and eat a Thai banquet for £7 from a set menu. It was small and intimate but with a crowd of students filling the entire restaurant it became pretty rowdy. She had made sure everyone had prior notice so I had a right selection of humorous gifts and silly cards. One particularly odd sentiment came from Dean and Diago. It was a card from the college shop, I knew because I'd seen them myself on those spinning wire things and giggled. The cover of it had a patient sat opposite a psychiatrist across a desk and the image was frozen in time as the doctor had pulled a level and the floor beneath the patient opened as a trap door. The line coming out of the shrink's mouth was in a speech bubble. It said, "You're too fucked up – next patient please." Inside the card they had both signed it saying, Dear Vic, You're certainly fucked up man, New Year's resolution, NO FUCKING WORK, stay cool and party on dude, loads of hugs, kisses and love. I took exception to that one because I knew they meant it but I couldn't stop the driving force to be the best. Nath cut and pasted my head onto a sexy woman's body he had found in a lads mag. The title of this piece was Northern Exposure, with a small cut out of Nath's head looking shocked in the corner saying, Southern Surprise.

Victor J Kennedy

Most of my class mates had turned up and a few of the fashion lot came along but after the toasting I don't recollect saying goodbye or thank you to many of them. Tanya dragged me up Station Road back to mine and put me into bed but after what felt like a short sleep I woke up feeling horny so I dragged her naked body onto the carpet and we fumbled around in the dark trying to find an orgasm through all the alcohol. We soon fell asleep where we lay in a heap but I woke hours later to Tanya shouting, "STOP IT! Vic!!! YOU'RE SOAKING ME!!!!" To my horror and shame I realised I had stood up in my sleep and started pissing on her legs as she lay asleep on the carpet. She had then sat up and tried to stem the flow, eventually having to shout at me to stop doing it. I was so embarrassed, I'd never ever done something like that before and I asked Tanya to keep it quiet, otherwise I would never hear the end of it. She kept her word. Like I said, she had a heart of gold. I was starting to drink far too much.

I used Tanya and Lewis in my first module of the year, Photographic Information 2. The brief was set by the tutors in the photography labs and it was the best one so far. We had to choose a well-known phrase, I chose "Make Love Pay" and then we had to create a subverted message by constructing a sentence with "the need to be" or "the need to be seen to be" and then make the story identify with a particular audience. So to subvert "Make Love Pay" I chose the need to be seen to be honest and the need for power. I chose to identify with men and women. I did a hell of a lot of research in the bar and around the refectory because I knew my choices were strong and emotive. My own behaviour over the last summer had prompted me to explore deception and because I had no models I used Tanya, Lewis and myself to portray a trist based on the results of my enquiries at the bar. My notebook was full of sketches, explanations and feedback about those sketches. It was also full of photography techniques and image manipulation to subvert the meaning of the original shots I would take. I was totally immersed in this one and it was all because it was such a juicy brief to get your creative teeth into. The final sequence went like this; 1) A hug between two lovers 2) A tube journey. He holds a condom behind his back 3) In a bedroom she performs a blow job, he yawns 4) In a kitchen she washes up, on her back a sign 'KICK ME' 5) A shot of her anxiously sitting next to the phone 6) In a bar the couple wait to be served, the camera catches him squeezing another girl's bum 7) Sitting round a table in the pub, he talks to his friend while she is ignored 8) Outside the pub she's upset, he says sorry 9) She puts his flowers in the dustbin 10) He leaves her cleaning the kitchen 11) In the pub toilets he boasts to his friends about his sex life 12) He leaves his friends after last orders and goes home 13) He puts the key in his front door 14) He walks in on his girlfriend having sex with another man 15) He cries 16) He's the clown (I put clown make up on). I then made cards based on my research, with a female response in pink and a male response in blue which were printed across each card under the photograph. This took the work to another level because it made the rest of the class divide into a gender war in the middle of the critique. All the girls backed the female character's comments and all the blokes did the opposite. I got 76% and came top of the whole year. I unintentionally pissed off Rory Clarke in the process because in the last twelve months he was reinventing himself as a photographer and had bought some fancy Nikon equipment and all I had was my Practica SLR from Foundation course. When I realised he was pissed off, I remembered him lauding it up at the start of the project, that he was in his element and would be doing easily the best work of his degree within this project. He made a few shitty remarks at my work and I realised what he was actually like after that project. I kept my mouth shut though. Let the work do the talking.

As it turns out, I teamed up with him, Nath and Twinkle for the next module; Sequential Information Design. We teamed up, then split into teams of two; Myself and Nath as concept, design and production. Carl and Rory as storyboard, direction and video editing. We made a video of Rory's mate getting drunk in the local bar Trinity, eating a Big Mac and then throwing up in the toilets. All this action played down half the screen. On the other half was the consequences of what the alcohol was doing to his brain during the six stages of his evening. Why six stages? Because there are six sides to a spinning cube, which Nath was repurposing from that project he did before Christmas. We edited the whole sequence to last exactly the same length of time as the rap tune, Insane in the Brain by Cypress Hill. We got 63%. Once everything was handed in to the tutors, I was on my way to Amsterdam for some fun and a bit of kaos.

Having collected enough receipts and rehearsed our story we set off from Harwich for what was the longest period of time I'd ever spent on a ship. To make the journey more pleasant they had dancing girls with lots of make-up on and gurning like they were on Es. I didn't have any drugs on me (yet) so I took Tanya into the duty free area and told her to point out her favourite drink. She chose Tia Maria so I bought a large bottle of it and a two litre bottle of coke. We sat down in the audience area and started drinking for seven straight hours as we watched the Can Can fortytwo times until we had to stagger through passport control. Once we'd managed to pull that off, we then had to try and find the train station. By the time we arrived in Amsterdam I certainly did not fancy spending time being interviewed in a Police station but old Tanya 'Ronnie Biggs' Baker was determined not to miss an opportunity so we carefully picked a tram stop to be the crime scene and then walked into the Police Station next to the Tourist Information Centre. I blurted out the rehearsed story about a guy talking to us about visiting a brothel, asking about our accommodation and then distracting us with a map for his directions while he grabbed our bag full of electronics and expensive items. The policeman didn't seem bothered to catch the alledged criminal or to fill in the form we needed. He'd probably seen this shit before and got on with it so we would leave and he could carry on watching porn or smoking spliff. It did smell funny in there!

Eventually he did fill out the form and in the end it contributed perfectly to Tanya's scam.

The next day we left our pokey hotel on foot and visited Van Gogh at the Stedelijk Museum and took a boat cruise around the Canals to some hilarious commentary that didn't quite sync with the position of the boat against the bank. We also got in trouble with our tram fare, only out of confusion but the driver still handed us over to the Police and I had to explain myself once again but this time in the back of a squad car. Once released we went straight into a cafe and bought some drugs, just to be rebellious. From the menu I chose an eighth of Nepalese black resin. We bought two coffees and sat outside in the wind while I helplessly tried to roll a spliff. We got stoned, got the munchies and then ate a meal. When it got dark we strolled aimlessly around until, after turning one corner I saw something out of the corner of my eye, "Did you see that Shroom?"

"See what?"

"There was a woman getting changed in that window just as we came around the corner."

"You idiot! This must be the sex district and she was a prostitute."

"I knew that. I was pulling your leg." But I didn't know. I was amazed because all the girls in Lingerie were at least a 9 out of 10 and I thought they would all be dogs if they were on the game. One of them even opened her window and asked me to join her. When I pointed at Tanya and said, "I can't, I'm with her. She's my girlfriend." she pointed at the camera around Tanya's neck and replied, "Bring her along, she can take pictures of me and you fucking!" She smiled and I burst out laughing. Tanya was also laughing her head off. That comment pretty much got us in the mood so we went back to the grubby hotel and did grubby things to each other and smoked spliff. Living that hedonistic lifestyle and all that shite.

Victor J Kennedy

The next day was more of the same, we shopped a bit, ate a
bit, smoked a bit and chilled out in museums. Apart from
that, there wasn't a whole lot more to do in Amsterdam so on
our last night we went to an Indonesian Restaurant called
Sarang Mas near to the Leidseplein nightlife district and we
had a lovely romantic meal which at the end I suggested we
split the remaining sixteenth of Nepalese resin and just neck
it. Down in one! Then we didn't have to smoke it or try to
sneak it back through customs either. I'd never tried
swallowing this amount before, only tiny amounts in cakes.
We both rolled our halves into a ball and before the waiter
could bring over the bill we knocked them back with our
coffees and finished our deserts. Then we strolled round to a
bar opposite The Bulldog pub, got two halves of lager so as
not to get drunk and waited for something to happen.
Eventually it arrived but the results were not positive, I just
felt really tired and heavy. It wasn't like getting high, it was
more like being ready for bed so that's exactly what we did.
Once back in our messy room we fell sound asleep, almost
instantly.
Eight hours later the alarm goes off to make sure we catch
our train back to Hook, in turn to catch our ferry back home
to England. I opened my eyes and everything was blurred. I
couldn't focus my eyes on the alarm clock but my ears could,
in fact, all of my brain could feel it ringing like a fucking
cymbal. I sat up and put my head in my hands, rubbed my
eyes and tried to focus them. There were clothes all over the
floor, nothing was packed and we had to be at the main
station in thirty minutes. As my eyes moved across the floor
at the debris and up the wall next to the basin I got really
scared. The wallpaper was crawling like it was alive. I
panicked and shook Tanya to get her up, "Somethings
wrong, the fucking walls are crawling! The whole room is
on the go. Look at the carpet!" It was making concentric
bubbling circles and the whole experience reminded me of
those 'monsters' that used to visit me in bed as a little boy in

the seventies. Tanya sat up and said, "Fuck. It's that resin we ate last night. It must be an hallucinogen."

"Fuckin yeah, you're right! I thought I was going mad! Grab your things we've gotta move or we're gonna miss the ferry."

"But I feel absolutely terrible."

"Look, I'm all over the place here too you know?"

"I don't think I can walk, never mind carry any bags. I'm so weak I just wanna sleep babe."

"You can sleep for seven fucking hours on the ferry, just help me pack all this shit in that bag please."

The following thirty minutes were absolutely horrendous. Paying the bill and feeling intimidated by the hotel manager, catching a tram while feeling paranoid about getting arrested again and then having to run for the train when all you wanted to do was lay down and die. This was all while your eyes fizzed away at brighter frequencies of light and bubbled concentric circles. I didn't know which was the more frightening of the two. I'd done LSD trips up in Carlisle on Foundation but nothing came near to eating Nepalese black resin and it never would again. I certainly learned my lesson from doing that. Me and Tanya didn't speak a word to anyone or even ourselves for the whole journey home. The ferry crossing was choppy as well, which made it even worse!

When I got back home I spent a couple of days in bed and then Nath came into my room, "You alright mate?"

"Yeah, just knackered. This weekend took alot out of me you know?"

"The weekend did or Tanya did?" He gave me a sly wink.

"Oh, yeah. Tanya did. She's the quintessential Essex girl. Loads of energy and a massive appetite."

"What was Amsterdam like then?"

"Drugs. Sex. Boats. Bikes. Lots of Bikes. There were a few trams too and some museums. You should go."

"I want to go to Liverpool. I've never been. Do you fancy coming?"

"When?"

Victor J Kennedy

"Now."

"Now!?"

"Yeah, why not. We can go in my car, get a hotel and go out for a lads' night out. Meet some scousers and show 'em a good time. That is unless Tanya has tired you out too much."

"I know what you're trying to do but I've actually got a better idea."

"Which is?"

"My Scottish mate Ray from back home, you know the one I went to Lanzarote with?"

"Yeah."

"Well he's now got a place at university doing Sport Science at Crewe and Alsager, which is about half-way between here and Liverpool."

"Which means what?"

"Which means we can stop off at his accommodation for free and have a night out in the process. Ray will introduce us to all his new friends who will also be on their semester break and in the party mood."

"Sounds good. And then we go to Liverpool?"

"Sure. But Liverpool is not all Brookside and Beatles you know. Be warned. You may not want to hang around and Ray gives us an option so you don't have to drive all the way there and back."

"I was thinking of sharing the drive with you."

"Am I insured?"

"Yes. Any driver!"

"You never told me that before."

"You never asked before!"

"I'll be asking to borrow it from now on, if I need to pop to Essex for Sunday lunch."

"Forget Tanya. Get on the bat phone to Ray. We need a place to sleep tonight. And tomorrow."

"Why tomorrow?"

"It's Valentine's day, stupid."

Even when he said that I didn't even think of getting a card for Tanya. I was totally seduced by another exciting couple of nights, having fun and getting off my face once again. When we got there Ray introduced us to his sporty friends who had far too many drinking games going on for my liking. They would drop a magic penny in your pint and if you didn't stop it hitting the bottom of your glass you had to down the pint. No drinking left handed or this big bloke they called 'the chairman of the committee' would order you a drink of anything he wished you to down in one for being 'soft.' He was a stupid fat twat and I told him to fuck off twice for attempting to 'discipline' me with a double Vodka shot. I also saw Ray do a 'tactical chunder' as they called it. This meant staggering to the toilets and sticking his fingers down his throat and being sick before his belly full of binge drinking made him too drunk to continue abusing himself. I couldn't get my head around it all but Ray was totally immersed in this infantile behaviour and the fact he'd paid for every drink he was forcing back out of his body to make space for more didn't seem to worry him in the slightest.

I woke the next day with a sore head, Nath was the same but he felt well enough to take a day trip to Liverpool. We knew we were coming back tonight because everyone was going on about this fabulous Valentine's disco at the local club and a series of buses were going to transport the whole campus to meet Crewe's non-student fraternity in this neutral venue for booze, sex and probably fighting. Me and Nath visited the docks. I took him to Ba Bar, the place to drink just before hitting the queues at Cream. We mooched around the shopping centre and I bought Tanya a Valentine's card, which made me feel guilty so I rang her from a phone box. It was a pointless phone call and just made her worry about this Valentine's Disco and what I was going to be getting up to tonight while she was on her own down there in Harrow. She had a point.

We got back to Ray's, had a brush up and jumped on the first bus to leave the campus. After twenty minutes we arrived at club Valentino's and flashed our photocopied tickets cut out of pink card. The ticket said NO RETURN TICKET, NO

Victor J Kennedy

BUS HOME! so I put it in a safe place inside my wallet. While Nath and Ray got the drinks in I nipped to the toilet to powder my nose. I couldn't tell either of them because Nath would not approve and Ray would do his nut, probably tell my mum. It was a good job I did because the music from DJ's Hugh Bryder, Skitch and Bendrix was not great. In fact, it was too oriented towards the Valentine's smooch and I just wanted to jump around now I was full of amphetamines. Nath didn't like the quality of women in the club either and suggested we play 'Pull a Pig' where each person gets nominated to snog an ugly girl of the other contestant's choosing. I got some real shockers courtesy of Nath casing the whole joint. However, even fast talking patter on Speed couldn't get me a snog, in fact I probably scared them to death while I chewed on my gum at fifty miles an hour. I was sweating alot too which was fairly unattractive and because of my dehydration I kept drinking more. The drinks were never water because I was speeding undercover so I had to drink pints of lager which made me gobby and slightly manic. It was the same Victor from that Benalmadena holiday all over again.

After a shitty bus ride back to campus I had a shitty night's sleep on the common room chairs. Nath was snoring and I was lying there stairing out the window at the sky thinking about Tanya, the universe and everything. It was the speed keeping me awake but my anxiety prolonging the pain. I woke in the morning feeling like I had about two hours sleep. We scoffed a few Corn Flakes and downed one of Nath's strong coffees and then set off back without even waking up Ray. I felt like it was a bit of a rush job and didn't spend enough time with Ray because I was with Nath all the time. I was unaware of what Nath thought because all the way down the M1 he kept asking questions about Ray and my life back home. Maybe I was still a bit high but I just talked and talked about anything he wanted to know. Maybe I was being self-centered but we didn't really talk about Nath

117

until just as we were approaching the M25 intersection when he said, "How would you like to see my parents house?"
"Yeah, alright?"
"We're about ten minutes away. My mum should be in but my dad's at work." He pulled off the M1 and onto the M25 westbound.
"I thought you were from Watford?"
"Watford?"
"On the first day at college you said 'Watford mate', when I asked you where you were from."
"I didn't."
"You fucking did Nath."
"I don't live in Watford. I live in Rickmansworth."
"Isn't that where Boy George is from?"
"I think you'll find it was George Michael."
"Is he your next door neighbour?"
"No he's not but Cliff Richard used to be."
"Fuck off. You're taking the piss now."
"Honestly?"
"Honestly!"
"We haven't lived here for very long. I was brought up in Weybridge and when my sisters grew up and got married my father didn't need such a big place anymore..."
"So he sold it to Cliff Richard?"
"No Vic, Cliff Richard had the next house along from us."
"No shit Sherlock! And I bet you had Elton John living on the other side of you?"
"If you don't believe me, ask my mum when we arrive in less than nine minutes."
"And your mum is French, right?"
"Correct."
"And that postcard you sent me in the summer from the South of France. Was that true?"
"We have a villa down there for holidays."
"No shit. Does Cliff Richard come?"
"No he doesn't Vic."

Victor J Kennedy

"And who pays for all this shit? The houses, the villas, the pop star neighbours?"

"My dad is the CEO of Muller Co."

"Really? So I bet your fridge is always full?"

"Actually Vic, right now he's brought some canned Iced Tea drink home that is being tested on your old stomping ground of Carlisle."

"Testing it? What does that mean? Is it not safe so you have to try it on Jocks and northerners before releasing it to the rest of the UK?"

"That's silly. He needs to find out if it sells. People might not like Iced Tea in a can. They might want to stick to Coca-Cola instead. So he doesn't want to waste money rolling it out over the whole country until he knows."

"That's smart."

"That's why he's the CEO." Nath pulled off the M25 at junction 18 and headed south on the A404.

"So you were brought up in Weybridge all your life?"

"Yeah, until I left school. That's when we moved here."

"So what was your school like?"

"Probably much the same as yours Vic."

"There you go again being evasive. My school was the comprehensive school in the film Rita, Sue & Bob Too. It was a shithole and I learned nothing apart from slamming, stealing and dossing! It's a miracle I've actually made it to university. How can your school be like mine?"

"Well, we also mucked about a lot. I played a lot of sport like you did. What's slamming?"

"You're off again being evasive Nath. It was a public school wasn't it?"

"Yes. Nothing to be ashamed about."

"I'm not ashamed of mine but I've not avoided any of it like you do."

"Vic, just because I don't broadcast it doesn't make me any less proud of who I am than you might feel you have to be."

"But I live with you and I don't know any of this. What about Mauli and Chris?"

119

"Well we all know Mauli's not the same as us yet we accept him."

"What Malaysian?"

"Wealthy Malaysian."

"Yeah but he's never been aloof about it."

"I haven't either. You just never asked until now. You've never asked Carl either."

"I've seen photos of Carl and his mates in a pool of mud doing stunts on their BMX's. They've even been up to London to visit. I don't feel like I need to interrogate him about his past. That's why I accepted you were from Watford, mate."

"I don't remember saying that and maybe I did but I was nervous of you. You had a skinhead."

"That wasn't my fault. My so-called mates shaved my head. You shouldn't judge a book by it's cover."

"My sentiments exactly, Vic." He turned left into a beautiful tree lined avenue.

"Is this it?"

"Yep, it's just up this hill." We pulled into a courtyard with a double garage and an L-shaped single storey barn conversion with beautiful grounds and a white lawn. I say white because there had been an inch or two of snow overnight in Rickmansworth. He pulled the key out and said, "We should have a snowball fight." I couldn't help feel like he wanted to exert some violence on me after I'd grilled him in the car. And after meeting his mum, having a freshly ground coffee and a tour of his palace, he gave me a thrashing at snowballs. Public schoolboy rules. I was told to be careful not to damage any of the exotic plants or the gardener would not be too pleased with Nath. After we'd ruined the idyllic winter scene we dried off, Nath swapped his clothes for some clean ones and we jumped into the electric blue Fiat Uno. I couldn't help feel it was a bit of a crap car for the son of a rich man but I didn't open my mouth. I'd had enough surprises for one day and at least he had felt he could trust me to reveal it all in the first place.

Victor J Kennedy

Unless he constructed the whole Liverpool trip to distract me as the car headed south on the M1. Then he could 'suggest' it and diguise his motives. But what were his motives? I had to stop taking the 'phet, it was making me paranoid.

Just before the semester break was over me and Nath were sat downstairs in his room. We were chatting under a dim light when there was a knock on his window. We both went silent and he jumped over his bed to catch a sneak at who was there through the curtains because number one, we didn't often get visitors and number two, especially at that time of night. The doorbell rang and Mauli sprinted out of his room to answer it. He did the same annoying thing when the phone rang. "IT'S SHUMANA AND RUTH EVERYONE!" Nath stared at me from the curtain and gestured with his spinning finger against his temple and whispered, "What do they want?" Mauli then burst in saying, "Look who's here guys! Who wants a cup of coffee? Or tea? I have green tea and I think there might be some Earl Grey in the cupboard from the people that lived here before." Twinkle walked in to see why Mauli was raising his squeeky voice at this time of night. The girls told us they were scouting around for a place to live in Harrow using Ruth's car and decided to pop in before they set off back to central London. It all seemed a little cagey to me and after we'd spent an hour chatting, flirting and having tickling fights on Nath's bed I knew that Ruth was after Nath and she'd brought Shumana along to give her some moral support. Nath was single now as Cathy wanted to concentrate on her studies, or some bullshit like that. I was glad really because in a twee foursome everything I said to Tanya ended up with Nath via Cathy and vice versa. A gruesome foursome. I thought the fact Ruth fancied Nath was really sweet and I could picture them together as a couple so I decided to help move things along and had a quiet word with Ruth one day at college in the refectory. After a long coffee it turns out I got it all wrong. It was Shumana on the hunt for Mr.

Mad in England - A memoir

Foreman and that she had felt like that since Barcelona when she was going out with Lewis! This was an entirely different outcome, one I wasn't sure I liked the thought of. Ruth painted a picture of this organised and single-minded approach to snaring him. Calculated. I didn't like Shumana and she was not a fan of me either. The recent revelations of Nath's wealth and her moves on him shifted sands under my feet. The repercussions were enormous especially as I was living with him. I'd chosen to take that path and now me and Nath were becoming close friends it gave me mixed emotions. I'd have to pay her lip service and spend more time with her than I wanted to. Her design work was shit. All she ever did was draw fluffy sheep in photoshop. Every project the same thing!

Things got worse the following Wednesday playing for the university. I got put through on goal and had the last defender sprinting alongside me trying to stop me reaching the ball first. Just as I moved to shoulder barge him, he made a sliding tackle so as my shoulder fell towards the hard pitch, my feet went up in the air to accelerate my trajectory towards it. When I sat up I felt and heard a grinding noise in my collar bone. The trainer ran over to me, "What is it Vic?"

"It's up here by my shoulder. Something's grinding inside. Just have a look down my shirt."

He pulled my shirt collar to one side and then said, "Yeah, you just broke your collar bone and it's sticking out of the skin."

"Errrrghh, fucking hell. Don't show me. What are we gonna do?"

"I'm gonna get you to the hospital before your adrenalin runs out and it starts hurting." We walked across the field and straight into Northwick Park Hospital in full kit. I was seen straight away by a middle-aged nurse with massive tits. She cut my shirt off and then grabbed my head and pushed it into her boobs, then she straightened my arm and pulled the clavical back into a normal position which was excrutiating. I screamed out in pain but her boobs did the trick and muffled it. She then put my arm in a sling and gave me a packet of Coproximol pain killers. "There's nothing more we can do love. Clavicals are always difficult to heal because we cannot put it in plaster, only a sling. The best thing to do is lay in bed for six weeks and disable your arm altogether, otherwise you might have complications."

"What about getting a shower?"

"Obviously don't get the sling wet and if you take it off be very careful to put it back on the same way. There's a leaflet with the pain killers that shows you how to do it."

"And how do I know when it's fixed?"

"You'll have to make an appointment with out patients after six weeks of rest. The doctor will assess it then."

So that was it then. No football for nearly two months meant I had to watch it instead. I went to Arsenal v Blackburn that Saturday wearing my sling and saw Kevin Gallagher break his leg. It's a rough game football. Later that night I saw Ray Parlour and David Burrows in the Epping Forest Country Club. I asked him to move aside at the bar so I could get served without banging my shoulder in the sling. When he turned his nose up I said, "It's okay I won't cause trouble, I'm armless!"

I also went to watch Terry Venables first game in charge of England against Denmark at Wembley. It felt good to have a decent manager again after Taylor had failed to get us to USA. I did spend a lot of time in bed around that time and Tanya was an angel looking after me, bringing food around and bathing me. She even slept on the floor next to my single bed to make sure I got a good night's sleep. I really loved her. Honestly. She was perfect wife material, so kind to me. Nobody had ever been this kind to me. She was kind to everyone. The kindness made me feel guilty about what I'd been up to last summer but I never said anything, even though at some point I knew I had to. I took her to see Schindler's List and Philadelphia over the following weeks at the cinema on Station Road and she took me home to Essex for a big Sunday lunch with her family. Towards the end of my rehabilitation I didn't need the pain killers anymore so I started going to the college bar again with my sling on. One busy Friday night I got really pissed and in the melee I ended up snogging Siobhan, the beautiful black girl from the first year. Even though we were surrounded by people no one saw us do it and therefore Tanya, who was somewhere near us in the bar, never found out. I don't know what I was thinking. I was happy with Tanya but I kept behaving like a twat. At the same time I felt my age justified the "I'll be monogomous when I'm married" philosophy and behaviour.

The fifteenth module Professional Practice was upon us and due to my collar bone and the fact I never fully learned Italian I was not going to Milan and all I had done to find a placement was send out some wacky CVs which looked like a collection of stupid passport photobooth shots representing my upbringing, my skills, my interests and my experience. I got nothing back until two London agencies I went after accepted to take a slave placement on for free.

Dear Eric,

As of Monday 21st March 1994, I will be working at the following addresses on the following dates. I've also given you the corresponding name of contact. If there is any problem concerning me while on the last placement then you can also contact me at my home number below.

21/3/94 to 26/3/94 (1 week)
Contact: Lisa Thorpe
Wagstaff Design
Crown Reach 147a Grosvenor Road London SW1V 3JY

28/3/94 to 8/4/94 (2 Weeks)
Contact: Diana Johnson
Carter Wong & Partners
29 Brook Mews North, London W12 3BW

Victor J Kennedy

11/4/94 to 6/5/94 (4 Weeks)
Contact: Reggie Murray
Goddard Murray & Associates
95a Stricklandgate Kendal Cumbria LA9 4RA

Yours Sincerely,
Victor Kennedy

The module overlapped with Easter so I sent one up to
Reggie to try and finish it off up there with some cash and he
accepted, like the gent he always was. This is how my diary
turned out.

Statement of learning objectives and goals:
• To create a good relationship with other designers.
• Get advice from them on how to get a full time job after
the degree.
• Get contact names of other designers or companies who
may be approachable.
• Have the responsibility to design my own work.
• To test my knowledge and skills in a real brief and studio
situation.
• Learn more visualising skills.
• Learn more Macintosh tips and tricks.
• Realise my shortcomings from opinions of senior
designers.
• Learn about any other technology I haven't used yet.
• Generally, just see what I learn when I get there.
--
Lisa Thorpe
Wagstaff Design
Crown Reach 147a Grosvenor Road London SW1V 3JY

Dear Lisa,
Prior to my phone call of last month I managed to break my
Clavical (Collar bone) in a football match. That was the bad
news! The good news is; it was my right shoulder and I'm

left handed. It was also three and a half weeks ago and I almost have full use of the arm again. The doctors have advised me not to lift anything heavy for two months so as long as I don't have to give anyone a fireman's lift then hopefully, no one will notice.

I've been given a list of criteria from the module leader that I have to conform to while doing the placement.

Unfortunately this includes a few things I must collect from you to pass the module. The list is below, I hope it's not too much trouble and I apologise if there is any inconvenience caused.

• Meeting with mentor at the start of the placement.
• Written report from the studio to the course tutor.
• Written responses from studios and confirmation of placement in writing.
• Record of first meeting with mentor and any subsequent changes to your goals and learning objectives. (aimed more towards me)

I will bring in my side of the criteria on the first day if you want to have a look at it, but it will not affect my performance through the day. I'm looking forward to starting and confirm my appearance at 9.00am Monday 21st March. If there are any problems ring me at home after 4pm.

Yours Sincerely,
Victor Kennedy
--
MY DIARY - Professional Practice 2

Wagstaffs Clients include:
Abbey National, Safeway, Spillers, Tetley, SKB, Masterfoods

Monday
Not much happened today just got an introduction into the company. I learnt about rubdowns as well today.

Victor J Kennedy

Tuesday
Got thrown off the Mac three times today. Had to develop
my idea for Safeways Crisps. i.e. visualising by hand! I think
my ideas are crap. Got sent out for six 2 litre bottles of coke
for a pitch.

Wednesday
Weird day! After yesterday's performance of collecting coke
bottles all day – I get asked to to do it again! 9am to 11am
running around Pimlico and Vauxhall to Tescos for more
stuff – a gofer! "Go for this - go for that"

Thursday
Talked to Kenneth the hand letterer. He helped me develop
my logo style for "Thick & Crunchy" He was about 60 years
old and a real fossil but really good at what he did. Steady
hand needed.

Friday
I went on a photoshoot to King Cross with a photographer
called John Merton. I met all his Home Economists and was
really surprised by them and the tricks they pull.

Carter Wong & Partners Clients include:
Sinutab, Boots, Safeway, Marks & Spencer, FIA, FIM,
Norwich Tourism, Design Museum, D&AD, Wheat
Crunchies, Shell, Woolworths, BAFTA, Flora, Champion,
Benylin, Alpha Romeo

Monday
Well, began the day by being introduced to the main man –
Phil Wong, nice bloke! It's a really nice studio and the
people seem quite friendly and it is ONLY my first day after
all! Lunches are paid for here aswell – Yippee!

Mad in England - A memoir

Tuesday
Got given some visualising to do for Phil Wong. A FIA
publication with a blend of photomontage to follow with my
own choice of photos. He's good and is teaching me (i.e.
giving me some responsibility and helping me to get it right)
I've also brought in my work to show him my portfolio.
Hopefully he'll find time to look at it last thing today but
we'll see.

Wednesday
Had to help Phil Wong again with the visualising in the
morning. A few alterations to the images to get the type in
position alright. In the afternoon got given a new brief from
Nick to design an Invite/Banners/Posters and Information
Cards for a Russian Avant Garde book exhibition for the
British Museum.

Thursday
Just a straight day being left to do what I wanted, to develop
the ideas I'd had on the Russian books brief.

Bank Holiday Easter Weekend.

Tuesday
Just did more of the same by developing more of my ideas
on to paper and through the Mac.

Wednesday
More of the same – developed another idea for a poster
using another book cover. It was difficult because the cover
was really busy with loud colours and a weird shape. I came
up with a block of information that looked like a stamp. It
was meant to resemble books on a shelf.

Thursday
While being on this placement I've really gone back to
basics with the procedure of visualising. They use omnicrom

here and pantone coloured paper plus all the markers etc. for visualising. As for the design work I've done, who knows? Will it go ahead or won't it?

Friday
Carried on working towards finishing off the Russian stuff. Phil Wong agreed to crit my portfolio and work I'd done so in the afternoon he did. He said some very nice things about my work and that it was good that I was in college for another year as he thought I needed it and the climate may be better then for a job.

Goddard Murray & Associates Clients Include:
Group 4, Summer Cottages, English Tourist Board, Cumbria Tourist Board, Reprogen, UCB Sidac, Brathay Developments

Monday
They couldn't find me any work to do for the full morning because they'd forgotten I was coming in! Reggie, the boss was away and Sally the secretary got me to sort out a transparency drawer all day. What a terrible start!

Tuesday
Just did exactly the same as the day before. Sorting out transparencies into a seethrough bag and filing it under a particular client. I'm really regretting this.

Wednesday
I can't believe that she (Sally) can keep finding me trannys from everywhere. I'm sure she's doing this as a test. Another crap day doing manual labour.

Thursday
I managed to sort the last remnants of the dreaded tranny drawer and finish the job off totally. Sally couldn't find any

more so she gave me an in house job for an order form for her.

Friday
Got two jobs from Reggie who is back today. The first is a development of an old logo into a new job – he calls it recycling old (good) ideas. The second is an advert for Creative Review advertising his College's reunion at Watford.

A Look Back at my Professional Practice 2

Wagstaffs
A good week which I enjoyed but I wish I'd been taken a bit more seriously and my designs had definitely been put forward because I have a feeling that they might not have been. At least some good has come out of it, in the job side of things.

Carter Wong & Partners
I enjoyed my time at Carter Wong but I wish I'd had some more time there. I preferred the agency to Wagstaffs because the work is more diverse and the studio is nicer. I was flattered to be asked to return next week to finish off my job completely but I just can't.

Goddard Murray & Associates
A bit of a strange placement with mixed feelings. I felt more used than any of the other placements. Maybe because I've worked there before. It was good to compare where I've come from and see the London companies next to it all. They really made GMA look drab. I know now I've got ambition to do better than that place and I will do better. As for the design work. It was enjoyable but not very 'juicy' due to the fact that they were all Reggie's little outside jobs for himself and it really got beyond a joke at times.

Victor J Kennedy

The term leading up to Easter had been tough, especially for Tanya. Something awry had occurred in a test with an anomaly on her reproductive organs. She kept it secret from me while at the same time leaking tiny details, which I could only presume was an attempt to shield me from feeling anxious about our relationship in the long term. During the initial weeks that I'd gone home to work for Reggie, she had to go see a specialist. She wanted to come up and visit over Easter after the check-up. I was looking forward to it and was blase about the whole thing until a card arrived for me from Essex with a starfish on the front.

Dear Victor
I just wanted to write you a short note to say a few things I have trouble saying to you.
Although I miss you a lot while you are away, I think sometimes a break is what every relationship needs.
The past term has been a bit of a disaster what with your shoulder and then my thousands of problems, I think surprisingly we've come out on top, but it certainly put a strain on us both and I really want to thank you for being so considerate, I'm sorry if at times I was overly sensitive, I hope I wasn't too unbearable.
I'm really nervous about next week, although I'm looking forward to afterwards when everything will be sorted out once and for all. I'm sure next term will be much better and problem free.
Anyway that's all really. I just wanted to thank you and say I hope you have a brilliant time back at home with your mum etc. I hope I'm well enough and can come up and visit you in a couple of weeks' time.
Anyway have fun.
All my love,
Tanya xxxx

We had a great couple of days together and she met most of my mates from the village again. She got on with the girls

131

while I got drunk with the lads and all that. She fit right in and we were a great couple. Everything changed after once again, I put her on a train heading south at Oxenholme, she cried her eyes out. Afterwards I span out of control. It was like an allergic reaction to undying love and devotion. That weekend Ray called a cheeky party at his mum and dad's house for a select few. Julie turned up. Alvin Drury was there too. He was also on the drugs periphery back in 1991 and was the driver of the car that nearly crashed into the farmer in Ilkley traffic lights on the way back from Leeds. He was now well into his medical degree and we chatted all night about becoming a GP and what Liverpool's CREAM was like. Before he left I got an invite to go down there the following weekend and meet up with some old faces, do some drugs and enjoy the full CREAM experience. CJ Mackintosh and Farley 'Jackmaster' Funk were playing and there was talk of my hero and favourite DJ Graham Park turning up to do a set. I had to go. The night at Ray's parents spiralled into a drunken game of pictionary with three contestants; me, Julie and Ray because everyone else had fucked off home in either boredom or the fact they had driven to Hale for Ray's social. Eventually even he got bored and dragged in some duvets, opened the sofa into a double bed and slurred, "I'm off to bed. I'm knackered." As soon as he flicked the light switch and it was pitch black me and Julie dived on each other in a drunken and confused, lusty romp. I awoke naked next to her in the morning feeling hung over and terrible about what I had done on full realisation. Julie was unbelievably nonchalant about it and said nothing. Even when she gave me a lift back to the pub she just said, "I'll maybe see you at Christmas Vic?" and then drove away. It kind of felt like, in some competitive schoolgirl sort of way, that she'd wanted to get back at Faye since sixth form and by shagging me (after all the fucking letter writing) she had confirmed she nailed me in the end. Or maybe she didn't feel like that and it was a stupid drunken mistake which has now fucked up our friendship forever?

Victor J Kennedy

After an emotional week of soul searching, I went down to Liverpool on the Friday and had a night of booze on campus to meet the people I was clubbing with the following night. It's always a good idea to meet them first. They told me of some bloke being taken off to hospital the week before, after making their own Microdots and he had an adverse effect to everything. Some of the girls were pretty concerned at what was happening to them all as medical students because they had access to labs and jars of stuff which, mixed together could save you paying £15 to an anonymous dealer for an ecstasy tablet. I worried about it for about as long as the conversation lasted because someone walked in who had scored some 'Tangos' or 'Disco Biscuits' as I was told when I handed over my £15 in return for this large, speckled, brown, sort of orangey coloured pill. I was advised to take half in the queue and put half in my sock for later. They were too strong to take the whole thing in one go. After the conversation we'd just had I wasn't going to question his advise, he was a trainee doctor after all. After a day on the lawns at the campus smoking weed and talking bollocks we started getting ready to go out. My mate Carl had come down from the Lakes on the Saturday and he was so excited about CREAM he kept shouting out, "Wherever you're from, be it Manchester, Liverpool or Leeds. Get it right on, right now!" until everyone was chanting it in the pubs and bars of the city centre before we got in the queue, which by now was massive. While we were waiting we all dropped half of the Tango monster. By the time I was searched and stood at the bar amongst this pumping sound I was up and buzzing. "You got yer Asterix in space, watch yer base bins I'm telling yer." (and all that shit)
To be honest the night was a bit of a blur. One rush into the next and drinking bottles of water to protect myself from how heavy this experience was turning out to be. The one thing that sticks in my mind was dropping the second sweaty, melted half of that ecstasy in the toilets and coming back to the dance floor to see the sun come up through the

plastic translucent corrugated ceiling. I was raving while I came up for the second and what would turn out to be my last time to Judy Cheeks' 'Reach.'

Chapter 6 - Falling Apart

The train slowly came to a halt at Euston Station and the passengers got out of their seats to congregate around the exit with their suitcases, like it was a race to exit. A rat race. I was back in the smoke, back in my other life. The clued up city lad back where he belonged. Once off the train I put on a fast pace to overtake all the twats who had been so anxious to get off. I could feel the competitive spirit rushing through my blood vessels as my heavy suitcase cut through my fingers. I shut out the pain with the satisfaction that I would be first to reach the tube ticket machines. But then I didn't have any loose change and the bastards overtook me. I could tell they were laughing inside as they strode ahead, looking back at the sweat dripping down my face and my impatient foot tapping as the queue refused to go down. I thought to myself; it doesn't take very long to get back into this way of life – this point of view. The thing is, as unpleasant and energy sapping as it is, I was engaged with it's flow and tempo. It had to be the only place in my country, if not the world, where you will accelerate your journey towards wealth, fulfillment and satisfaction. That's what Dick Whittington said, right? The streets were paved with gold. After a ten minute walk from Northwick Park station with my suitcase pulling my shoulder out of socket, I got back to the house and dropped off my things. Everyone was out and all the internal doors were locked, apart from the toilet, the kitchen and the pantry under the stairs. Nobody trusts anyone in London either. Especially when you're in competition with each other on the same degree at university. There's a gaping void between the need for privacy and the need for secrecy. My lack of sensory stimulation, combined with the muted buzz of the returning hero meeting a wall of silence, quickly sent me into anxiety and my need for attention had to be satisfied. I grabbed a jacket and walked across the cold playing fields at Northwick Park to Tanya's. When I arrived I got the reception I was looking for with a Sunday dinner on top. Cathy was out but Lewis and Ross were upstairs in their equivalent of our living room, squeezed on to a couch playing Mario Kart. It was almost a carbon copy of our house, only they didn't argue or squabble about the results. I sat down to watch and soon enough Tanya arrived with a tray of chicken, roast potatos, broccoli and hot gravy straight from the oven. I chowed down while the racing continued. I was so fucking bored of watching Yoshi versus Toad going around the same bends, doing the same things again and again. I was feeling anger and a lot of disdain towards Nintendo for inventing the SNES and subsequently, designing a multi-player game that was so good it was scorching my retinas, not to mention dominating the behaviour and spare time of my friends who had turned into sheep with DISCIPLE branded on their woolly hide. After having his arse kicked by Ross for the third time in a row Lewis held a contol pad out to me, "Fancy a crack at Nigel Mansell?"

"I'm still eating."

"Ooeeerrr, somebody's not in a good mood."

"Why is it you two never fall out?"

"Eh?"

"You and Ross. You never seem to get agitated after the chequered flag like we do."

"What, you and Nath?"

"Not just him. The whole house is in uproar. We can't even turn off the Snez and watch The Bill until Mauli gets his revenge. It's a good job I've got my portable in my bedroom."

"Me and Ross have known each other for a while, haven't we mate," he gestured across and then affectionately put his arm around Ross. "Devon boys. Through and through."

"I don't want to know about your sexual experimentation in the countryside, lads."

"Oi, leave it out! You know that type of talk upsets Ross, he's misunderstood." Lewis joked.

"But it's refreshing to see some unity. Some peace."

Ross interjected, "It's probably because Lewis is stoned."

"I'm not! I've rolled one all afternoon. Do you want one Vic?"

"Nah mate, I don't feel like smoking right now. I took a really heavy E this weekend and I've hardly slept."

"Ahh, that explains it all now. I thought you were a bit techy when you got here."

"A bit techy?"

"Yeah. Edgy and broody. You've been a bit too quiet for my liking. A normal Vic would be telling us all about what he did over Easter."

"Bollocks. What am I supposed to talk about while you're playing that?"

"Cheer us on!"

"Fuck off. I just told you I've escaped the whining Mauli to find some peace down here and you lot are doing the same thing I'm trying to avoid."

"But you just said we don't fall out. Didn't you?"

"Yeah. But..."

"Well that's a contradiction Vic. I told you, you're edgy. Take a chill pill my friend."

"I'm fine."

"You're not."

"I am!"

"You need a chill pill and I've got some down stairs in my room. I'll go and get them if you want? I fancy having a Temazzy Party!"

"Temazepam?!"

"Yeah, I've brought some jellies back from home. We had a road test on Good Friday at a party and they are super chilled. Properly chilled out my friend and no smoke involved whatsoever."

Victor J Kennedy

"I've never tried Temazepam before."

"I'll go get 'em!" He jumped out of his seat and ran as quick as he could to his bedroom downstairs. I could hear him speaking to Tanya, who was doing the washing up in the kitchen. I couldn't quite make out the exchange but whatever was said I felt jealous and suspicious of their relationship. I knew what he was like but I couldn't mention anything because I wasn't sure in my mind. Part of my brain disagreed with the other. I was telling myself that I was paranoid at the same time as feeling anger and resentment towards Lewis. Not to mention the fact he was bringing some green 'poison' up the staircase for me to kill myself. Tanya followed him up and stook her head around the door, "Is that it then babe? You finish your dinner and then knock yourself out?"

"I won't go to sleep."

"How do you know?"

Lewis tried to appease her, "Tanya Wanya, we won't cause any trouble on these babies. They're really nice. Just mellow. Perfect for getting ready for bed."

"But I've hardly had a chance to talk to Vic about Easter and I want to have some time with him on my own, without a Nintendo or one of my house mates taking him away from me."

"Tanya! I'm not taking him away from you. I'll go get one for you too and then we can all watch the film at 9 o'clock?" He jumped up and followed her downstairs to finish off his art of persuasion. He was a master of peer pressure and his art was perfected during the first year in halls of residence. He would make a great pimp and that was why I didn't like Tanya living with him. To be fair to Lewis though, he always appeared to have the utmost respect for my relationship with her. Similarly, he was about to feed the three of us prescription drugs when he wasn't even a qualified doctor. The Temazepam took the edge off my anxious mood. It was like inducing relaxation. Forcing yourself to calm down. It seemed like an option to escape the darker places. A way out. Amphetamine on the way in,

Mad in England - A memoir

Temazepam for a way out. Control. As innocent as drinking a coffee to wake up in the morning.

I stayed at Tanya's that night. After a coffee, a kiss and a dash across the playing fields to the new term it was the 10am briefing for the Design Futures module. It was quite an open brief. We had to choose something like a cash machine, for instance, and then develop the concept to suit a 21st century audience. We could go as far as twentyfive years into the future but no more than that. During the first week I'd seen some printouts of Nath's metallic looking 'information donut' around the house. When I'd asked what it was he told me he was mucking about with Photoshop filters and he stumbled across this funky looking donut so I knew he'd applied and embellished some bullshit to this accident in his unformidable style. I'd been thinking about Creative Review magazine for a while now and the fact that some of it's sections I always made sure I read and some were irrelevant to me as a student. The following synopsis along with my prototype mock-ups of how the CD-Rom would work, earned me 75% for the Design Futures Module:

My Brief - May 1994

Design a monthly interactive multimedia magazine on the internet that is modified each day of the month by the users as they choose to read, watch or listen to it. Concentrate on a new system to move through the magazine that has no metaphors or links to the 'traditional' format of the magazine but still holds it's structure and juxtaposition of each section. Improve on current interactive magazines on CD-Rom. The main goal is to be totally USER FRIENDLY and embody the user with total control. Personalise each person's issue for their specific needs, yet still keep Creative Review's current identity throughout all copies sent through the internet.

Victor J Kennedy

Background
Creative Review is a magazine. It's a pile of bound paper
that is filled with articles about the creative world. It can be
picked up from a shelf and flicked through by hand. It has
sections that people look for when they read it regularly and
specific pages for services to its readers.
With the current trend of CD-Rom conversions and
replacements of today's magazines (Emigre) and newspapers
(The Guardian) the future of these printed publications are in
doubt and the subject is surrounded in clouds of controversy.
Adding to this digital revolution is the internet. A modern
network computer highway, linking every computer in the
world to each other. Already 20 years old and growing
bigger every year. It uses each national telecommunications
company from each country to form a global information
web.

Aims
My proposal for Design Futures is to redefine the
'Traditional' magazine somewhere in an uncertain future,
however near it is. The magazine in question is Creative
Review and the environment is the design world. A place
where designers, around this planet are linked by their
Macintosh or PC screens through an opticle fibre to the
Creative Review Database in Poland Street, London.

Interviews and other Research
6/06/94 Interview, visit and research with Glenn Oliver -
Design Editor of Creative Review, Poland Street London.
16/06/94 Exchange of ideas and concept in Hackney,
London with Isaac Bishop of 3W Global News Letter (A
current magazine produced purely for the internet today)
No.1 in this month's Wired "What's Hot"

I guess meeting Isaac Bishop while working on that project
changed my life because although I only sat in his basement
and chatted informally for about two cups of tea, I came out

of his house and rushed back to college to open an email account so I could talk to him through the internet. It was like discovering CB radio or the same excitement you had as a kid about walkie talkies. The weird address given to me by the IT department was xjbld@wmin.ac.uk and apart from a guy sat in the same classroom as me, Isaac was the only person I knew who had an email address. Over the coming weeks and months Isaac would drip-feed knowledge to me over email about browsers and the world wide web. I felt so excited about it all. I felt like I could be a pioneer of this new medium just like Isaac had. He was the most well-known Englishman on the internet in 1994, apart from Tim Berners Lee; the bloke who 'invented' the world wide web protocols. I got so excited that I was determined to buy my own computer so I didn't need to borrow Mauli's any more. Mauli's was a bit shit anyway, it was an LC Performa and was really slow when you used Photoshop. I wanted to do it all, especially video so I set my sights on a Quadra 840av at an unbelievable 40 Mhz, 32 bit data path, 32 MB of RAM and a further three slots to expand into later; 500 MB hard drive, 1.4MB SuperDrive and an Optical 2x speed CD-Rom drive. It had millions of ports for ethernet access to the internet and a SCSI drive for my portable 120MB Optical disc drive. You always need a back up! I took myself down to a computer fair at The Royal Horticultural Halls which was advertised in Creative Review. I spent the whole morning gawping at stuff and collecting crap marketing freebies to stick in my prized Apple carrier bag, with a big logo on the side. The computer was way out of my league at a staggering £1,800! I went back to college with just the carrier bag and my tail between my legs but as I got off the Metropolitan train at Northwick Park, Aaron from Illustration stopped me on the platform just as he came up the stairs. "Alright Aaron. You skiving off again? Oooeerrr, I can't talk! I've just slammed off myself to go the Apple show instead." I held up my trophy carrier bag as his face went all somber and serious.

Victor J Kennedy

"You haven't heard then?"

My heart sank, "Heard what?"

"Tanya's been rushed into hospital."

"You what?"

"She collapsed on the stairs outside the art supply shop."

"Fuck. What happened?"

"Not sure but you know Celine from behind the counter in the art shop? That one who looks like a bloke?"

"Yeah, go on..."

"Well she said that one of the lads from our third year found Tanya on the floor holding her stomach..."

"Shit!"

"...and that loads of blood was coming out of her."

"Out of her stomach?"

"No, no. From between her legs."

"Fucking hell. Is she alright?"

"Apparently, he picked her up and carried her all the way round to the hospital next door and got her in A&E. Then they took her in and he came back."

"What time was that Aaron?"

"This morning mate, about 11ish."

"Cheers for that fella, I've gotta go."

"No worries mate. Send her my regards will you?"

"Will do."

"Later."

I sprinted across the field, over the exact same pitch I broke my collar bone and followed the same steps as I did that day. I found myself in A&E again, sweating and stressing out just like I was last time I was in there. At the information desk I found out which room she was in and made my way there. Through the glass door I could see Cathy but there was a curtain around the bed obscuring Tanya and I could only see half of the nurse treating her. Before I could put my hand on the door handle Cathy spotted me and came to the door. She had her index finger to her lips as if to indicate that Tanya was not to be disturbed. She came out, quietly closed the door, clocked my Apple carrier bag and grabbed my arm as

she frog marched me down the corridor. "Where the fuck have you been Victor? When she needed you the most!?"
"Just a minute, how is she? And what's happened to her?"
"She's going to be fine. No thanks to you."
"Whooaah! Hang on. This isn't all my fault, you know."
"Oh really? And how would you know that? You weren't even here when she collapsed." She looked through her nose at the carrier bag and gestured her head towards it.
"She collapsed on the stairs in your teaching block Cathy. If I was in college I would be in the design block anyway. It's not even two o'clock. This happened less than three hours ago and I only just found out from Aaron at the tube station. I've ran all the way here. Look at me. I'm sweating!"
"Well you are responsible."
"Tell me."
"Do you know what an ectopic pregnancy is?"
"Oh no. She's been pregnant? Aaron said there was alot of blood."
"She's alright Vic. She's got through the worst part. The doctors have removed the fetus and stopped the blood. She could have died."
"And it was my baby they 'removed'?"
"The baby was already dead Vic. An ectopic pregnancy is when one of Tanya's eggs begins it's journey down the fallopian tube but is fertilized by your sperm before it reaches the womb. The baby has grown until it tore her cervix at 11am this morning. So you are responsible."
"Hold on a minute Cathy, that's not fair. She was on the pill. At least that's what I thought."
"Well something's obviously gone wrong."
"Have you spoke to her about all this?"
"No. I don't think it's appropriate. Do you?"
"Where's her mum?"
"She's been stuck on the North Circular. She'll be here any minute. You made it just in time."
"Look, let's try and put the comments to one side and make this less stressful for Tanya's sake. She's my girlfriend and I

want to go and see her now." I walked off, back towards the room Tanya was in and got to her bedside. The nurse gave us a minute together.

"Oh Shroom, what's gone on luv? You ok?" I grabbed her hand and sat on the bed.

"I'm sorry babe. I got pregnant and it died."

"Don't apologise. It takes two to tango."

"I feel really sore."

"I bet you do."

"What's in your bag?"

"Computer stuff. Don't worry about me babe. Are you alright? That's the important thing."

"Of course. It was just a bit worrying seeing all that blood come out. I've never seen so much come out of there before." She smiled, but the whole thing was just alarming me.

"Are they keeping you in overnight?"

"I hope not. I asked Cathy to ask mum if she can get me in at Buckhurst Hill. My dad's got medical insurance at the place I went to over Easter. It's lovely."

"And if she has found a bed there, do you feel well enough to get in a car and travel back round the north circular?"

"Oh petal, I just don't want to stay here. Anywhere but here."

"Do you need anything sorting out while you're away?"

"I think Cathy is gonna do all that stuff. You just concentrate on your work and don't worry about me. I'll be fine."

"But that's the thing Mushroom. The more you say 'don't worry' the more I do the opposite."

"I love you Vic."

"I lo..." Tanya's mum, Carolyn, walked in accompanied by a stone-faced Cathy. I shut my mouth instantly and stepped away from the bed to allow a full mother-daughter interaction. Tanya started to cry but Carolyn held firm, showing only loving support and affection. I could see as they held each other that this relationship was a very strong one. Mother and first born daughter. A nurse soon followed and after much deliberation, Tanya was allowed to get dressed and leave. I held her bag all the way to her mum's car. Cathy said her pleasantries and left me to see the car off. Tanya cried again. Carolyn said thank you to me but I didn't do anything apart from carry Tanya's bag. Then they drove away and once again I walked back across the playing fields. Being alone on that football pitch thinking about personal injury sent the altruistic thoughts of Tanya to the back of my mind. This allowed the egocentric thoughts to resonate through my head. For instance, I could have been a father. Or, I hope it was mine. Not forgetting the classic; at least I know my balls work properly.

With Tanya out of the picture, I spent the next few days trying to apply to Bunac and teach kids football in American Summer Camps. I'd been thinking about it since I saw the leaflets when I did the parachute jump in the first year. I think my mind subconsciously wanted to be far away from here, from London and the mess I felt I was in. I was trying to do it through Bobby Jindal, my football manager and the campus gym tutor. He had all the forms and was prepared to lie through his teeth about my capabilities as an adult and as a trained football coach. My big motivator was the USA'94 World Cup. England were not going to take part due to Graham Taylor's use of over well over fifty different players during qualifying. Gazza was injured for most of it too although I wasn't going to recreate Italia '90, I still wanted to be there in the country where it was taking place. Bunac would give me the perfect solution, a break from college and a summer filled with football.

The English football season had come to an end, United nearly did the domestic treble. Only losing to Aston Villa in the League Cup final at Wembley, which Nath was working at – behind a counter, dishing out plastic cups of coca-cola for £4.50 an hour. Admittedly, I was going to do it because money was too tight to mention and I'd never been to a final at Wembley before. Mind you, it was better to try the FA Cup final and that's exactly what me and Diago tried to do when United destroyed Chelsea in the pouring rain. We

Victor J Kennedy

rocked up pissed ten minutes after the kick off, after legging it from a washed out barbeque a couple of miles from the stadium. We watched it on the monitors inside a BBC van and then when the coast was clear we hurdled the barriers around the televsion crane at one end and opened the first door we found. A couple of stewards saw us and started chasing us around what turned out to be the offices of Wembley PLC. Eventually we got caught, hiding under someone's desk like the Red Hand Gang. The twat who picked me up, span me around into a half nelson and nearly broke my arm as he and his fellow cronies frog marched us off the premises. On exit there was a loud sarcastic cheer from the crowd of lads trying to do the same thing as we'd just tried to do.

After the Cup Final there was just the play offs and then pretty much straight into the World Cup. My mate Mark from Foundation course was a massive Preston fan, so was his brother Gary and all their mates from the Lakes School near Windermere. I've got no idea why it was PNE they supported but he rang me and offered to get me tickets to watch them contest Martin O'Neil's Wycombe Wanderers for a place in the second division. I asked him to get two tickets and then Nath could come along and experience some proper northern banter. I didn't consider that jaunt to Liverpool as being the baptism of fire he was going to get from this lot. We met in a relevant pub called The Preston (geddit?) on Preston road, one stop away from Wembley and myself and Nath were scared when they all bounced in wearing face paint, already drunk and singing noisey abusive stuff about southerners. They were all hugging me and a lot of banter was kicking off about Bradford City being crap and what a brilliant suggestion to get them in this particular pub. It was going to be a symbol of good luck and they bought me lots of pints for helping them find it. Nath wasn't mixing at all. He was laughing along but he seemed vacant amongst all the neanderthal testosterone, not to mention the chips and gravy. We got to the ground and ate pies, took

145

photos and larked about in high spirit but not Nath. He did
enough to take part but I could tell he was observing and
recording the behaviour. It all went downhill for Preston as
soon as we took our seats.They eventually lost 4-2 and all
the grown men who'd come all the way down to meet Mark
at Wembley and witness a piece of history were crying their
eyes out. Face paint everywhere! Nath was amazed by this
reaction to such a ritual and gleefully pointed at the sobbing
giants and silently grinned. It was the first time throughout
that day I saw him enjoying himself. Part of me agreed with
him and laughed at the jokes he made at their expense
afterwards. But at the same time, a big part of me has origins
in that type of honesty and belief. Nath was green. He was
not a football fan and after that day, I knew he wasn't taken
by spawn of the north either.

We left the real fans at Preston Road tube station and made
our way home to find Mauli firing an air rifle in the back
yard. He had bought it from some dodgy fire arms shop in
town and was shooting a crappy target he'd drawn on the
cardboard box at the bottom of the garden. Nath instantly
relieved Mauli of duty and began firing needlessly around
the neighbour's things. I asked for a go and Nath passed it to
me at the kitchen door as he went inside. Mauli explained
how to use it's compressed air with greatest effect. I pumped
enough in to send the pellet to the moon. Nath came back
outside holding his trusted camcorder, it was already rolling.
"Go on Vic. Kill something."
"How about you?" I pointed the weapon towards the camera.
"Easy! Not me. Take out a slug or something. Mauls, have
you shot yourself with this yet?"
"No Nath, I haven't turned the gun on myself yet. Why don't
you volunteer and stand at the end of the garden? Gimme the
camera and I'll video Vic from behind him. Bullet eye view."
I spotted a small starling watching us from the top of a tree
in the opposite garden so I raised my aim, "It's ok, I've got
my target."

Victor J Kennedy

Mauli thought he knew the range of his new toy, "Dude, you've got no chance of hitting that from there."
I took aim as Nath kneeled in front of me and continued filming. I didn't believe for one second that I would hit the bird but I did! I was horrified seeing the bird fall from it's perch and hit the floor. The gun shot evidence and the reaction on my face was all caught on film. Then Nath proceeded to play it back to everyone who visited the house over the coming days so everyone knew I was a 'bird murderer.' All very funny for everyone else, especially Nath but I felt like it was a set up. Because there was hardly any project work left in the year, he was increasingly observing and filming everything, like he was documenting something. Once filled, all the video cassettes were thrown in a cardboard box next to his bed to gather dust and wait to be edited or used as evidence sometime in the future when they may come in useful.

A couple of days later, after Tanya returned fully recovered from hospital, Nath invited me and Lewis to Rickmansworth to enjoy the freedom of the Foreman's empty house. His parents were in the south of France at the villa for an early summer break so we all jumped in the electric blue Fiat (with the video camera of course) to get drunk and misbehave in the lap of luxury. We stopped off at a supermarket and stocked up with cans of Stella and Apple pie. When we got there Lewis was really taken with the grounds and the interior. He took his shoes off as a mark of respect while Nath did the tour of the house. It had French polished wooden floorboards throughout and Lewis's furry socks were causing him to slip and slide around. As the evening wore on and the drink began to take effect, Lewis would start running down corridors and doing long 'skids' into the back of a sofa and then dive into it. By midnight the sliding theme had become raucous. The camcorder was out and we were pulling each other across the floor by our feet whilst the person on the floor being pulled on their back filmed the other one dragging them along. Nath upped the

147

stakes by taking off his shirt, then challenged me to drag him along while he was 'bare back.'

I had to, even though I knew it was going to hurt him. His skin made a horrendous high pitched squeak noise across the open floor boards until I stopped at the door to the kitchen because I saw a metal strip dividing the rooms which would've really hurt him. I dropped his legs and they fell to the floor with a bang. Lewis was squeeling with delight. Then obviously once Nath did it, everyone had to follow. So me and him swapped places, only this time he took me right over the metal strip. I stood up amongst the laughter and tried to make a joke, "I will tell you, that's fucking painful. Fucking painful!" Then it was Lewis's turn. He lay down with the camera and Nath grabbed his legs at the door of the kitchen. "Hold on, you're pressing the red button. The light's come on. That's it. Okay, follow me for pain." Nath started running and Lewis began screaming in pain, his back making a horrid shrill against the varnish. I shouted, "Byee Byee!" as he flew off through the lounge but as Nath manoeuvred the furniture Lewis slid outwards and hit his hip against a radiator with a huge bang and then really screamed out in horror, "AAAARRRGGGHHHH, AHHHHH, HAA, HA, FUCK!" He was in alot of pain but was also laughing. Me and Nath were silent until Lewis clearly sounded ok. Then I picked up the camera and filmed him while he wriggled in pain in front of his two giggling mates at midnight in a converted barn on the outskirts of Hertfordshire. "TAKE THE PAIN! TAKE THE PAIN!" I shouted. "NATH, BITE IT AND SUCK THE POISON OUT!" Lewis stuck two fingers up at the camera as he struggled to stand up. Nath was laughing, "Get it all on tape." You'd almost think he'd planned everything. We giggled at him limping into the kitchen. I followed him in saying, "Wounded soldier!" I turned to Nath, "You should've seen it man. He twatted it full on, right in the middle of the thigh!" Once we got in the kitchen Lewis started cooking the apple pies and we all filmed our pink backs and Lewis's wound, which was pretty bad. All the skin was broken and bruising had already appeared. Then we did the obligatory moonie and when the food was ready we went outside in the garden to eat. Two minutes into the feed, the drunken banter started.

VIC: "What sort of custard is that?"

LEWIS: "It's ASDA."

NATH: "ASDA"

LEWIS: "I nicked it from Anthony's locker before I left."

VIC: "ASDA? Fucking Thurston-Coe custard. Can I have some more then?"

NATH: "Have another piece Vic." He gestured at the last piece on the table.

VIC: "That one or that one?" I pointed at the other one behind Nath.

LEWIS: "Mmmbpphh. He he." He giggled as I stood up to get it.

VIC: "What's the crack with this one then?" I got suspicious they'd put pepper in it as a joke.

NATH: "It's fine."

VIC: "No, you're alright. I'll have that one I think." I sat back down as Lewis started laughing.

LEWIS: "What is wrong with you!" He giggled.

NATH: "You sound a little defensive Vic?"

VIC: "No! Notice how much I trust you?"

LEWIS: "He's very paranoid all the time isn't he?"

VIC: "No I'm not. It's only 'cause I'm round that cunt all the time." I gestured towards Nath and he gave me a wink.

Once we had finished eating, Nath brought up the subject of next term and who had plans to live with who. We had an hour of deep and meaningfuls but it was too late in the night and we were all knackered. Nath set up a makeshift bed in the lounge on a sofa and Lewis kipped there in front of the TV. I got the spare room and Nath tucked up in his own bed. In the morning I found Lewis snoring away with the TV still switched on. Nath came down and mustered up some coffee with croissants, then we spent the rest of the day watching

Mad in England - A memoir

Nath's home movies from sixth form. They were really
revealing and personal. Loads of stuff with his ex-girlfriend
in. She was absolutely stunning. Very exotic looking and she
had an unusual name to go with it. Her type very much
reminded me of Shumana. Then I wondered if Shumana
reminded Nath of his ex. I was putting a picture together, a
viewpoint I didn't have before. He kept a video diary. He
was keeping one now in that box at the end of his bed in
Harrow. If he was always conscious of keeping the diary
then his on-screen behaviour would be capped, whereas
everyone else's behaviour was not capped and neither had
we signed any disclaimers or given him permission. It gave
him power now and in the future, should he need to release
any of it. After he had spent the afternoon introducing us to
all his schoolfriends through his parents huge television set,
he asked me and Lewis if we wanted to see Weybridge. We
both wanted this to continue, I did anyway so I said yes.
Lewis agreed and we jumped in the Fiat to spin around the
M25 and visit the driveway of Sir Cliff Richard. We also
toured the village knocking on doors and chatting to his
various mates, then onto the local haunt and met lots more
posh people in a beer garden. It was then that I became
conscious of myself and my accent. This was the big
difference between me and Nath. Lewis being from Devon
just polished his vowels and went undetected as a farmer's
son and GID student. I was wearing 'chips and gravy' on my
face. Nobody gave me more than two minutes of interest. I
spent most of the night listening and hardly any of the night
talking. Shandy drinking, southern . . .
Keeping up appearances was a theme right up until the end
of term after Tanya bought tickets for Royal Ascot. The
tickets came through from an old colleague of hers who had
become a close friend. His name was Paul. I had to get
dressed up and I was looking forward to getting drunk on
Pims and Champagne with some Essex girls (and boys). I
wore my crappest check jacket from Next, which I'd owned
since I was sixteen, together with a pair of sunglasses, a

flower in my lapel and a smile. We did get drunk, very drunk and disorderly but then so was everyone else apart from the Queen. It continued all the way back to Waterloo where on saying goodbye to the rest of the gang, me and Tanya found a disgarded wallet. We started mucking about trying to buy CD's with it in Our Price but I was too drunk to forge the guy's signature so we spent his cash in a passport photobooth and took numerous filthy photos of each other then took them home to Essex in a black cab. I don't know why we went back to Tanya's parents but we did and in the morning she left the photos all in a bedside drawer before we made our way to the Islington Design Centre for the third years' fashion show. I hadn't seen Twinkle or Mauli for nearly two weeks and it seemed strange meeting them both there with Dean and Diago who were both now dating fashion girls and had also got dragged along. Jeff Banks was there again and The Clothes Show's Caryn Franklin was sat next to him looking over-dressed. It was basically the same shit as last year but only not quite as good. None of this year's lot had the personality or verve of Seth and his bondage S&M collection but then again, how do you top that? Afterwards the GID and fashion gang sat outside a bar in the hot sunshine over Upper Street for a last drink before we all went home for the summer. These past few weeks had been fragmented and because of the ectopic pregnancy, I'd inadvertantly thrown myself into the Design Futures module and I hadn't seen anyone to speak to properly. The whole episode had been forgotten. Dean knew how hard I worked and took me to one side for a chat. He told me how much he cared about me and handed me a piece of paper with a wave drawn on it. I unfolded it and read the letter.

Friendship
Your friend is your needs answered.
He is your field which you sow with love and reap with thanksgiving.

And he is your fireside. For you come to him with your
hunger and you seek him for peace.

When your friend speaks his mind you fear not the 'nay' in
your own mind, nor do you withold the 'ay'.

And when he is silent your heart ceases not to listen to his
heart;

For without words, in friendship, all thoughts, all desires, all
expectations are born and shared, with joy that is
unacclaimed.

When you part from your friend, you grieve not;

For that which you love most in him may be clearer in his
absence, as the mountain to the climber is clearer from the
plain.

And let there be no purpose in friendship save the deepening
of the spirit.

And let your best be for your friend.

If he must know the ebb of your tide, let him know it's flood
also.

For what is your friend that you should seek him with hours
to kill?

Seek him always with hours to live.

For it is his to fill your need, but not your emptiness.

And in the sweetness of friendship let there be laughter, and
the sharing of pleasures.

A couple of empty weeks passed right at the very end of
term inside a vacuum of no work, all deadlines had been
met. People went out and enjoyed the first part of summer.
The rotas at the empty shell of 34 Crofts Road had slipped
beyond comprehension. The contract was coming to an end
and our landlord, Mr Fenchurch was going to have a lot of
cleaning to do over the summer. The cupboards were bare
apart from some of Mauli's dried seaweed and a tin of Heinz
beans. One day after mucking about in Harrow's new
shopping centre, me and Nath sat down in a cafe outside the
tube station and watched some shit World Cup build up and
Nath could have a ciggie. After some serious scheming we

Victor J Kennedy

decided on an exit strategy to avoid any entanglement in the organisation of tying up loose ends of bills, council tax, water rates and gas. Not to mention the pig sty issue staring us in the face and polluting the atmosphere amongst the four of us. Nobody wanted to admit it and neither did any of us confront it. There was an opportunity here for a sting. We returned to the empty house and quickly emptied both our rooms into Nath's Fiat with it's seats down. In three sweaty trips to Rickmansworth all my stuff was in the garage of Nath's dad. All Nath's stuff was back in his own bedroom. During the two hours at his parents' we sat down with all the bills and a calculator, dividing everything by four equal ways. Once we knew how much each person owed 'the house' we returned to Crofts Road, via a cashpoint withdrawal to bring our contibution to the table. We knew Mauli would not be around but Twinkle had kept popping home sporadically from wherever the hell he had been. Both our rooms had been unlocked with the doors wide open to display the emptiness. Mauli's bedroom door was now open and his room looked like a bomb had hit it, everything strewn everywhere like somebody couldn't find what they needed in time for a flight. The kitchen was still the same stinky, rancid mess as before. As we walked up the stairs to knock on Twinkle's bedroom door, the house felt sad. It was the end of our second year. He didn't answer. Nath didn't mess about and tried the door handle. It opened and we found Twinkle in bed. He sat up startled and dazed from being in a deep sleep. Unprepared, he was in a perfect position, on the back foot. He couldn't get away, this was it. Nath explained everything to him regarding the bills and the protocol when Mr Fenchurch came round for his rent and the keys. We were living out our deposits as the last month's rent. Fenchurch had no choice because he didn't fix the broken oven until Christmas so Twinkle was briefed not to take any lip from him. Nath handed over our cash. Twinkle counted it in front of us. He also agreed everything was fair and that Mauli had already caught a flight home leaving him

153

in charge of his belongings, apparently they had already arranged to live together next year. By the look of Mauli's room Carl had a lot of work to do. We said an edgy goodbye. I could tell he wasn't best pleased but then no-one enjoys getting shafted, do they? Especially not at the exit as well as the entrance. The only question was who would eventually take the blame for the sting?

Nath very kindly dropped me and my remaining bags off at Tanya's parents. We said our goodbyes and promised to sort out a place together with Lewis nearer the start of the third year. I didn't tell him, but I felt like Twinkle. Like I'd had enough of me and Nath. I felt like I wanted to live with Tanya next year but then again, I was in Essex amongst future in-laws. Off he went for a summer in the beautiful south of France with Shumana. All I had to look forward to was working like an idiot again for zero money in the not-so-sunny Lake District. I phoned Smudge back in Millhead and asked him to organize a weekend trip to London with a few mates. It was Tanya's mum's birthday and they were having one of their monumental barbecues in the massive back garden. I told the lads to bring sleeping bags but leave enough room for my stuff as I was hitching a ride back north with them on the Sunday. I rang Reggie during the week for initial talks to sort out a job but Tanya overheard me and had other plans. I spent the week watching the World Cup while Tanya proposed various schemes for me to stay in Essex over the summer. She knew I had to make about £2000 to buy my beloved Quadra 840AV. One of her suggestions was for me to become a postman around Buckhurst Hill. She had a mate who had a boyfriend who was a postman and could 'get me in' under the radar. Then she had me doing data entry at her mum's estate agency and finally pushing me to do her old bar job at Fairlop Waters. She also typed up and embellished my CV and sent it off to Copycats, a sort of imitation Prontaprint shop in Walthamstow. By the time the lads turned up on the Friday evening I was stitched up good and proper. I told them and they all looked me in the eye and

asked if I was sure. I wasn't worried about being under the thumb but I'd done my maths and if I got the Copycats job along with the bar job at night I could raise the cash in twelve long weeks. It was the only weekend I would spend with the lads so we made it a big one, going to Walthamstow Dogs and impersonating Take That and East 17 at Charlie Chans cool nightspot. The next day, after recovering, we clubbed together and bought Tanya's mum a fifty quid bottle of red wine for her birthday and to say thanks for putting us all up. We handed it over at the barbecue and she put it in the kitchen behind all the other booze on the kitchen top. Out in the garden, Tanya's dad was cooking away as the guests arrived. He had those large scented candles lit to keep the flies away. All us northern lads were huddled together early on, just consuming cans of beer and giggling at all the folk interacting in the garden. Tanya was milling about, making sure everyone had what they needed and was having a good time. Carolyn was doing the same, like mother like daughter. She came over to us and had a laugh with the lads and that pretty much broke the ice (and the booze had begun to take effect). After that point we all split up amongst the crowd, laughing and joking about everything under the sun. That was until the sun went down and Tanya's sister Jennifer turned up, with a selection of 'orrible stinking drunk mates. One lad of about eighteen, made a bee line straight for us. It was like he already knew northerners were present. As he stood in front of all five of us; me, Smudge, Gibbo, Mitch and Ernie, his head was wobbling on his shoulders, his eyes could not focus in the darkness and he pointed his finger,
"Who won the World Cup in 1966?"
"England."
"Who won the World Cup in 1966?"
"England!"
"Who won the fucking World Cup in 1966?"
"England won it."
"No they fucking didn't."
"Who won it then? Go on, tell us."

"West Ham."

"How did they manage that then?"

"Bobby Moore, Geoff Hurst, Martin Peters and John Byrne."

"Who the fuck is John Byrne?"

"On stand-by mate. Who do you support?"

"Man Utd. He supports Liverpool. He supports Carlisle and them two are farmers, so they're not arsed about football."

"Scousers eh?"

"Not necessarily, no. Cumbrians."

"Cumbre-whats?"

"Cumbrians"

"Cunts more like. I remember you scousers coming down here before they got rid of the chicken run."

"Chicken run?"

"Yeah. Chicken run. Main stand on one side. Wall on the other. Away fans on one end and the faithful on the other."

"The West Ham faithful?"

"Who do you fink, you fucking northern monkey?"

"Eh, there's no need to talk to us like that."

"I wasn't talking to them. I'm tellin' you a fuckin' story, now listen muppet."

"Get on with it then."

"I'm at one end, with the lads. You scousers at the other and we run. We all run. Then we clash, I was right at the front and this big fat cunt stands front. He puts his fist in the air to give me a whack but before he can do that, I pulls out my screwdriver and with my fist clenched I stick it right in his forehead. Fackin' claret every fackin' where! He didn't know what the fuck hit him." he started laughing, just to himself.

"Look mate, thanks for that. We're off inside for a drink. See ya." We went in doors and came to the conclusion he wasn't dangerous but it was best to keep away. The music came out and we all had a boogie into the night. The last thing I remember was Smudge dancing with Tanya's mum and complementing her on having "such a wonderful pair of breasts."

Victor J Kennedy

In the morning we all woke up in Tanya's, now smelly
bedroom, with groans and moans about sore heads and being
thirsty. I was in bed with Tanya and they were all flat on the
floor in sleeping bags. Tanya nipped downstairs and quickly
mustered up some bacon sandwiches and coffee. As soon as
they were down, the bags were packed and then carried
downstairs to the awaiting black Ford Escort RS Turbo
waiting outside. The amazing thing was that Gibbo came
back up stairs with a tale. "That twat from last night is lying
in the grass asleep outside the garden gate. You will never
guess what he's got in his hand? Only our birthday present to
Carolyn – that bottle of £50 red wine, half drank. He
probably bloody spilled it!" All of us helped carry down the
remaining cases and sleeping bags to the car. As each of us
passed him we kicked him in the head, just once each – if
only for that scouser with the screwdriver scar in the centre
of his forehead. As soon as the car was packed, we all had a
hug and said our goodbyes. Smudge had spent the morning
trying to convince me to 'come home' but it was too late, I
had been convinced into staying down over the summer by
Tanya and her hospitable family – my family. Now there
was a thought. He tried one last time before he got in the car
but it was no good, I was staying down south with an
unconscious hooligan laying on the grass behind me. They
drove away super quick, I could hear the turbo come in as
they disappeared around the corner.

I spent the following week doing more database work at
Carolyn's office and waiting to find out about my application
and interview for the Graphic Designer position at Copycats
in Walthamstow. I had lied in the interview and told them I
graduated in June with first class honours. They obviously
liked my college portfolio and gave me the job for £12,000 a
year. I did my sums and that paltry wage wasn't going to do
the job in twelve weeks so I accepted the barman position at
Fairlop Waters on Thursday, Friday and Saturday nights.
Fairlop Waters is an old quarry hole which had been filled
with water to create a 'Lakeside Leisure Resort.' What

worked out nicely was the outfits for both jobs involved black shoes and black trousers. Both employers supplied a polo shirt, Copycats in bright yellow and Fairlop in bright red. Both had a beautifully embroidered logo on the breast. It was like working for McDonalds from 8am to 5:30pm through the day and when Tanya picked me up from Walthamstow and drove me to Fairlop for my £3.50 an hour, I would quickly eat a sandwich in the car, change shirts and my evenings were spent looking like I worked in Pizza Hut. I got a lot of shit for being northern from all the Essex boys, especially when I couldn't understand orders like 'Light and Ale' or 'Whiskey American', which eventually turned out to be dry ginger from the brand Canada Dry. But I wasn't to know this because I was a 'northern monkey'.

After a few weeks of abuse I just started thieving from their change, just a pound coin on each round. I'd only do this at the end of the night because they were all so pissed they never checked their change. To be honest, I started thinking about it and there have been many times that I've woken up with kebab on my face next morning and been shocked at how much money I'd spent in those clubs up north. I started to think my pound coin thieving antics were a national epidemic because you had to make sure the till was straight or you were escorted downstairs by a bouncer to see the management in the basement. Who was probably the son an an East End bank robber and one of his henchmen would have knee-capped me with out blinking. The rest of the staff were okay though, that's because they were all my age and all getting paid £3.50 an hour. The DJ 'Rob' was funny though, he couldn't help but play Waterfall by Atlantic Ocean three or four times a night. He fucking loved that tune and every other member of staff hated it by the end of the summer. What a scorcher it turned out to be too! On Sunday afternoons I had to collect all the glasses from the parched grass surrounding the Lake. I had to run through a gauntlet of Wasps, buzzing around the sticky lager pots and being threatening as well as annoying. Not to mention the

Victor J Kennedy

dickheads on jet skis who would spot my bright red polo shirt and give me a spraying as they 360d in the shallow water next to edge of the Lake. Absolutely fucking hilarious, that was.

At Copycats there was no spraying of water but a lot of larking about with the two print lads in the back print room. They were a bit older than me and loved their Madness. They played the greatest hits every day, dancing and jumping around the machines, singing their heads off having a right laugh. I could hear all this from the front shop while sat in my yellow t-shirt at the computer making business cards and logos for local builders who'd just walk in off the street. It wasn't just builders. They had solicitors, hairdressers, estate agents even a member of East 17 came in, John Hendy, and asked for photocopies of some photos he had taken of himself with his top off! I had to serve him and thought it was odd because I didn't recognise him due to the fact he wasn't one of the main two singers. When a bunch of twelve year olds wearing East 17 t-shirts ran in after he left, asking all sorts of questions about what he was doing, I realised that he was famous. That explained why he was dressed even more ridiculously than I was. During that earlier part of the summer Tanya asked me to do some 'work' on the side by giving me the responsibility of designing and printing her parent's 25th Wedding Anniversary invites. For free! It was going to be in The Bald Hind in Chigwell on 10th September at 7.30pm. Tanya was sorting it all out, the food, the DJ, the surprise guests, the lot! She loved them both so much that she was prepared to put herself out so much to make it really special. You only get one 25th Wedding Anniversary after all.

In what little spare time I had over that long hard summer of 1994, I read the papers on a Sunday morning in the Baker family garden, in the sunshine with a bacon sandwich and a coffee. One Sunday in mid July I read this huge double page spread by The Sunday Express Astrologer Joseph Campbell entitled 'The Jupiter Effect". I've been a bit fickle in my life

Mad in England - A memoir

since my mum christened me a Methodist, took me to
Sunday school and taught me a lot of the stuff her mother
taught her. When I was a little boy I would pray by my bed
every night and the whole family, apart from my dad used to
discuss our horoscopes in context of the Daily Papers. Then,
as I got older and discovered football, masturbation and
thieving I got confused by all this religion and horoscope
stories. Eventually I decided it was all bollocks and was
going to slow me down so I dropped it all in the eighties.
Five or so very productive years had passed and I was about
to enter my final year at university but I accidentally
bumped into this double page spread. It stopped me in my
tracks and got me thinking about 'The Jupiter Effect' on my
own life. That big bastard planet was moving into some part
of the universe which will bring about 'an amazing turn of
fortune to all of us in this planet as we move towards the
next Millennium'. I admit, I was drawn in. I was so
captivated by it that I tore out the pages and kept them in a
secret place, waiting for it all to come true. I didn't tell
Tanya or any of her family what I'd experienced on my own
in that garden but it felt magical. Like I was being visted by
a spirit. I carried on reading the predictions about Brazil
winning the World Cup. The Jupiter Effect no doubt. Then
Tanya brought a letter out for me that had arrived on Friday.
I was surprised I had a letter, postmark said Eastbourne and
only my mum had this address. It was from Twinkle's dad. I
say, from Twinkle's 'dad' but what I mean is that his father
wrote the letter in his own handwriting and then Carl signed
the bottom of it. His signature looked angry.

Re Gas Bill 34 Crofts Rd
Messers: Forcett, Kennedy, Foreman, Song
a/c 100 9 82 60034 0036

Dear Victor and Nath,
Having received the gas bill, copy of which I have enclosed
for £62.49.

Victor J Kennedy

I have informed the gas company that it is to be split four ways @ £15.62 EACH.

Having sent my cheque off to cover my share and Mauli's together with the amount you owe me on account Total £41.25.

This leaves a balance of £13.62 (VICTOR) and £7.62 (Nath) to pay. I will be grateful if you can settle this amount due with the Gas Company when contacted.

I have given the breakdown to the account dept.

Best Regards,
Chris

Well, this was extemely bad news. Short term and long term. What disturbed me was that after thinking about it, Nath had been to Tanya's parents many times so he knew the address. Carl had no idea where she lived outside of college time. So Nath must have spoken verbally to Carl. Then I checked it again and noticed my name was in caps with the largest so-called debt and Nath owed half my amount and got off scott free with upper and lower case name. Then I post-rationalised further and thought back to mine and Naths conversation in Harrow the day we did the runner and left Carl in the house to face the landlord alone. I knew I deserved it but all of a sudden the blame seemed to be on my doorstep (my girlfriend's parents' doorstep) and Nath gets away scott free, with a clean pair of heels. And it was his idea! As for Carl, I was massively disappointed because we were proper mates in the first year before Nath came on to the scene. I was done up like a kipper. The more I thought about it, the more I couldn't avoid the blame so I paid the whole bill and got it over with. I would get it back from Nath later on and it was not worth upsetting British Gas now that Carl had grassed me up. I would've preferred him to leave his dad out of it and paid the fucking bill and then bollocked me to my face, then take fifteen quid cash off me for being a shit housemate and running away at the end of

161

the contract. But I guess if you dish some shit out you get some shit back. Unless your name is Nathan Foreman.

The rest of the summer continued to be as stressful and as equally tiring due to these two jobs totalling around 13 hour days. After speaking to my mum on the phone every Sunday and telling her of my stress, both her and dad decided to pay me a visit to see if I was alright. They visited Warwick and then carried on down to Loughton, pitched up in a hotel and then both families met in a gastro pub halfway between Buckhurst Hill and Loughton. This was serious. This meant I was in marriage territory, if the in-laws were having a pow-pow. Even her grandparents Edna and Cyril came along to have a look at my mum and dad. I just got drunk to try and hide my nervousness and then started making jokes and trying to take the weight of attention off my parents. I thought I was doing alright until Tanya whispered in my ear that her Gran was cleaning her bedroom the other day and had found the pornographic photos we took of each other in Waterloo station on Royal Ascot Day. I shut my mouth after that.

After a full inspection, my parents left without a worry. I appeared to be coping with it all. But I wasn't. I was waking up in the middle of the night all hot and sweaty. Tanya just said it was a really hot summer and wasn't normally like this. I felt I wasn't getting enough recreation. It was all work, work, work. I needed some football to release my tension. So she obliged and behind my back got in touch with Mike, her ex-boyfriend and he came round the house one Wednesday night to pick me up and play in his team. They played in a summer-night league down Coppermill Lane in Walthamstow. I jumped in the car with only a pair of airwalk trainers and no shin pads to play in. The whole night was bizarre spending time with him, especially in the showers after the match. He was even telling me in the pub about all her bad points so I could look out for them. We even joked about the weirdness of the situation at one point. Fair play to Tanya though for doing that.

Victor J Kennedy

Even though I was absolutely shot, I was loving Essex.
Especially Essex girls. They are the best looking women
crammed into one county that I'm convinced there has to be
something put into the water and it's not just fluoride.
Ninetynine percent of them at Fairlop were fit. I went to The
Epping Forest Country Club with Tanya, her sister Jen and
their mates (one of which was Mark, who a few years later
got his 15 minutes in that boy band Another Level) who
were all fit. Even the blokes. The only ones to let the place
down were the professional footballers from West Ham and
Spurs. To be honest, you could walk around the club and
they all looked exotic, like they were from another country.
The illusion works until you walk up to a girl who looks like
Sade and then she opens her mouth. That's when it all goes
wrong. You expect some deep sexy latino drawl and she
shouts, "HIYAA! You alright treacle? Get us a white wine
and soda will ya?" I remember getting a Day Rover ticket for
50p back in 1980's West Yorkshire, to travel across the
county. At 13 years old I could tell the girls in Leeds were
fitter than the ones in Bradford or Wakefield.
Nip across the north circular from Woodford into
Walthamstow and something happens to the faces too. I very
rarely saw a nice looking lady go past the window at work
all day. That was probably because they had MTV in the
shop to entertain the customers as they waited for their
photocopies to finish or their business cards to be sliced.
Towards the end of the summer I'd managed to find a good
mate. Roy, manager of the Barking office, who made
frequent visits to our office. He was from Enfield, a Spurs
fan and a player himself. That was where our friendship
gathered pace. He was older than me and used to go out with
a "lass from Barnsley, eee-by-gum lad! Bratford." He liked
to do his northern accent and he was quite good at it too. I
was kind of like his emotional punch bag and it reminded me
of being bullied by Reggie and his cronies in Kendal. The
two Madness fans in the printers out the back didn't care for
Roy too much and they told me to watch myself. I thought

he was okay and one night when I wasn't working at Fairlop,
I joined him for a game on the astro turf at Market Road.
When he saw me play he asked me to join his Saturday team
called Winchmore Hill. So I bought myself some £7 boots
from Stead and Simpson and borrowed some shin pads. By
the time preseason was done and I'd played for the second
team it was time to return to Harrow and finish my degree.
At work Roy had asked me to be drafted to the Barking
office to supposedly help out while his designer was on
holiday. There wasn't that much to do in Barking. Certainly
not as much as in Walthamstow. So during my spare time I
wrote a letter to Hopkers, my old mate from Dermont
borders. His dad was in the army and could afford to put him
through a proper school but that didn't stop Hopkers doing
all the drugs under the sun with me back in 1991 when I was
in Carlisle. Hopkers had got his grades and gone to do a
Pharmacy degree in Sunderland.

Dear Matt,
How are things? I hope they are fine. I'm okay but just
pissed off at my current situation. In fact I'm completely
arsed, right off with it all! I'm working at a sad company
called Copycats in the East End of London where that
famous, contemporary, musically genius band East 17 come
from! Walthamstow is the place and it's the most depressing
place in the world. The freaky thing is the group members
come in this shop for press release photos copying for their
walls at home. NIIIIICCCEEEEE!!! What fashion kids they
are too!
I got this job after I decided to stay in London or should I
say, forced to stay in London by Tanya (Chick), who
promised me a £300 a week job at the post office and then
the whole thing fell through as it was organised and
promised to her by an idiot who couldn't tell his arse from
his elbow!
Anyway, by the time I'd realised that I'd been conned it was
too late, my old job at Goddard Murrays in Kendal was gone

Victor J Kennedy

as I lied to the boss and told him some big design company in London had taken me on for £18,000 a year NICE ONE Vic! I'd also turned down a lift home to Millhead from Smudge, who came down for a party at Tanya's with various mates from home, which was a good night! So, I was stuck down here and had to look for a summer job that paid well enough to get what I want for my third year.

After not getting work in America in May of this year I'd decided against trying to have a laugh all through summer of '94 and just work my bollox off for a new Power PC Apple Macintosh which just happens to cost a mighty handful of rio de janiero! I couldn't afford to get a holiday so that was out of the window as well. Basically all I had to do was dig my heals in, get my head down and work hard. Tanya's mum and dad said they would let me stay at their house, rent free! So that has helped me a lot by getting paid the high wages of the south and the MAM N DAD's house syndrome of free food, cleaning, washing etc. of up north. I haven't taken the piss though, as me and Tanya have spent over £300 between us to give her parents a surprise 25th wedding anniversary party. I designed and got printed the invites at work and Tanya's sorted out the venue, balloons and Karaoke etc. It should be a really good night as we got hold of their old school friends etc. About 70+ people! Tanya's got to do all the food though, hopefully it keeps me as the 'Blue-Eyed Boy' they think I am!........Which I am!!!

I've also have a job in a mad bar called Fairlop Waters. It's an old water-filled man-made quarry that people windsurf on and the bar is at the foot of the lake. It's like Pine Lake in Carnforth but the bar has a lot more interesting "young" people in it, not your usual sad "DAVES DISCO" or "JEFF DUNCAN'S QUARTET - LIVE" say no more.

Anyway, I get so many direct offers for sex – it's unbelievable! I never thought doing a bar job could pay well and be such a laugh. I haven't taken up any of the offers though. Got to think about who I'm going back home to! Or have I? No, honestly I haven't been bad at all.

Mad in England - A memoir

So I work for Copycats through the day for £220 a week and Fairlop Waters at night for £75 a week and because it's a bar job I don't get chance to spend money on drink. I've lost a full stone in weight because of it! I'm starting to reach breakdown point though as I get so knackered if we have a party after work on Saturdays and I miss a night's sleep. I've had some good laughs and stuff this summer but I'm looking forward to getting back to University for a rest!

Anyway, I've saved about £2,300 and I've got my grant and third year loan to come which are £1,000 each so I should be okay for my final year. My rent will take a lot of it this year though because we've decided to go for home comfort and not wallet comfort. I'm living with Nath and Lewis in a 3-bedroom bachelor palace (47 Manor Road, Harrow, Middx) with walk-in kitchen/lounge for £54 a week and only 4 doors down from Grandma Tanya's Sunday lunches and all her home comforts etc. etc. I have a feeling this is going to be a good year!

I've played a lot of football this summer as well, squeezing them into my tight working/sleeping/working schedule and met a lot of Tottenham fans who live around Walthamstow who I've played with and against. We play at Leyton Orient's training ground who Bradford City hammered at the start of the season. Other than that all I've done that is anything decent is go see Galliano at the Town & Country, Camden and have lots of tacky Italian meals at small restaurants on Sunday nights, my only night off.

I'm going home on the 14th September and will be around Millhead until Sunday and then I'm coming back down here for my last week's work and start back at university. I will probably go to Bradford on Thursday until Friday 'cos it's my mum's 50th birthday party that night. And then that will be it until Christmas.

Well that's about it really, by now you've probably guessed that this is a standard letter that I've sent out to all my mates but ask me if I'm bothered! Sorry for bursting your bubble if you hadn't realised.

Victor J Kennedy

Take it easy,

Victor 'The' Kennedy

After finishing the letter, which had now become a circular, I printed them out and nipped down the post office to get them delivered before I appeared up north for that tiny window around my mum's 50th birthday. When I got back to the office, Roy was back from one of his 'meetings' and looked pissed off. He confronted me straight away, "Where have you been?"
"Post Office."
"I do the post. You do the logos."
"It was for me. I just posted a letter to a mate Roy, relax."
"Did you send it up north to Bratford? Baarnsley, Waakefield, Batley, Leeds, Bratford! Ay up! Yorkshur!!!"
"No Roy. They've gone to Cumbria."
"Nay lad, not to Yorkshur? Tha's betraying thou's roots lad."
"Fuck off Roy and start speaking English."
"That's what we speak darn 'ere."
"It's spoken all over the country."
"Yeah but this is where it's spoken the best mate, innit. Queen's English."
"Look, can we talk about something else? Is there anything for me to do?"
"Just those cards for that Balti House in Chigwell. You set 'em up wrong and the boys in Walthamstow have sent 'em back to Yorkshur to be done again. Correctly!"
"Let me look again, where's the job bag?"
"Don't need a fucking job bag, it's on the computer. Sit down son." Roy dangled the bag in front of my face.
"Just give me the bag you prick."
"Oi oi! Monkey just called me a prick!"
"Roy I'm not into this, just let me look at the set up and stock details. There might be an explanation to all of this."

"The explanation is on the computer." At this point I lost my patience and my cool. I sat down by the computer as if to start doing the work. Roy sat down at the front desk and as soon as he turned away, I rang the print boys back in Walthamstow. I knew they didn't like Roy and I smelled a rat. The phone rang and one of them picked up the phone which displayed my office's caller ID He answered, "GEEEEEZER!" I could hear Madness – House of Fun playing in the background.

"Who's that?"

"Matty. Who's that?"

"It's Vic down in Barking office."

"GEEEEEZER!"

"Alright mate, just a quick one. Has Roy just been up there?"

"That cunt is always round here mate. He's worse than a stray. What's up?"

"He's just bollocked me about that Balti House job."

"What's he said now? He was rabbiting about it in the front office."

"He said I've set the artwork up wrong and told me to have a look at it. I've brought the Quark file up and I did 'em 8 up with cut marks on A4."

"Yeah, they're on the same beige as that taxi stuff so we were gonna use the off cuts and put 'em through the machine again. What colour is it?"

"It's not black mate, if that's what you're asking?"

"Bollocks. It's single colour though?"

"Yeah, a sort of burgundy. Pantone 181U."

"That's alright, tell him to fuck off."

"I did already but he's got the job bag in his hand. Have you made a plate yet?"

"Fuck no. I've been rushed of my feet mate. You'll have to tell him to bring the print out back over here. Dickhead."

"Can you tell him? He won't listen to me. He never does."

"Alright, put him on the phone."

"Roy! Come here a minute!" I shouted over and he frowned as he came across the shop.

Victor J Kennedy

"What the fuck are you doing on the phone? Shouldn't you be sorting that artwork out you fucked up on?"
"It's Matty from Walthamstow." I held out the phone.
"He didn't ring here did he? Because I never heard the fucking phone go." He took the receiver and proceeded to have it out with Matty, who just happened to be the same age as Roy – somewhere in their early thirties. They had a right ding dong until Roy slammed the phone down and turned to me and said, "You fucking grass." and threw me against the wall. Very quickly I was held by the throat with my feet on tip toes, in the front shop window at Barking's Copycats. I was pretty scared because he had lost it. "Don't you ever make a mug out of me ever again you fucking northern monkey. I've taken you down Winchmore Hill you little twat and now you're taking the piss out of me? Bet you think you're fucking smart, with your degree and your fancy fucking logos. You're just a fucking snitch and I don't trust mouthy cunts who go running to their mums." At that point the phone rang and he went to answer it. I could breath again but my heart was racing because I'd just realised there was only me and him in this office. I felt hugely threatened and was considering doing a runner out of the front of the shop and leaving my jacket in there. He answered the phone, "Good afternoon, Copycats Barking. Roy speaking, how may I help you." He paused for a second. He said, "Yes, he's here." and then handed me the phone. "It's your mum." And for a split second my heart and spirit lifted until I put the receiver to my ear. "Hi mum. How did you get this number?"
"We've been trying to get hold of you all day. Tanya gave us the number for work but when I rang there they didn't know where you were. I've been worried sick. Tanya drove to your work this afternoon and then she found out you'd been transferred to another office. She just rang me from there and gave me the number just now."
"So what's the matter mum?"

"It's your gran. She's in hospital and it's not looking good luv."

"What's happened?"

"It's a lot of different things. I think she's been poorly for quite some time but you know how much she gets scared about going into hospital. She's been avoiding it by hiding things from us and not telling the doctors."

"Is she gonna die?"

"Let's just say, it would be a good idea to go and visit her when you and Tanya come up for my birthday."

"Sure. I'll borrow your car?"

"I think me and your dad will be visiting quite often so we'll take you down to Bradford quite early on the Saturday morning. We'll go to Bradford Royal Infirmary first and then have a cup of tea at your sister's."

"Well, I was thinking of staying at our Jan's on the camp bed and show Tanya a night out in Bradford."

"So you'll need my car?"

"If that's alright?"

"Just be careful with your drinking. It can still affect you in the morning."

"Okay mum, I'll be careful. Tanya's with me anyway, she'll keep an eye on me."

"Okay luv, see you next Thursday. I hope the move goes well."

"Thanks mum, tickets are booked on the 12.15 from Euston so that's a fixed deadline. If we get the keys for the new place before Wednesday then I'll take my stuff round and leave Wednesday free."

"I think that's a better idea. You know what you're like with bloody trains."

"I don't have a choice mum. The new landlord has still got to fix some things which we complained about so if he finishes early, we get the keys early. Anyway, I only have to put all my boxes etc. in my room and then it's done. I won't be unpacking until nearer the start of term." I lowered my voice so Roy couldn't hear, I didn't want to blow my cover.

Victor J Kennedy

"Fine. Your dad will be at Oxenholme for half past four, on the Kendal side – not in the car park."

"Thanks mum, see you next week. Give my love to gran."

"Bye luv. I love you."

"I love you too." I put the phone down and quietly went back to my desk and set the business cards up exactly the way Roy wanted them. We didn't really speak for the rest of the afternoon but I made sure he knew what was going on with my gran and hopefully that would make him give me a break. He gave me a lift back to Walthamstow and all I could think of was handing in my notice and getting back to college. I'd had enough of working like this. Two jobs for twelve weeks was very tiring emotionally as well as physically. On top of this I was now deeply concerned about my grandmother. Before me and Tanya made the journey north I had to put my problems to one side and help Tanya get through her parent's surprise 25th wedding anniversary. I threw a sicky from Fairlop Waters and spent most of that Saturday blowing up balloons and putting streamers throughout The Bald Hind function room in Chigwell. I helped Tanya display the buffet on a trestle table. She did a fantastic job and I still felt envious of how much she was prepared to do for her mum and dad. I'd never gone this far for my parents. After it was all set up and ready to go off, we went home and pretended to get ready to go out on our own. We said goodbye to Carolyn and Bob, who were going out for a meal at The Bald Hind in Chigwell, apparently.

I spent the first hour before they arrived at the pub being introduced to all the relatives and friends from way back as "Tanya's boyfriend from university" like she had another one somewhere else. My new housemate Lewis and his ex-housemate, Ross turned up as they were already back at Harrow. Lewis told me that nothing had been fixed at the flat and he had been chasing Mr. Kapoor, our new landlord, since Thursday. He'd also brought me my keys so I could take my stuff around before Thursday.

Mad in England - A memoir

At 8pm on the nose, the lights were dimmed and everybody was told to "Ssshhhh!" Carolyn and Bob walked in and everyone shouted "SURPRISE!" and popped their party poppers. It was amazing. Tanya's mum burst into tears but her dad, Bob, well he looked more shocked than surprised. Alot of flash bulbs went off and I never saw the results but I bet his face was a picture! The night was full of photos and Tanya's mum made sure she got a photo of me and Tanya, just before midnight. I was pretty drunk but I gave it my best smile.

On Monday morning I gave my notice at Copycats, which was supposed to be one week because I was still inside my three month probationary period. They took it well but asked if I could stay for two weeks and then I had to make up a bullshit excuse that I had another job to go to. I couldn't tell them I was going back to uni so I lied again instead. The next couple of days were tough, working all day and then travelling around the north circular with my life in boxes again. The flat was a shit tip from the last tennants. It looked good on first inspection but the shower had not been fitted, there was no washing machine and the taps in the kitchen didn't work properly. The drainage from the sink was crap too and the storage heaters annoyed me. The landlord didn't put one in the bathroom so in the winter it was going to be freezing. Apart from that, it was a lovely flat. Lewis was installed in the little room next to mine. Me and Nath had found the flat, saving Lewis the trouble while he worked on his parent's farm in Devon. He took the smaller room as recompense for the supply of somewhere to live. It was in an ideal position. Only 500 yards from our home on Manor Road from last year, with Twinkle and Mauli just over the railway bridge. Good for Nath, as Shumana and Ruth had moved in there too. The best thing about my new flat was the fact it was practically next door to Tanya, Cathy and their new housemates Miriam from ceramics, Sam who lived with Tanya in the first year and another fashion student Shelly, who was now Dean's girlfriend. Lewis again promised he would keep chasing Kapoor, our new landlord, about the minor issues that felt pretty major to me. So I said goodbye and got in Carolyn's Escort, which she now let me borrow, made my way back to Buckhurst Hill and packed my bag for the weekend.

The morning of my mum's fiftieth birthday my dad quietly entered our bedroom at 7.30am, slowly opening the door he muttered through the gap, "Come on you two, I want to be off by 8 o'clock. You've got thirty minutes." He would always do this. He took pleasure from setting deadlines and barking orders. Thirty minutes of rushing around and we were on the A65 again heading for Bradford Royal Infirmary in about an hour and a half's time. Tanya did her best to appease me during that time but I was apprehensive to say the least. By the time we got to the hospital, hearing my parents tell the stories of her deterioration, I was really nervous about seeing my gran. As we walked up the staircase to the ward, Tanya said she wanted to stay back by the doors so as not to interfere. She had never met my gran and this would not be the ideal circumstances for introductions. As I got to the doors I was greeted by a ward sister and asked who I was here to see. "Marjorie Philips." I answered.

"Ah, she's been sleeping but I think she's awake now. It's that bed over there." She pointed towards the second bed next to the window. The first thing I noticed was that there were no bed covers on my gran. She was lying on her side in her nightie with no slippers on. Her feet were bruised and there were lesions on her elbows, shoulders and her poor cheek bones. Her hair was unkept and made her look like Don King. As bizarre as it sounds I just couldn't work out what the hell had happened to the woman I knew who had helped bring me up for the first sixteen years of my life. What had the nurses been doing to her? I knew her as a strong woman with a hard opinion of people and of life. All I saw before me was a defeated human being, on every level. It was severely upsetting. I knelt down next to her bed so my head was level with hers. "Hello Gran, it's Vic. Are you awake?" She stirred and slowly opened one eye.

"Go away. I don't want to see you." My heart sank. That was devastating to hear her say that.

"Why? What have I done?"

"Just leave me alone. I want to die." she whispered.

"Oh come on Gran. You've got more fight in you than that?"

"No. Go away."

"But what about this Bird's Trifle? I know how much you love your cream. Just try some." I picked up a plastic pot on her bedside table and offered it with a spoon.

"No. Just go."

"Ahh, come on Gran. You can do it." But she wouldn't reply. In fact she found the strength to roll over and face the other way. She had given up. I didn't know what else to say or do. I felt hugely self-conscious, like all the nurses were watching me so I stepped away from the bed and stood back against the doors with Tanya while my parents comforted her. I lasted ten seconds before I had to go outside and stand in the car park. That was it. The last time I saw her alive. That night, my mum's birthday party in the Cricket Club came and went, I couldn't tell you what it was like. After travelling back to Euston, Tanya's dad dropped us home to Essex the next day. We had hardly had a cup of tea when the phone went. Tanya's little brother, Luke answered the phone. It was my mum. Gran was dead. I got on the train the next day and went back for the funeral. I saw my dad cry. I saw my older cousins cry. I cried after looking at my cousin Martin's face as they walked out of the service. I felt sorry for him. I'd never seen all my family so upset in the same place, all at the same time before. It was too much. I realised I was mortal.

I drank Tetley bitter at the wake and pretended to be a proper Yorkshireman again, like I'd never left at 16 years old and London had never been a part of my life. I felt a fake, it was something to do with my identity being split between the north and the south. It was also more than that. I knew I had many identities for many different occasions and for lots of different people. Today I was playing the good son. The family guy. Tomorrow I was back to being the over ambitious student who was going to come first. All these events, these things that occur in your life and the time that they appear is the key. It is like a game of mousetrap. All set up at the beginning and there is nothing you can do to stop it catching you. One trap sets off the next trap etc. You're always heading towards your destination. It's all set up. Even when you realise it's too late. I already had a rocket up my arse in terms of trying to escape what I'd become by the age of 19. I'd felt I was on a catch-up and the rocket was fuelled by the ambition to be transformed into something else. The death of my grandmother just before the start of my third year and the mayor part she had played in my upbringing had significantly increased the amount of emotional traffic passing through my subconscious. Bereavement should be recognised as a mental illness. It's like a cold for some people, for others flu even pneumonia, sometimes even finishing them off! 'They' call it "dying from a broken heart" when what you actually die from is a broken mind.

I actually thought it didn't bother me, my gran's death, but it must have. As soon as I got back to Harrow I threw myself into sorting out all the problems of the flat. I unpacked my boxes and my suitcases. I even bought some cheap, dark, blue fabric from the market off Station Road to hang over my ceiling and create a moody soft den which would help me sleep during all the stressful times ahead. My drawing board fit perfectly at one end of the room facing the window. I also had the water boiler in my room which heated it up nicely and I had extra room to put things above it on a makeshift shelf. I put my hand around the back of the boiler and found more space to put portfolios or large pieces of card and my cutting mat squeezed in nicely. I bought a cheap wooden shelving unit and put my ghetto blaster on it and all my tapes. I now had six Compact Discs; Prince, Stereo MCs, The Future Sound of London, The Prodigy,

Mad in England - A memoir

Carleen Anderson and not forgetting Jam & Spoon who
were the crisp perfect electronic trance sound you would
expect from a Panasonic XBS. The Stone Roses were about
to release their hugely anticipated second album, cunningly
titled The Second Coming and I had my eye on the release
date to add it to my collection. Between us we only had one
TV, which turned out to be my portable so I never had
anything to retire to if I didn't like what they were watching.
I wasn't bothered because I knew we would mostly be
working and if I had a computer in my bedroom then I
would be sat watching that monitor instead. We mounted it
on the coffee table in the lounge but it was only a 15" screen
so a box was added and a spare piece of dark blue fabric was
laid over to hide the Kelloggs logos. We assembled a 'babe
wall' up the staircase and landing area using images cut out
of FHM and Loaded magazine. Nath unveiled a drawing he
had done called 'The Three Amigos' after the recent comedy.
I wasn't sure which person was meant to be which because
Nath had written a different name under each head. Under
my head was Lewis's name, Lewis had Nath's name and
Nath, who was in the centre with his arms around the other
two amigos, had Vic underneath. First of all we laughed and
took the piss out of ourselves but the poster stayed on the
wall. It was just at the entrance to the lounge at eye level.
You couldn't miss it. Well, I couldn't miss it and the eyes
followed me around as much as the swapped name tags got
inside my head. We went shopping together in the Fiat Uno.
Me and Nath imposed the shopping rules from the second
year on Lewis while on the way to Tescos. Lewis craftily
turned this to his advantage and put all manner of rubbish in
the trolley which we all argued about. He had a massive
addiction to chocolate in all it's manifestations. Our first
weekly shop for three amigos came to a whopping £82.43. It
concerned me that we were setting a precedent and that
Lewis's addictive personality was going to set the tone going
forward. My anxiety led me to the issues unsolved by Mr.

Victor J Kennedy

Kapoor, our invisible landlord so I drafted a letter and got those two to co-sign it, showing our solidarity.

47 Manor Road
Harrow Middlesex
HA1 2PF
081 861 5294

27.9.94
RE: let property 47 Manor Road Harrow

Dear Mr Kapoor / Mr Humphries,
Further to our phone calls of 19.9.94. 20.9.94. 23.9.94. 26.9.94 and our meetings at the time of viewing and payment of rent (with deposit), the following items have still not been fixed or produced as promised before we moved in:
Shower and shower curtain.
Fully working washing machine.
3 original keys.
Fully working taps.
Decent drainage from the kitchen sink.
Working electrical heater in the bathroom.
As you will be aware we took on the property on 15.9.94 and you had at least a week's notice before this date to sort these problems out. It was not our responsibility to check that the taps, drainage and the electrical fan heater worked before the 15th. This is clearly unprofessional business practice. We refuse to be taken advantage of and as of the above date you have 5 working days (7 days' written notice) to sort out the above problems before we take any further action. We need not remind you that we pay £150 a week for a fully functional flat a further 7 days could pass before they are sorted out which will be 3 weeks = £450. We are also unable to get to the electric meter on the side of the house to read and thus change our names to the bill. We have had to pay £10 for electrical points for a joiner who also took a £5.00 hammer from us that he borrowed. We have also had

to buy batteries to make the door bell work, and the vacuum cleaner smokes through bad wiring when we use it. Our housing officer will receive a copy of this letter as proof of this notice although we hope this matter will be resolved without delay and the need for further action.

Yours Sincerely,
Victor Kennedy, Nathan Foreman, Lewis Thurston-Coe

We didn't do the Freshers' Week stuff because we thought the propect of pre trials piss ups, a pop quiz, a sports disco, and hypnotist were too naff to waste money on. Me, Tanya and Lewis went along to watch a banjo performance by the frizzy haired actor who played Nigel in Eastenders but it was terrible. That was it really, just straight into the work. We were pretty much mobbed with briefs at the beginning of the year. One full module and two half modules, not to mention the dissertation or contextual study to start planning for. Apart from the dissertation and the Information Application module, every other brief was working in teams. This had the obvious effect of a scramble for places, just as it had done in the second year but only this time it was more intense because of how it would impact on the degree. We weren't messing about any more. People were looking for allies and talent. I instantly noticed Twinkle avoiding me in the scrum. That stupid gas bill had come between us which really disappointed me not just because he was a mate but because he was talented. He would've been great to partner with as we were both looking to apply to The Royal College of Art. (We had both coincidentally turned up at the same RCA open day without telling each other.) Obviously, Nath was still sweet with Carl though. On this evidence Nath seemed to be sweet with everyone and had spread himself evenly amongst the group for these initial pair ups. Eric had added a little extra incentive on his Typolinguistics 3 module. He offered £50 to the winning team. I joined up with Nath, Rory, Alan and Jahan. We were very strong and also had flair. Alan was hugely analytical and extrememly funny, to the point of doing stand up comedy on-demand during the brainstorms. I was convinced he was wired up to a comic genius who was feeding him lines through an ear piece. Most of the Typolinguistics 3 work was done in our flat and because Alan's old man worked at Smithfield market he would bring around massive packs of bacon. The big running joke was to get Jahan, who was Hindu, to eat some of it. Eventually he succumbed and then Alan never let it lie – all just healthy team bonding. Nath and Rory were spending a lot of time hanging out together during the first few weeks and they'd decided to pair off on the other two half modules; Numeration and Representation & Mapping, both 7.5 credits each. I was in a bit of a panic because deep down I wanted to work with Nath and his choice of partner had surprised me to say the least. I felt rejected by him especially due to the whole stitch up on Twinkle. Shumana was living in the same house as Carl so Nath had to show solidarity. But he also lived with me. I didn't understand what was going on and everything seemed confusing because I no longer felt in control. At that time I couldn't put my finger on it, I just had to get on and find myself a partner. I always new Alan was good at what he did, not that good executionally but that didn't matter to me. I could do all the bells and whistles so I thought we would make a good team if I approached him to do those two half modules together. At first he was delighted and surprised that I'd asked him to be my partner. I found that dynamic pretty weird to deal with as the more I worked with Alan the more intimidated I got about how brilliant he was. I could hold my own with him but the irony was that he considered the executional stuff that I could do, as more important than the planning and idea generation which he was strongest at. He constantly surprised me to the point of scaring me with his talent and observations during those two projects. The other slightly unnerving thing was how much I was relying on his input and he was relying on mine during that first term up to

Christmas. We were together all the time. Not only due to the intensity of the work and the increased amount lecturing from the course Professor Raymond Beattie, I seemed to be finding a new level of understanding about Information Design and it's significance to my role in 1994 both as a creator and a consumer of life on this planet. For instance, Raymond was so impressed by the research gathered and presented for our response to the Representation & Mapping Module that he continually showed it to students long after we had graduated University.

Traffic Lights - One Interface, Two Users, Two Sets of Rules.

The traffic light is an interface for two sets of users, the driver and the pedestrian.
Both the driver and the pedestrian wish to reach their destination. This means they must navigate through the area controlled by the lights. (the Zebra crossing, for example.) Traffic lights work by alternatively holding back one user and allowing the other user to have access to the road. The interface works by the use of three colours which stand for three commands, stop, prepare for next command and go. The important element of the traffic light is that the driver and pedestrian both attach different meanings to the colours on the interface. For the driver, seeing the red command means they must stop and the pedestrian can now cross. In essence, for the pedestrian the red command means go. In the traffic light, we have an interface that can be used by two sets of users at the same time and still be effective, as long as the users obey their set of rules. If the two sets of rules are mixed or swapped between users groups it will result in stalemate or an accident. Our booklet represents and maps the chain of commands given by the traffic light, showing what each command means to the different user. It also illustrates the resulting action of these commands which

Victor J Kennedy

determines who has control of the road area or right of way
at any one moment.

The praise we received for the accompanying piece of work
on Traffic Lights did not go down well with Nath. The
reason I know this was due to the amount of digs he gave
Alan whilst me and Nath were chatting around the flat. He
even made a cartoon of Alan with a huge overbite and squint
eyes. He even stuck two wonky teeth coming out from his
lower lip. Admittedly, it was a clever representation and the
speed at which he could draw it made it even more funny.
The tactic was one I had seen him use before in the first year
and now I was aware he'd had a competitive upbringing
inside Public School I began to side with Alan. Me and Nath
were turning into a warring married couple. I didn't like his
relationship with Rory and he hated me doing well with
Alan. Having three people in one flat doesn't help either
because although Lewis was savvy, he was easily used as a
weapon. In that scenario there'll always be one person left
out. Not really the three amigos after all. Most of the time it
was peaceful and I always had Tanya to pop round and see
for a break.
It was during the pressure cooker moments before a deadline
that things seemed to get tricky. As an early adopter, Nath
bought a big black mobile phone when absolutely nobody
else owned one. It wasn't long before Lewis followed suit.
Then, at least they had one another to send text messages to.
Same thing happened with the computers. I finally managed
to buy my beloved Quadra 840AV for £2,873.70 from
Central Systems Ltd. in Milton Keynes. This included
£940.00 from my student loan. After enjoying his summer in
the south of France and with no money to spend, Nath
agreed to do the Information Application module as a front
for a commercial project managed by his close friend from
school, called Norm. His father's model making company
bought Nath a top spec PowerPC with a huge monitor to
produce an interactive map called Light-Up-London. A

week after that computer was delivered, Lewis spent the money he raised working on his parents' farm, on a low spec Apple Centris 610 with a built in monitor, which couldn't fit in his tiny bedroom so it sat next to my portable TV in the lounge. The flat became an instant office. Computer equipment everywhere and now the lounge felt like Lewis's studio and drug den.

Lewis had an extra curricular group of mates linked to his social stature in the Harrow bar with the drug supplier/friends that helped get him high. A lot of the time this included me and my financial contribution because he was always smoking in his bedroom and the smell made it's way into mine. Like a good pimp he never asked if I wanted any but he always gave me a toot if I asked him. This resulted in a half-ounce-a-week habit for the pair of us. Nath never bothered. Nath was not a drug man. He got his kicks from people and from games. For a start, he made sure we all got tickets for the new National Lottery game that was starting on BBC1. It was exciting times as all three of us sat there after Baywatch had finished with our tickets and fingers crossed. We talked at length about what we would do if we won that night. We believed we would win. They were both going to throw in the towel as far as university goes and disappear travelling. I couldn't understand that. There were things to do; a degree to finish. Not to mention gaining as high a mark as possible. Then who knows! But none of us did win and the Lottery has not had the same appeal or raw potential since that first night.

Nath also introduced a more sinister game to the flat. Walking to college one morning he noticed a replica Ruger P89 Silver Spring Airsoft Gun, complete with gas cannister and plastic pellets. It looked like a real gun. We went in the shop and on inspection it was of the kind of weight you would expect from a real firearm. Quentin Tarrantino had just released Pulp Fiction and Nath was all over the lifestyle when the Ruger sparkled at him from that Toy Shop window. It was retailed at £44.95 and he told the guy he would come back. All the way to college he tried to convince me to get one but after what happened with that bird and Mauli's air pistol I didn't fancy it at all. So as soon as we got to college he convinced Rory to do it. It didn't take much convincing because Rory had spent £2,000 plus on his Mountain Bike so £50 for a gun was peanuts. They brought them to the campus and shot people with the coloured plastic pellets, which really hurt. They would break your skin if shot from point blank range and would probably take your eye out if someone were careless enough with their aim. After a few days of terror in the computer labs. Lewis joined the 'crew'. They spent lots more money on new pellets and new gas propellant, whilst scaring the life out of me at home in the flat. This was classic Nathan Foreman power games. I had expressed a serious opposition to using the flat as a gladiatorial gun-fighting ring when I was trying to work but that just made them worse. If I closed my bedroom door they would open it and have a gun fight at each other from close range on my carpet. If I closed and locked the door then Nath would turn the electricity off to the whole flat and they would gun fight in the dark (extremely dangerous) while I would lay on my bed in silence, unable to do anything without electricity. I hated him for doing that. I felt trapped on every level. I couldn't even jump out of my bedroom window because it was too far to the ground. I found all that gangster gun thing really disturbing and it made me think about real guns inside the jackets of young men on the streets of Harrow. It was a really bad time for bringing guns into our lives. I didn't care if they were 'toys' or not!

Me and Tanya were having a tough time too because of what had happened with the taboo of her womb anomaly earlier in the year and our ectopic pregnancy, not to mention the workload and stresses of our final year had brought a persistant thrush issue into our sex lives. We had tried our best using Canesten to clear it up but we kept passing it between us, so we made an appointment the GUM clinic again at Northwick Park hospital to get rid of it once and for all. They told us we had to refrain from sex for quite a while. Practically until Christmas. When we walked home I told her it meant we could spend more time working and therefore get better degrees. We would then find great jobs and get a better flat together once we graduated. I was trying to make her feel better by finding a positive out of all this but she was not impressed. She said she would need a holiday after all this. Somewhere hot.

I got home to find Gideon Barnes sat in my lounge having a chit chat with Lewis. Nath was out so I stook my head round the door of the lounge, spotted him and then put my bags in my bedroom and got changed. I didn't know what the fuck Gideon was doing in my flat. I didn't like the bloke whatsoever and he couldn't have been drug dealing for Lewis because he was your quintessential working class hero. A true northerner. He was twice the northerner I could ever be. He wore megadeath teeshirts under the nastiest skin tight denim with hob nail boots. He had long black greasy hair and he drank bitter. Nothing else. Just bitter. He was a tall bloke and had an intimidating presence. He had given me a few stern stares in the bar before now but I had never done anything wrong to him. In fact I stayed away for two reasons: 1) He was the complete opposite of me. 2) He was a walking cliche and he gave a misrepresentation of northern people to a London campus. There was only me, him and my tutor Noel from north of the Watford Gap so we had a job on our hands to offset Gideon's PR machine, which sometimes involved punching people and being 'hard' in general. He would offset that by sitting in the refectory openly reading Shakespeare like he was broadcasting the fact. But that was his trick, he was on CMP (Contemporary Media Practice) so he was going to move into telly. Panto if he was crap. I put on my AIR JESUS teeshirt to grate on his ACDC one and then I went into the lounge walked past him into the kitchen to make a cup of tea. Lewis piped up, "Viciee. You've met Gideon before?"

"Aye. How's it going?" in my best northern accent.

Victor J Kennedy

"Not bad marra, and yer sel?" in his best northern accent.
"Alright yeah, anyone want a brew?"
"We just had one Viciee. I've been keeping Gideon warm while you got home."
"Oh yeah?"
"It's not me he's come to see. He wants to ask you if he can borrow something." Lewis winked at Gideon.
"Oh yeah. What's that?"
"Well it's a funny one really. I'll get straight to the point. Can I use your girlfriend in my film for my major project?"
I was on the backfoot after that one, "Sorry? Use Tanya in a film?"
"Yeah, I've written the story and it's been approved by my tutor and now I'm casting it. One of the characters will be of a similar type to her. I'm shooting it in December and possibly a bit in January if I don't get it all in the can before Christmas."
"Is it a major part?"
"It's the female lead."
"What makes you think she can act?"
"I've got no idea mate but if she can't do it then I'll have to find someone else who fits a similar description."
"And what has Tanya said?"
"I haven't asked her yet."
Lewis interrupted, "He thought he better ask the boss first. Didn't you Gideon?"
"Look Lewis, I've got a chance to get a first if I get this project right. If she is no good in front of the camera then I'll be finding another lead."
"And are you the male lead?" I quickly asked.
"I'm the director."
"But you're not gonna be snogging my bird on screen, are you?"
"There's no snogging in the story. It's a thriller."
"And how long will you need Tanya for?"
"On and off during the next six weeks or so. I go into post production after Christmas so that'll be it."

"What does on and off mean exactly?"

"It means I brief her on each shoot and give her some lines. We might catch up a couple of days later to see how she's getting on before we shoot each segment."

"So, about three times a week."

"Yeah, not more than that."

"Is this gonna get in the way of her fashion stuff."

"No. Not at all. Most of the meetings will be at college in the refectory at break time or during lunch. Obviously the film is set on campus so she won't be far away."

Lewis interrupted again, "So, can Gideon borrow your bird then?"

"Yes, Gideon can borrow my bird but he'd better go round and ask her now because I don't want to look like I'm leasing her out or anything."

"Cheers mate, much appreciated." Gideon tipped his imaginery flat cap and left the flat. I turned to Lewis.

"Do you know him?"

"Oh Viciee, stop worrying. He's harmless mate. He stinks of patehouli oil anyway and I bet he hasn't washed his cock since sixth form. Tanya will probably say no anyway. To doing the acting, I mean."

"She won't. Tanya will help anyone out. She's too helpful! Sometimes to her own detriment."

"Fancy a spliff?"

"Go on then, roll one up while I make another coffee."

I was drinking quite a lot of coffee and due to the amount of different blends and types we bought each week it was possible to vary the intensity of boost. I preferred Nescafe Gold Blend with one sugar and a sprinkle of milk. As the term progressed and the deadlines appeared we were all staying up later and later through the night. This doubled our consumption of coffee so to supplement and for emergencies I went out and bought a packet of ProPlus. I'd heard from Melanie, my old housemate from Carlisle that some 'phet and six ProPlus were known in Bournemouth as a 'poor man's E' which had stuck in my mind for twelve months.

Victor J Kennedy

When I returned with a packet to the flat, the three of us took one each and explained the effects as they happened. We all agreed they were great for emergencies but to go easy with them alongside the coffee. There was a warning on the box. I didn't read it all.

As well as working with me, Alan was also up against me on the Information Application module. The brief was set by the RSA student competition for 1994. It was open to all university student's countrywide to supplement the research already being done by British Telecom. They were testing a video-on-demand system on the townsfolk of Ipswich during that year. It was a customer facing, on-screen application that according to the brief should be an embodiment of the three Es: a) entertaining b) engaging and be c) easy to use. The brief stated the user had to 'stumble' upon new, undiscovered movies and sell lesser known titles. It should be constantly available, have a vast catalogue of film and television. The main aim of this interactive film companion was to draw users into the exploration of the wide choice of catalogue. I had to show evidence of a different approach to the problem and put the ideas down on paper to convince the RSA jury it would work 'In an ideal world'. I produced the screens in the latest version of Photoshop which had just been released and installed on the computers in room 309 of the teaching block. Photoshop 3.0 had layers. They were amazing when I actually found out how they worked. You could make them transparent and place objects in the middle of the screen over the top of another layer and then move it around! It was like having another dimension. I mocked up the interface in the drawing program Freehand, then I imported the vector shapes into Photoshop and added effects using the new filters available. I lit the shapes and then added drop shadows to create depth. The blobs were done using Infini-D which was 3D modelling software. I didn't know how to export them into Photoshop so I took screen shots of each blob after rendering then and then cut each one out, which took me ages. The results were amazing. It was a breakthrough piece of visual work but it's strength was in the idea.

Blob TV Video-on-Demand interface.
Deselection is the key idea here. Thinking along the same lines as walking through a physical video shop. If you know there is a genre of "Comedy" then you walk towards that shelf to find something funny. Everything else has been ignored and you have narrowed your choice to that single shelf. But what if the film you want is not on that shelf? If "Comedy" is part of the GENRE paradigm then what other paradigms do people rely on to choose a film?

Blob TV is a chooser driven by seven paradigms:
1) ALPHABETICAL BLOB - meaning "a to z"
2) ERA BLOB - meaning time set or made "1974" or "1934 to 1962"
3) HUMAN BLOB - meaning actor/actress/director etc
4) TITLE BLOB - meaning "Batman"
5) GENRE BLOB - meaning "science fiction"
6) ARTICLE BLOB - meaning subject or thing "motor bikes"
7) EXPANSE BLOB - meaning place set or made "america" or "human body"

If you choose the Genre Blob of Westerns then you instantly lose all the other Genres. Perhaps, add another Actor Blob of 'John Wayne', mix the two Blobs together in front of your eyes and you get closer towards what you want as well as what you need. Even if you're not sure what it is that you are looking for, you will stumble across something within your personal classification or mood. All dressed up in a 'Forbidden Planet' theme, get out there and search the movie universe using the Blob TV cockpit.

To me it sounded really simple and straightforward but to get to that point I had to burn the midnight oil and go on the

Victor J Kennedy

research journey of a lifetime. Within the first ten weeks of my final year I had tripled my awareness of interactive video design, the interactive learning revolution, satellite technology, hyperdocuments, flow visualisation, 3D interactive computer graphics and most important of all, I had discovered the true importance of the internet. It was my breakthrough. My realisation. I felt empowered. I decided not only to do my dissertation about the future impact and social effects of the internet but I was also going to make a stand alone interactive contextual study piece using the authoring software called Director. I wanted to show my research in a more entertaining way. A way that a 10,000 word essay cannot achieve. I didn't care or think about the task I had set myself over the following twelve weeks because I was absolutely convinced I would achieve it now I had my own computer. I was extremely focused at this point and spent most of my time in my bedroom. I didn't need to go to college unless I needed the research facilities in the library. I felt liberated and extremely streamlined and accelerated. Nothing was going to slow me down, especially not sleep. So I started using ProPlus without telling Lewis and Nath. I read white papers, technology magazines, which led me to books like Neuromancer by William Gibson. I read while they slept. I became captivated by conspiracy theories I found during my discovery of the birth of the web, a US military facility called ARPANET and the fact it was created in the same year Neil Armstrong supposedly set foot on the moon. In 1994 the internet was full of geeks and geeks possess inspired imaginations which are usually fuelled by science fiction. I was five years old when I was inspired by Star Wars. I was brought up on Commodore 64 computers. I actually started to feel like I was part of a thick plot in a best selling thriller. I just wasn't sure what my role was going to be. I just felt that in November 1994 I was in the right place at the right time. My thoughts were fleeting and the ideas were flowing. It was a wonderful time to be alive, even though I was completely broke and in trouble with the bank, not to mention my mum.

Cheque enclosed for £10
I couldn't sleep last night for worrying about you.
I have dipped into my balcony fund for the £200 and I know you'll pay me back as soon as your grant cheque comes through, which I hope doesn't take too long!
I will ring as usual on Sunday.
I love you
I care about you
You are very precious to me, so look after yourself.
All my love,
Mum xxx

Inspite of my money situation I needed a couple of things to make my life complete. I went out and bought the new Stone Roses album The Second Coming after Ruth McGregor had given me a thorough review. Five stars. When I got it home I was blown away. It was everything I expected and more. It was hardly off the CD player in the run up to Christmas. I also found out the hard way that I had bought a computer with too little RAM inside it. I was constantly having to 'Purge Memory' whilst using the Director software and the amount of layers I'd created in my Photoshop files meant either flattening the layers or making one change at a time, saving and then restarting the software. I regularly couldn't copy and paste because 'the scratch disc is full' or there was 'insufficient RAM to complete task'. My new baby which had cost so much sweat and toil over the summer was sick and I needed to make it better. I had to perform an operation and install another 16 megabytes of RAM into it's hardware. I found an article in a magazine that showed you how to install it and I travelled down to Techworks in Shoreditch to buy two third party 8mb 72 Pin 60ns Simms. Bit of a mouthful. They were sealed in their own static bags and the bloke behind the counter advised me NOT to touch anything metal, only touch the green plastic. The magazine had warnings about static and it had diagrams of people wearing a plastic wristbands to earth themselves. Because the RAM was so expensive at £44.95 each, I couldn't afford a plastic wristband and I went home shitting myself that I would break my precious computer. The most expensive thing I had ever bought in my life. When I got back to the flat Jahan was round our flat working on the signage project with Nath and Rory. I asked if anyone could help me fit the RAM and the only response I got was from Jahan. I took him to my room and instantly made him strip to his underpants, which put more than a smile on his face until I explained we could not have any static while we did it. I stripped too after I'd carefully taken the Quadra apart. As it turned out, I wasn't quite sure of a certain component opening fully so Jah held the box as wide apart as possible while I contorted myself and put the Simms into their resting place. It was so stressful even though we giggled about it. I had sweat dripping from my forehead which made me stress even more, thinking it would land inside the computer and fuck everything up. We must have looked like a couple of semi-naked bomb disposal experts but we did it! We put the case back on the tower and started it up. It seemed to take too long and I started to shit myself again, expecting smoke to come out or worse, an explosion? But no, it was fine. Everything worked and I quickly checked the system preferences 'About This Mac' and it told me there was indeed 32mb of RAM installed. I turned and hugged Jah. We both laughed and I sighed a huge sigh of relief.

Now I'd got the computer working properly, I decided to capture some video on it for my interactive contextual study piece called Internet Or Not. I'd identified three protagonists: A Technologist, A Psychologist and A Sociologist to make credible comments based on my questions on the social issues and social effects of the coming information revolution driven by the internet. I compared what was about to happen with the communications revolution in the 15th

Mad in England - A memoir

century when Johannes Gutenberg invented the printing
press. At first, I was going to have four protagonists using
The Sunday Express Astrologer Joseph Campbell who wrote
that Jupiter Effect article which got to me during the summer
but I spoke to his secretary and she said he didn't fancy
contributing to such a project. It was a shame because the
four opinions would have made better TV. I managed to get
Isaac Bishop to be my Technologist, Esther Potocki, lecturer
and owner of London's first Cyber Cafe 'Cyberia', to be my
Psychologist and Natalie Wade lecturer of Sociology at
Sheffield University to meet me in central London, be
interviewed and filmed for my contextual study. It was
amazing because all these people agreed to meet me over
email before they knew who I was. All of them apart from
Isaac, that is. He actually put me in touch with Esther
Potocki, an entrepreneur and pioneer of the commercial
aspects of the internet. I borrowed a camcorder and tripod
from IT for fortyeight hours and shot them all straight onto
VHS in quick succession. I bought different coloured fabric
for each person's background. Isaac was yellow, Esther was
red and Natalie was green. Everyone was cooperative but
Esther lost patience with my 'negative' questioning and I
took a beating for dissing the future of the internet.
According to Esther, the internet would be nothing other
than great. Fabulous in fact, darling! I didn't really like her
attitude because if she was a lecturer she should have known
I had to create and structure an argument. That was why I
called it Internet Or Not? From all my theoretical research I
discovered around twenty key questions for part 1) Social
Issues and a further twenty questions for part 2) Social
Effects. They say in life it is not the right answers you
should try to find, it is the right questions. During my time
comparing concepts and theories from various sources, past
or present, everything I discovered had a profound effect on
me. The amazing part of my contextual study was going to
be 'dialling up' each protagonist's response or answer to each
question on-demand. As the videos played back their

responses I was demonstrating the message as the message was being delivered. The presentation itself started with a passive explanation of the birth of the internet and a potted history to the present day. It then quickly covered how the internet works and gave a tour of the basic protocols, what email was, File Transfer Protocol and the world wide web. After that came the introduction of our three protagonists and the twenty questions on Social Issues and Effects, then the presentation became interactive. Pick a question and the three video opinions would play back the answer to that question so you can see the responses side by side. There was also an abstract and bibliography to take a look at if you wished. You could even go back and watch the passive presentation again.

During my research for this project as well as the Blob TV stuff for that Information Application module, I started to think about how human beings find and store things on screens. The seven paradigms I'd put together for the Blob TV interface wouldn't leave my brain and even as I walked down the street instead of humming a song I was thinking about the problem. The thing is, I didn't know what the problem was apart from the fact that in the future people will need to organise themselves and their lives inside a screen or through a window in another place. I found the following piece of research in the pink newspaper Mute Digital Art Critique. Mute was a periodical written by Cyberpunks and artists from London which I'd picked up on my travels around Old Street. It was dripping with forward thinking. It made me brainstorm about being published and what that actually meant. My mind was also cast back to the summer and my work for Creative Review on that futuristic interface for a CD-Rom version of the magazine. I knew that Glenn Oliver had now commisioned a real CD-Rom to be produced and stuck it on the front of every subscriber's issue. The article spoke about Cybersex. Sex across a network:

Mad in England - A memoir

Today when people get very ill and need very special treatment they need to be rushed to the nearest specialist, surgeon or doctor. Sometimes they have to raise money to fly themselves to another country where the specialist lives and practices. If before they can raise the money, things become an emergency and it is then impossible to get a patient to a specialist in time, then today in 1995, the patient may die.

Internet evangelists are predicting many brilliant things to come in the future and one of these will be Telepresence. Telepresence is a form of virtual reality but in this case only for one of the users. This form of Telepresence is called virtual medicine and has two users - a patient in Britain and a surgeon in America. The surgeon is the only user who sees a virtual reality through the head set and gloves that he or she would be wearing.

Now, the patient in Britain is lying on a bed in a hospital's surgery with various nurses and doctors around the bed keeping an eye on the robotic arms above the patient that will perform the operation. These robotic arms are connected to a computer terminal that is logged on, through the internet to the American surgeon's computer terminal. The surgeon's computer terminal is connected to the virtual reality headset and gloves. The operation can now begin. The surgeon in America feels like he or she is actually in the same surgery as the patient and the robotic arms take the place of the surgeon in Britain. If this happens in the future then it would revolutionise medicine and the idea of the 'local' hospital. It could improve mankind for the better.

I noticed the word Teleprescence. Then I chased the meaning through the dictionaries of the University library. I couldn't find it. It didn't exist in a dictionary. It made me feel paranoid that I couldn't find it. Like someone was having a joke at my expense, while I wasted all this energy chasing answers. I thought it might be made up by the bloke who wrote the article but then why did that matter? Best not get paranoid. Most product names are made up or are a fusion between two existing words to make a one which that helps explain what that product does or is. After a long period of getting quite anxious about such a stupid thing, I breathed a sigh of relief when I found an entry in an encyclopedia:

Telepresence is the experience of being fully present at a live real world location remote from one's own physical location. Someone experiencing transparent telepresence would therefore be able to behave, and receive stimuli, as though at the remote site.

I added two questions to my contextual study after reading that.
1) Have we created this 'safe environment' because the real world is a horrible place?
2) Can you see any effects of Cybersex/Cyberrape over the internet? Could it happen?
I knew that as pioneers of this new place, as town planners, we had responsibilities to make it accesible for everyone and that meant it had to be easy to use. People had to have as much, if not more control over this as they have over their own lives. A sense of order. A sense of control. Going to new places represent new dangers as much as new oportunities. That is why we explore. That is where the science fiction comes from in every geek. That night, as I walked home from college I saw a huge poster on Station Road for an upcoming movie called Stargate, an ancient human transmitter discovered in the Egyptian desert. It was a portal to travel light years from earth to another planet. The poster had a massive circle with hieroglyphics around it's perimeter. In the centre was a pyramid with two silhouetted explorers walking through the Stargate. The observation, even if only of the movie poster caused neural sparks in my head based on the ancient Egyptian's system using pictorial symbols to represent meaning or sounds. Not

to mention, a circle or bounding 'gateway' to another dimension or world.

The screenwriter Dean Devlin's observation of current events in 1993 when he wrote the screenplay could have lead to the key theme of the story – the human's journey to find 'truth' this side of the grave using science or religion. Ancient Egyptian semiology is always there for the taking, especially concerning a commercial audience. Most of us have little or no understanding of hieroglyphics but we know they can be decoded if we took any time to bother studying. So the commercial screenplay adds the aura of myth and plays on our lack of real knowledge. I was hooked, line and sinker. But not of the movie. It was the significance of that poster as a 'sign' sent to me by someone or something from somewhere else to help me solve this 'problem' of the internet. It felt magical and I thought to myself, I mustn't tell anyone from college that I'm tuning into this stuff or they will steal my advantage and my edge. This was my little secret I was having with myself. Sort of like an imaginary friend that a small child might have but not tell anyone about.

Another reason for all the secrecy was due to the final module of that year Professional Practice 3. It was all about being professional and how copyright can protect you as well as destroy you. That was only if you do not protect your work and the intellectual property of what you create. We were lectured in quite a military style by a Barrister friend of Elena's called Herman Lindenbaum. It was a half module but his booming authoritative voice made it feel like a full module. He frightened the life out of all of us. Especially me, with his warnings about the future and the past, especially if you were 'borrowing' other people's work that IS protected by copyright. He reassured that as students we were protected and could rip off anyone's stuff willy nilly but as soon as we leave the academic environment we had to be super careful not to get screwed by a highly paid lawyer like Herman Lindenbaum because he would take you to the

Victor J Kennedy

cleaners. I have to say that he put the fear of god in me. He also affected my behaviour because I started writing 'Copyright VJK 1994' on every single piece of work or scribble that I produced, just in case someone might be thinking of stealing it. I even added a section to my dissertation at the beginning and was so paranoid that I filmed myself reading it out and added it to the contextual study at the beginning.

Disclaimer (c)VJK 1994
Today's date is: 23rd November 1994
I, Victor Kennedy of 22 years of age, understand that my rights as a student protect me under the copyright act of 1988. So that, as a full-time member of an educational institution I am allowed to use copyright protected material in my work that is marked towards gaining my degree in Graphic Information Design.

I got worried even my flat mates would steal my ideas so I began hiding my work behind the cistern in my bedroom so especially Nath didn't walk into my bedroom when I wasn't around and gain any advantage or pass my work off as his. I knew what he was like. He'd passed off those colour holiday snaps as black & white for that project in the first year. He was clever enough to be getting paid for that Light-Up-London work while passing it off as a study for his degree at the same time. Raymond had no idea what Nath was up to and I felt it was wrong. I was really resenting Nath for his behaviour towards me when Rory was in the flat. He would ignore me and treat me like I was beneath him, often locking Rory in his bedroom with him and the computer, leaving silly messages on the door like 'do not disturb.' He got an obsession with Star Wars figures and began buying the original seventies Palitoy versions, second hand from a guy with a stall in a tube station near One-to-Onehundred, the model makers he was doing Light-Up-London for. I remembered watching him at my parents' home at the end of the first year while he enjoyed looking through my collection of Star Wars figures, kept in a box since 1977 along with my Lego which I showed to him, Cathy and Tanya as my parents told them about my childhood.

In the flat, Nath left a message on the door saying "DARTH SAYS FUCK OFF" and stuck the Darth Vader figure to the door using blue tac. During that evening Lewis drew another comment, "MASTER LUKE SAYS THAT'S A BIT RASH. WHO FINISHED YOU IN THE END - DARTH." Then later on, Rory came out for a piss and added, "RAYMOND TAUGHT YOU WELL, BUT NOW?" As I made my way to the kitchen for another coffee, I read all of this tomfoolery and got angry because I felt the last comment had negative undertones and was not funny anymore but slanderous and belligerent because of it's implication of people's education outside of that room containing those two people inside and whatever they were making. I wrote under Rory's comment, "GET THE MASSAGE." to cloud the issue and hint that something else untoward was happening in their room if the door had to be locked and they had to be left alone. This pathetic game continued late into the night as the next time I walked past Nath had added a little drawing of a Millennium Falcon, Darth Vader wearing underpants and Luke Skywalker on his knees, as his hand was chopped off. Speech bubbles leaving the Falcon said, "QUICK, SWITCH TO HYPERCUBE CHEWY." More speech bubbles from Vader announcing, "I AM YOUR TUTOR!" And Luke Skywalker shouting, "NOOOOO" The problem was in decoding it, on analysis I thought the Skywalker character was representing me and Vader was supposed to be Eric Glaser, the tutor I least got on with. The whole thing got to me big time. I felt like it had opened up a big wound in our relationship and this competitive thing was getting to all of us. There were wedges getting driven in between me and Nath left, right and centre but I blamed him for it all because he had hoodwinked me about the whole public schoolboy thing. Deep down I just found him to be untrustworthy. That night I went up and stayed at Tanya's after venting my spleen to her about all these goings on. She was a great listener, her advice to talk openly with him about it was simple but brilliant and that gave me comfort. I slept deeply and at length for the first time in quite a while.

The next day I spent at home on the computer but on return from Tanya's the flat was empty so I was alone with my thoughts which made it difficult to focus on my work. I couldn't really concentrate on one thing for very long without walking around the flat and staring at things and analysing why they had been left that way. I wondered which of those two were playing these little tricks on me and leaving me these cute messages. Neither of them locked their rooms so I had a nosey, just as I had imagined them to have done in my room. Then I would go back to my room and arrange things in 'traps' to catch them snooping when I wasn't around. This involved carefully displaying objects in memorable positions so if I returned and it's position had moved then I would know I was under surveillance by one of my two flat mates. It was like living in a cold war. No trust whatsoever. Or at least that was my perception. We were no longer mates, we were competitors and Nath wasn't playing by the rules, Lewis didn't realise there was a competition and if he did, he sure wasn't outwardly showing that behaviour. I could only come to the conclusion that Nath had hoodwinked Lewis the same way he was chameleon-like with me. I felt Lewis supported Nath more than he supported me and that made him offside. That also meant it was two against one. Nath just had to 'massage' his relationship with Lewis and I was a goner. My brain spent the day working out connections and scenarios to arm myself for when Nath got home and I would confront him about that "DARTH SAYS FUCK OFF" poster on his door from last night. He arrived just as I was watching Countdown on Channel 4. There was an instant atmosphere as he walked in the lounge. "Alright."
"Alright."

"Good day at college?"

"Where were you?"

"In here again, trying to work out what's gone wrong?"

"What's gone wrong with what?"

"With you and me?"

"I'm not with you Vic?"

"Ah, come on. Let's not play games. I'm trying to level with you here."

"I haven't noticed much wrong. You spend quite a lot of time on that computer so it's difficult to know if there is something wrong."

"What, with me?"

"I don't know Vic. You're the one levelling with me. You seem to know what this is all about."

"What's with the posters on your door?"

"They're a bit of fun. Remember that Vic? They are meant to lighten the load a little bit."

"They're designed to marginalise me."

"Marginalise?"

"Yeah. They're your propaganda and your cloak. That is the way you get into people's heads. That's how you control your court once you've got inside people's heads. Divide and conquer."

"Who are you to point the finger?"

"Exactly. You don't need me any more so nothing I say or do matters."

"Vic, you've misunderstood me. What I meant was, who are you to talk? Because you draw pictures of people at college all the time. Your layout pad is full of cartoons of Alan and you are supposed to be partnering him. What is that all about?"

"Who exactly invented that cartoon of Alan?"

"Ok ok. Fair enough but I didn't force you to keep drawing it did it? Take responsibility Vic."

"Fair enough. Take responsibility for that." I pointed at the Three Amigos drawing on the wall.

"What?"

"You drew yourself in the middle with your arms around me and Lewis."

"Which means what exactly?"

"That you're the centre of attention. The guy pulling the strings. The most popular."

"It's just a drawing Vic. If it bothers you that much then take it down."

"Why do you do all these drawings and leave these messages on the walls?"

"To pass the time? They're a bit of fun. They're meant to lift the mood a little bit, but obviously not for you."

"So I'm the odd one out then? This is my whole point."

"Vic, have you ever thought that all this might be your problem?"

"No."

"Does that mean that none of this is because of the way you treat people?"

"I don't understand?"

"Let me put you in the picture, excuse the pun. Vic, what you don't realise is that you compartmentalise your life."

"Which means?..."

"You put people in pigeonholes."

"Sorry?"

"You do it with everyone. You put Tanya in the 'girlfriend' pigeonhole. You put Dean and Diago in the 'free spirit' pigeonhole. You put Twinkle in the 'Royal College of Art' pigeon hole."

"Talk me through the 'Royal College of Art' pigeonhole again?"

"In general, you don't speak to people unless you want to be associated by what you think they can give. You hardly ever sit down and talk to me about anything other than Photoshop or Director lingo. I'm in the 'Apple Mac' pigeonhole and I'm just bored of it. Everyone is."

"Everyone?!"

"Look, let's just say that a few of us have been talking about it and we all feel the same way. It's quite funny really because I thought it was just because I lived with you but it's not. You do this to a lot of people Vic."

"Has Lewis said anything?"

"No. But he thought what you wrote on the door last night was a bit odd."

"Shit, I'm sorry."

"It's okay but don't say anything to him about it. It's best for all of us that we just move on from this. It is a very small flat for three people anyway."

"You're right. I shouldn't have said anything."

"Look at it this way, at least it's out in the open now and we can both do something about it. I'm gonna try and keep the drawings to a minimum but if I do a drawing you have to understand it is not about you, ok?"

"Agreed. Thanks Nath, please don't tell anyone else about this conversation."

"It's just between me and you."

"Nice one."

"Oh, and Vic can you try and make more of an effort with people at college?"

"Anyone in particular?"

"No one specifically, just speak to the rest of us in GID as a friend, not just as a student rep."

"Eh?"

"Just be friendlier to your classmates."

"Will do." I got out of the chair and went into my bedroom, closed and locked the door, then burst into tears on my bed. Those comments completely destroyed me. I didn't even realise I was like that. I just thought I was a normal friendly lad from up north who said hello to the security guards on the University reception at the front door and continued to talk to everyone in between. I never knew I pigeonholed people and that really frightened me. It made me feel like a monster who believed he was one thing but in actual fact he was something else. Dr Jekyll and Mr Hyde! Worse than Dr Jekyll! At least Dr Jekyll knew he was experimenting on himself. I didn't even think about the drugs or the fact that

Victor J Kennedy

Tanya and Nath both told me I'd been 'odd' since returning from Liverpool at Easter. I just lay there and cried until I felt better, then I took all my woes up to Tanya's to see if she could make sense of it all. She couldn't. Not only that but she lost patience with all my quivering and wimpering. She shouted at me to pull myself together and then became really dismissive of it. This led to another argument and eventually I left. I didn't want to go home and face Nath so I thought I would find solace with Dean. He would help me. He was a true friend. He told me the opposite of Nath's story, that a lot of the class did not like Nath and the way that he undermines people using humour. Dean said Alan hated Nath for creating that caricature and I agreed to stop using it whilst working with Alan. I felt terrible because I remember actually laughing in Alan's face when he took exception to it. Dean also suggested it was Shumana talking to me through Nath. That the words were all her words. That she was more manipulating than even Nath. It was all dark forces at work. The worst thing to come out of my chat with Dean was that he told me 'something really important' that could be major or it could be minor but he had to say something. He had taken his girlfriend Shelly, who lived with Tanya, to the cinema to see Interview With A Vampire a couple of nights ago. After the film had ended and they headed for the exit, on the way down the staircase Dean spotted Tanya leaving the same film but she was with Gideon Barnes! Not only that but they were arm in arm. Dean felt terrible for telling me but I reassured him that it was for study and research purposes. Although, inside I was even more battered now. And isolated. Apart from when I was with Dean, I was totally self-conscious from then on. I developed an obsession about how I was perceived by others. Psychiatry states that a poor or abusive upbringing can lead to insecurity in adult life. In the space of three hours I had experienced enough bad news to turn my weakened mind into a complex web of unassisted self-analysis. It was like a roller coaster had been constructed inside my skull and Nath had just pressed my 'go' button. Scream if you wanna go faster.

Tanya's mum had a great upbringing. She was the daughter of a Leeds teenager and in those days it was considered shameful to be with child outside of wedlock so Carolyn was put up for adoption. At the same time, down south in Essex, Edna and Cyril were longing for a child. The authorities matched up the family and Carolyn grew up as an Essex girl, rather than a Yorkshire girl. Cyril and Edna gave the young Carolyn full visibility but it wasn't until years later that Carolyn's daughter, Tanya, met a Yorkshireman called Victor. When their relationship was over two years old Carolyn decided to talk to her daughter about finding her real mother back in Leeds. Tanya being Tanya decided she wanted to help her mum trace her blood grandmother so I was then involved in a search through the Salvation Army family tracing service. All of this seemed to be at the absolute wrong time for me but I didn't want to say no because of everything Carolyn had done for me during the summer. She was a wonderful caring woman and I thought her face would light up if we found her real family. After spending much of the early part of December doing that instead of my work I got anxious and tried to accelerate the process to get rid of it and concentrate on my studies but it just led to further arguments with Tanya.

The work I was trying to finish was for the campus signage project and the other tricky little half module Numeration with my new confidant, partner and close friend Alan. We came up with an interactive multimedia presentation called Your Number's Up. We created a scenario of a bus driver and his awaiting passenger. The bus journey and the time it took were represented as numbers with no meaning attached to them. We chose seven number types: Departure, Distance, Speed, Arrival, Destination, Capacity and Money. We said that by understanding these representations of numbers (values, amounts and labels) will determine and affect a person's ability to reach a goal. The user was prompted to choose a path, either the bus driver or the pedestrian. Once the bus driver's pathway was chosen, the numbers were displayed. After the user chooses a number, a segment of his story concerning that number, was displayed. For instance, the bus driver might get 'two bloomin' punctures'. That information would display when the meaning and importance of that number was revealed. We did it as a cartoon, funnily enough. It looked like something you could use in a school maths lesson. We got 73% for that one. The campus signage project was also a success. So successful we won the £50 prize as Eric's favourite solution. I couldn't believe Eric gave me his best mark so far with a whopping 78%. It did surprise me because I thought Eric disliked me, just as I felt everyone else did at that time. Jase and Scott from the other side of the room were really peeved about not winning and the fuss they caused split the classroom just before we broke for Christmas. Eric was even shouting his mouth off and being an idiot. He shouldn't have offered £50 and then the competition would not have been as fierce. He took me to one side after the melee had calmed down and said, "Victor, your group's answer to this problem has been outstanding and the signage contractors for the development firm would like you to join them in a top level meeting after Christmas to decide a wayfinding solution for this campus once the redevelopment is complete in 1996. Well done. Shall I tell them you'll attend? You are the Student Representative after all."

"Sure. I'll do it."

"It would be a great mark to leave on the University, in more ways than one."

We took the money and had a night out together as a team. All the animosity disappeared, mainly because Rory knew about a Sunday Sport glamour girl show at a bar in Raynors Lane. We spent the £50 on entrance and drinks. The strippers were free but they made money from a raffle (we got ticket 69) and £5 to have your photo taken on a crappy polaroid with the topless ladies. It was utterly cheap and

Mad in England - A memoir

Tanya wasn't happy when I told her. Lewis tried his best to get in the strippers' knickers but failed miserably. He had been on form recently with a tall leggy blonde girl who I felt was a stalker from the Ceramics course. She'd been hassling me for weeks about his availability, as if I'd know, but that didn't matter to her. She had a strategy to hassle the flat mate instead of the target. She was like an assassin. One Friday night after the bar finished, she invited herself back to a GID party at Ruth and Twinkle's house just because she knew Lewis was there. She told me on the way there that she was going to "fuck him whether he liked it or not but he was gonna like it". At the party I proceeded to tell everyone this quote in the front room whilst sitting at their dining table. Unfortunately, she was standing behind the door and overheard everything I said. She burst in and yelled at me shouting, "thank you very much for that Victor." I didn't even realise she knew my name. I couldn't forget hers; Lyndsay. I did feel terrible for what happened at that party but in the end she got her man because she would regularly eat my Bran Flakes in the morning after a good night before. I knew she was a screamer because our flat had thin walls and Lewis's bedroom door was opposite mine. All that shagging led to one thing. I was looking in the fridge for something to eat on a Thursday, late in the week anyway, because there was nothing left apart from some natural Bio Yoghurt. I didn't recognise it from our weekly shop so I picked it up and opened the plastic top. I peered in. It was three quarters full but with an indentation in the centre so I put it back and got a biscuit. Lewis came home and I asked him, "Is that your Bio Yoghurt in the fridge?"
"Yeah man, I had to sort a little problem out."
"You what?"
"I've got thrush and my mum told me to use Bio Yoghurt to get rid of it."
"Is that indentation from your cock then?"
"Yes mate, I'm sorry. I should've said but I was a bit embarrassed."

Victor J Kennedy

"Fucking hell mate! I nearly ate some of that."
"But you would be ok, the culture eats the thrush."
"Lewis, it's just not nice."
"Well, at least you know. Never touch the BIO baby."
"Very funny. Does that mean something floral will grow on my tongue if I do?"
"Get back to work."

I didn't really have any work to do after I'd sealed my Blob TV entry to the RSA that afternoon. All I had left to do was pack my bags and get ready to go home for Christmas. This year however, was going to be a working Christmas due to the fact I wanted to write a dissertation. The contextual study was almost finished. I'd practically done enough research already. All I had to do was organise it into a stream of text and type all 10,000 words in January after we got back from Christmas. Tanya came back with me to Millhead this time and we had a mixed holiday. The snow fell over Shap and I took her up to see it with Ray and his dog. We had a really good laugh and the winter environment with the blue sky was perfect for retaining bright loving memories. The rest of the holidays were tough for her because of my drive to complete my research. She spent a lot of time downstairs with my family while I sat in the centre of my bedroom, surrounded by paper and putting little red marks or numbers next to each piece of handwriting. I was lost in my own categorisation system and I wanted to find my way out of it. Christmas day was wierd due to the fact Tanya bought me a pair of pink furry handcuffs which I opened in front of my mum and dad. Another present, this time from Carolyn, was a framed photograph of me and Tanya at The Bald Hind pub in September, the one Carolyn took of us on her twentyfifth wedding anniversary. It seemed to bear a certain significance to me. I felt added pressure to marry her and become a solid part of her family. Maybe that wasn't Carolyn's motivation. The photo obviously had a different significance to Carolyn otherwise it wouldn't end up as a gift at Christmas time.

Mad in England - A memoir

Jesus Christ was born almost 2000 years ago. Because of the Numeration project, I fully understand the implications of that round figure. I know those numbers have meaning and huge significance to the human race who understood them. Nice and neatly brought together with four digits, three zeros and the number two in front, like a Swan's profile carrying three eggs and heading west. Maybe the internet's development towards the close of this century is going to save us? Maybe messages were left in the past for people in the future to decode. Maybe I am on to something?

My mind had wandered off there for a second and my dad was calling me downstairs to go for a Christmas day pint. It's a family tradition to go for a drink so I grabbed my new Christmas sweater and my wallet to go and join him. The studying was taken away and my mind was rested using alcohol.

New Year's Eve was really bad. We actually spent it in the village at Millhead. There were no parties on at people's houses or farms. Nothing exciting or out of the ordinary was going on so me and Tanya joined my parents in the Institute, a sort of working mens' club come British Legion. They had a couple of entertainers on there, a man and wife I think, who sang songs from a bygone era and maybe something by Wham or Duran Duran if we were lucky. Because I was feeling agitated by what a crap New Year I was showing Tanya, I couldn't sit still. I was experiencing a really short attention span. I had her moving from pub to pub and we were having more and more serious conversations until it had got to that drunken time of the evening and an argument ensued about me and my work. I couldn't understand her ungratefulness because all I wanted was to show her a good time and all she was doing was having a go at me. Once back at the Institute, right in front of my parents we kicked off again and I just stood up and walked out. I went home in a fit of emotion and went to bed in tears. I was deeply upset.

Victor J Kennedy

More upset than I'd actually been about anything for quite
some time.

We talked about what had happened rationally on the train
back down to London and I decided I needed some self-
analysis to find out where in my life I started to be such a
workaholic. What is it that makes me like this? Why do I put
work before all my other relationships and end up putting
people in pigeonholes? We got back to the flat and before
she had time to put the kettle on I sat her down with a pad
which had every year of my life on it so far, 1972, 1973,
1974 etc. to 1995. I lay on my bed as if I was the patient and
she was the psychiatrist. Then I asked her to read out
random years to which I would answer the first thing that
came into my head about that year. It was bound to bring
some interesting results because those thoughts, the first
ones to arrive in my head, would be the most important thing
I can remember of that year. Here are the results:

Victor Kennedy's "Life" 1972 to 1994. A profile of 22 years
of learning and experiencing
1972 Born St. Lukes Hospital, Bradford, West Yorkshire
1973 Don't remember?
1974 Matthew Kerr's mum
1975 Don't remember?
1976 Hot summer
1977 Queen's Jubilee
1978 Lord Mayor's Parade
1979 Auntie Caron
1980 A new decade
1981 Begin school, FA Cup Final. West Ham
1982 Spanish World Cup football
1983 Mrs Atkins, French teacher - first crush
1984 Bad year – Got the pump Mr Rochester
1985 Change schools – Buttershaw Upper Comprehensive
school
1986 Mexico World Cup, Jodi Brown
1987 Discovered women

Mad in England - A memoir

1988 Left school, bad results, left Bradford, Big change!
1989 Butterfly. Left emotional baggage behind in Bradford
1990 Italia '90 World Cup. Westmorland U18 team. Finally accepted
1991 Acknowledged
1992 Indifferent year, left Reggie, left Faye
1993 Hit London. Tanya
1994 Bad year. England don't qualify for World Cup in USA

Tanya didn't say a word. She just sat there and did what I asked her to do. She had no opinion but looking at the results I knew it was all about 1988 to 1990. The two years following my move away from Bradford. Moving out of the shadow of my best mate Dale Ryeland and finally being recognised as a good footballer, I qualified to play county level at 17 years old. 1990 was the year when a P.A. to one of the Director's at Duke Brothers, had told me I had enough talent to go to university. That was the spark. Her name was Cathelyn. Nobody in my life had said I was any good at anything until then. I always had the belief growing up but I could only watch Dale Ryeland from the substitute's bench or my sister enjoying her piano lessons while I went out and pretended I was Luke Skywalker escaping the trash compactor in the local mill's cardboard filled skips. I had a massive score to settle and that was the rocket up my arse. That's what propelled me. The desire to prove to people I was not a loser. The only question now, after take off, was which planet would my efforts guide me to?
As I beavered around the campus I noticed nothing and no one other than that which mattered towards achieving my deadlines, which were less than one month away at the semester break. All universities understand that this time of year for third year students is especially stressful and many posters regarding help and information for them are placed on the walls of the campus around these vulnerable periods. At Westminster are in bright red or yellow so as to attract attention to issues such as stress, rest and relaxation or tips

to help you sleep – 10 point plans, that type of thing. I never saw one of them. No one seemed to see me either. Every other student is looking inward at that time or, is worried about the looming deadlines and how this important time may affect the rest of their lives. They are not necessarily looking out for anyone else. It's all about numero uno.
The deadline for submitting your portfolio and application to the Royal College of Art was here and I wasn't quite ready. My portfolio needed adjustments but my forms were complete.

I have chosen Computer Related Design to enable me to develop my current interest in Graphical User Interfaces and how information can be displayed on screen. I am concerned with exploring the potential uses of technology, mainly concentrating on screen design. I want to develop my knowledge of current authoring software and new media applications to help me further understand the totally different set of rules and values that screen design has. At the moment I am unsure of my role within the design community and feel I need more time to experiment, explore and find myself within a team. I know from various visits to Computer Related Design that group work is an integral part of the course and I believe it is crucial to the development of multi-disciplinary skills.

At college a van had been organised that would drive every student's portfolio to the RCA's front door at Kensington Gore irrespective of which discipline. I was in the CRD pile. I was fairly agitated that day because in the morning as I awoke, after spending half the night selecting my best pieces and mounting them neatly on A3, Nath walked into my room and asked, "Have you got one of those forms for the Royal College going spare?"
"Yeah, why?"
"I think I might give it a go."
"Give it a go? You're a bit late aren't you?"

Mad in England - A memoir

"I'll be ok. I had a little root around last night and I'm in pretty good shape. So have you got one then?"
"Here." I handed him a spare application pack I was keeping in case I made any mistakes on any of my first one. He returned to his bedroom to fill it in. After ten minutes I packed up my folio and my bag, ran down the stairs to set off to college when I heard him shout, "Vic! WHAT'S THE NAME OF THE COURSE AGAIN?"
"COMPUTER RELATED DESIGN!" I slammed the door furious. First of all, he had expressed no interest whatsoever over the past twelve months during the time me and Twinkle went to those open days. Or even visiting the shows for the last two years to see the kind of work they do there. It was my future not his. I had been working harder than him and preparing more than he had without a doubt. My god, he didn't even know the name of the course he was applying for on the day of the deadline. This behaviour and attitude was everything I hated about him and it was crawling all over me on that ten minute walk to college. By the time I got there I just thought he was taking the piss and winding me up. But he wasn't. He got there and sat at the back of the class next to Shumana, his keeper of the leash. His seat was opposite me, next to Lewis. He couldn't sit there because I was struggling with all the labels. RCA applicants must put a description of the project and their name and address on every piece of work. The labels are official with a logo on and the actual number code of the applicant. I screamed when I realised they were missing and about four people, who were not applying, jumped up and started to help me. I was amazed and humbled by it but Nath got angry. I could hear him at the back of the class. He wanted me to hear him. He spoke loud enough to Shumana about what a tosser he thought I was and how much he hated me. He then proceeded to slag off the people helping me for being slaves. "Don't they see what he's doing." All sorts of expletives were being used by him and I was laughing inside at the fact that after all these years he was showing his true colours at last.

Victor J Kennedy

He hated me. He had always hated me and he couldn't help himself in this moment of pressure. Shumana tried her best to calm him down and shut his mouth, like she was his PR but he was like Mount Vesuvius. No matter what he said throughout that tirade, I never aknowledged once that I heard any of it. I just continued to stick those labels to my work with the help of Jahan, Anthea and Suzanne. My three angels. Between us we met the deadline. Twinkle, Estella both finished and so did Nath. They were all in the van before it drove away.

I stayed with Tanya that night to avoid Nath but mostly to make sure she was okay before her operation the next day. From what she told me it was a very straightforward piece of keyhole surgery to remove some foreign cells on her womb. This was the problem she had had last year. The gravity of this had still not hit me, partly due to the way Tanya dealt with what she perceived to be the prospect of death. Even before I was around she had this looming over her and it had manifested psychologically into a person who is very giving. She always wanted to make the best of now. She lived short term not long term. But she never said any of this and because of it, I never realised I had to ask the question. I'd not really taken the monogamous part of the relationship very seriously but I did love her. Deeply by now! Her father picked her up at 7am to beat the A406 traffic back to Essex. She was going private on his medical insurance. He would come back for me after work around 6pm and take me to see Tanya post op. I arrived at Tanya's bedside around 7pm. It was clear from the pain etched on her face that the air which had been pumped into her abdomen to carry out the procedure, was taking a while to dissepate. She didn't want to stay in the hospital and was adamant that she went home and stayed in her own bed that night, so that is what she did. It reminded me of when I broke my collar bone and she slept on the floor next to my sick bed only this time our roles were reversed. I lay there all night listening to her breathe, just to make sure she didn't die. I was like a sentry, guarding her life whilst she rested and got her strength back.

I went on a journey that night. I saw the sun come up. They say the brightest dawns follow the darkest nights and when her dad quietly came in to her room around 6am to get me ready for my lift I was already sat there reading a magazine, dressed and ready to go. In the car he told me how much he rated me and that he looked at me now more like another son. I felt priviledge to be so accepted and I told him I cared not just for Tanya but for the whole family, Luke, Jennifer, Carolyn and him. It was a good chat and I felt charged as I got home.

It was a Wednesday and that meant football at Chiswick. I was really in the mood even though I had been awake for twentyfour hours. I got on the coach at Watford Road and by the time we got to the ground I had kicked every ball and knew what I was going to do in that game. I was going to score and we were going to win the game. I knew it. I believed it. And the frightening thing is, it all came true. I scored a header and we won 2-0. I ran the game from left midfield. I never actually stayed in left midfield. I was all over the place, running and running and running. I was shouting a lot too. I've always shouted but I was really shouting, almost growling. I knew I was intimidating the opposition players and my own team also responded if I demanded the ball. I was probably quite scary that day but I didn't care. I was superman and after the game I told Bobby the same thing when he praised my performance in the changing rooms in front of the lads. I actually felt like I could become a professional if I wanted to. It was just a matter of choice. University or Premiership. My belief systems were skewed by this absurd euphoria and boundless energy that was impacting on my confidence so much that I found it hard to think straight or at least concentrate on one thing at a time. The Premiership would have to wait because I had so many amazing ideas bubbling up in my brain and I had bigger fish to fry.

Victor J Kennedy

Ruth managed to wrangle some tickets for the live transmission of Channel 4's The Word at Teddington Studios on Friday the 13th January. I made sure she knew that was my birthday and then an impromptu piss up occurred in the college bar on the afternoon before the show. Lewis brought some spliff to college so we hammered a lot of that outside under the staircase of the teaching block. At one point Jahan was unconscious with his head on the metal table. Everyone giggling at him and trying to wake him up. Eventually I became unconscious too. To my dismay I woke up on my back at the top of the stairs of our flat around 2am with The Word ticket still in my pocket. I'd never made it. I was gutted but I was still drunk and sloped off to bed.

The next day Tanya had organised a surprise party for me at her house. She made the classic English party spread with sausages, pineapple and cheese on sticks. Egg and cress sandwiches, vol-au-vents, the lot! Everyone she asked to turn up, made the effort to come. Some of them bought presents. Most of the gifts were simple and straightforward, others were more complex and ironic. It was really difficult for me because a) I had a massive hangover and b) I had to stand in front of these people and open them to applause or big laughs. I was over a barrel. Rory, who I was feeling threatened by at that time, handed me a parcel. I opened it to find a book on How To Be Cool - The complete handbook. It told you who invented it, what the cool rules are, how to speak cool, how to look cool and of course who to invite to make your parties cool. He gave a little comedy speech while he handed over that book which seemed to be funny to only a select few and then when I queried why I needed such a book he said, "Oh, no Vic. You don't need it. I just thought it might help you." I still didn't understand but then I wasn't meant to. The joke was at my expense and maybe it was pay back for being top of the photography project last year? I felt really stitched up because Tanya had tried to organise a surprise party. I felt uneasy for the rest of the evening. Nath and Lewis got the same card as Diago & Dean bought me the year before. That one from our college shop where the patient is being ejected through a trap door of the psychiatrists surgery by a lever under his desk. They both signed it, "You're fucked up Dr. Kennedy. Patients Nathaniel and Lewis x" That one hurt too.

I tried to talk to Dean about it at the gym on Monday lunchtime and I tried to mention all the stuff going around in my head but I was way too embarrassed to just come out with it for fear of further humiliation so I spoke in riddles. We both talked in a strange third person kind of way to try and disguise or at least avoid moving into deep territory. When I referred to Rory's Cool book indirectly, Dean didn't quite understand me and began talking about a book that his mum gave him when he was a kid. He spoke elaborately about it without even mentioning it's title. It spoke of someone appealing to the people in the late twentieth century. Someone who would lead them out of trouble, as well as save them from the bad things that happen and balance the world. I got confused and thought we were referring to the bible and I mentioned my mum had introduced me to the same book. But then he thought I was talking about the same book as his mum gave to him. It was a stupid conversation because it was not an authentic communication. It was like a game of hide and seek. We were playing with words while we pumped iron. We were training the same way we had trained for two years and this was the furthest I ever felt from him. In fact, it was the loneliest I had felt for my whole life. Nobody understood me and I wasn't prepared to tell them how I felt for fear of ridicule. My birthday party just proved that. I left the gym and went home.

On that ten minute walk off campus I was looking at cars, shoes, clouds, trees, basically everything and anything was a sign or a bridge between the past and the future. I felt my heart beat, I thought about the cold air passing over the orifice of my ear. I could feel the temperature of the concrete through my trainers and socks as I walked. I could taste the

exhaust from the planes flying 30,000 feet above my head. I was the second coming. I was the person in that book that Dean's mum gave him. She made sure he was at the university in this year so he could meet me and tell me that now. He'd just confirmed that all my studying had been to get me ready to invent something for the internet that would change the world. That will help people. Make everyone's lives better and rid the world of oppression, of evil.
I got home feeling exhausted so I opened a half empty wrap of speed from inside my secret Body Shop container under my bed and poured it onto my tongue. It tasted really sour and off. I had not touched any since Liverpool in April. I then made a coffee to take the taste away, popped a couple of ProPlus and pressed play on the CD player and again enjoyed another performance of The Second Coming by The Stone Roses while I worked. My energy was back, my thoughts were clearer and more focused. I worked for most of the afternoon and then took a break. I walked into the lounge and spotted some mail. One of them was for me and it had an RSA franked envelope. I opened it.

RSA
The Royal Society for the encouragement of Arts, Manufacture & Commerce
Founded in 1754

26th January 1995

Dear Victor Kennedy,

RSA STUDENT DESIGN AWARDS 1994/1995 - Multimedia

I am pleased to inform you that you have been shortlisted for interview in the above-named section of the RSA Student Design Awards. The interview will take place on:

Mad in England - A memoir

Thursday 23rd February at 10.00am

at the RSA, 8 John Alan Street, London WC2N 6EZ. It will last approximately twenty minutes. We suggest you arrive fifteen minutes before your interview time.

Please arrive at the RSA's main entrance in John Alan Street. The nearest tubes are Charing Cross (Northern, Jubilee and Bakerloo lines), Embankment (District, Circle and Northern lines), Leicester Square (Piccadilly and Northern lines). A map is enclosed.

INTERVIEW

It is essential for you to confirm, by telephone or in writing, that you are able to attend the interview. Please reply as soon as possible to Sybil Harries, Jacklyn Bates or Catherine Kirkwood, for if we do not hear from you, it will be assumed you will not attend. If, for any reason, you are unable to attend the interview on the day arranged, we are afraid that an alternative interview date cannot be made. In such case the July's decision will be based on your competition entry alone.

At the interview you should be prepared to discuss your entry and show models or other work which you have developed from it. Please come with a minimum of two 35mm slides/prints of your work and your models. These will be retained by the RSA for publicity purposes.

All students: Please bring your portfolio as the Jury will also wish to see a selection of your other college work.

EXPENSES

All students who attend interviews are asked to pay the first £5.00 of their travelling expenses. The RSA will then reimburse the balance. It is essential that you take advantage of student reductions and saver fares where possible. (Taxi fares will not be reimbursed.) If you are travelling overseas, the RSA is only able to cover travel expenses from your UK landing point (unless entering the New Design for Old Section). Please bring receipts with you.

AWARDS * Please read the enclosed sheet for details of the available awards *

TRAVEL AWARDS In each section, sponsors have provided funds to allow winning students to make overseas study tours, to research their chosen design area. At the interview the Jury will wish to discuss any ideas you may have for such a study tour, and in the event of your winning a Travel Award, the RSA will help make more detailed plans and provide a list of useful addresses.

ATTACHMENT AWARDS If you are interested in any of the Attachment Awards on offer in your section (if applicable), the Jury will wish to discuss the implications of taking up such an award. Please bear in mind that a representative of the company sponsoring the award is likely to be on the Jury and will be able to answer any questions you may have about the award. In most cases you should be free to undertake an attachment during the summer/autumn 1995.

If you accept the offer of an Attachment Award, you must understand that you have made a commitment to the sponsoring company to undertake the placement, which must be completed before you start full-time employment. If you are in any doubt about your availability in the summer/autumn 1995 or your ability to undertake a commitment to an Attachment Award please let the RSA (or judging panel) know.

Mad in England - A memoir

It is very important that you make it clear to the Jury whether you are interested in a Travel Award or an Attachment Award, to prevent confusion when the Jury decides on the allocation of awards.

Two important conditions of either a Travel or Attachment Award are:
* The award should ideally be taken up within six months of the announcement of the competition results (especially Attachment Awards) and will be withdrawn after eighteen months.
* A written report must be submitted to the RSA within three months of completion of the study tour or period of attachment.

Finally, I should like to take this opportunity to congratulate you on reaching the final shortlist.

Yours sincerely

Sybil Harries

I was absolutely delighted! Totally over the moon. I rang Alan's house but he wasn't in, he was at college obviously, but I asked his mum if a letter had arrived with RSA printed in red on the front of it. She confirmed that it had arrived. Again, I was really pleased for him but at the same time I hoped he didn't win. I knew he had a great chance of winning because of all the time I'd spent with him witnessing his clever thinking first hand. The only advantage I had was my finish was more polished but then again, never trust beauty. To celebrate, I took Tanya to the cinema on Station Road to see Shallow Grave, which turned into one hell of a fright. It was an awe inspiring film and we could not stop talking about it all the way home but it did freak me out. All because of the flatmate who moved upstairs into the attic, then drilled the holes through the ceiling to keep an eye on the other flat mates. It was very much like that experience I'd had around the house with Nath drawing the picture messages and leaving them around for me to find. All my traps I'd left in my bedroom had been going off regularly and he kept borrowing my Jam and Spoon CD without asking. I wasn't seeing much of Nath or Lewis at the moment. Nath was avoiding the flat by staying around at Shumana's all the time. Lewis had found himself a new stunner called Justine, from the fashion course and he was in love. I think she had a better bedroom than Lewis so they stayed at her's all the time. I was left alone in that tiny flat and I had stopped tending to it, as a protest to my isolation. I hardly slept, although I was really productive and had typed around seven thousand words into my dissertation. I did miss their company when I took my breaks. I wasn't having a laugh with anyone because no one was there. I spoke to Dean about it and he invited me down to their house to watch Disney's Aladdin which had just come out on video. He now not only lived with Diago, but also Jase, Anthea and Sharon. They all welcomed me in and we sat down and enjoyed it. I found it really comforting to be accepted by them. The feeling of underlying hostility in my own accommodation was not present and I enjoyed their company. They made me feel relaxed and I realised I hadn't been relaxed since before Christmas. The film was affecting me spiritually as well. All the symbolism in it was amazing and the bright colours stopped me analysing it and made me just enjoy it. It gave my mind a rest.

At the end they all said goodbye at the door and Dean gave me hug. He whispered in my ear, "I will be your magic carpet forever."

"Thank you." I whispered back. Then I waved to them all and said goodbye, before making my way through the darkness of Northwick Park and back home. He set my mind off thinking stupid thoughts again. Did he mean that I'm Aladdin? Or that I'm like Aladdin? Or did he mean I'm the hero. Was he trying to offset Rory's joke with that Cool book on my birthday? On and on and on... ...all the way home. I never gave myself a break from this constant analysis. I was like a dog chasing it's tail. Or tale, depending on how you analyse it.

I knew that none of us were getting along at college and that we had a show to put on in July to try and get everyone a job; I took it on myself to knit everyone back together and create some kind of realisation of the gravity of the consequences if we do not work together. We were the first student's in the history of this country's higher education establishments to undergo a modula degree. The results were fascinating because there were around six or seven students with the potential at this semester break to proceed and gain First Class Honours. Last year they didn't get one. The year before there was one person. The prospect of almost a third of the classroom receiving First Class Honours, I believed to be unfair and a complete failure of the new system. I spoke to the tutors about this and obviously they disagreed. I had a heated argument with Eric and Raymond told me he thought this was the most talented group of people he had been lucky enough to teach in his time at The University of Westminster. Noel took me to one side and spoke off the record. He said he thought there were failings and that it would look bad if in the first year of the new modula system so many Firsts would be produced by it. People could suggest standards had gone down. However, he told me that I needed to back off and think about myself for a change. He said I didn't need to get involved in these kinds of issues because that was his job. He also disturbed me when he said he was worried about me. I felt he was trying to spoil my attempt to put things right so I went ahead and did it anyway. First of all I made posters on the computers in room 309 and plastered them around.

Thursday 9th Feb 1995
1pm 'till he shuts up!
It's payback time you mothers!

Victor J Kennedy

The Famous Group Hug 3rd Year Student Meeting
Evangelist Victor Kennedy and his infamous crisp, will give
their Graphic Information Superdesignway speech!!
It's time to tell the world we're here!
Join me and my crisp and become: "In yer face," "No Frills,"
Raymond has taught you well, use the crisp Lewis.
Plenty of cheese guaranteed!!!

Then I went home for two days and wrote the speech based
on what had been going on recently. On the second night I
didn't sleep and woke Lewis early to check it for any
mistakes I couldn't spot myself. He made a few amends and
sense checked parts of it but overall he said it was, "really
noble of you". I'd also decided I needed to wear something
special so I put on a black teeshirt that had 'Mad in England'
on the rear collar and the word "Armed' on a pocket over the
left arm. I also pinned a Gold Heart badge from Esther
Rantzen's Variety Club campaign to help disavantaged
children. The strapline was 'Wear your heart on your sleeve'.
So I did. It would give me the strength to talk. Lewis left
without me and Nath wasn't there so I walked to college
alone with my thoughts. This was going to be the biggest
speech of my life. I composed myself and prepared for any
possible disruptions or hecklers. I had Rory down as the
major spoiler but when I got started everyone went silent. It
was 1pm, Thursday.

Ideology can be shared and given to others, the same as a
biological order or disorder passed between human beings.
Today, I'm giving blood to those of you who have bothered
to turn up!

I wear a mask and my mask is a comedian's mask – I try to
make you laugh if I feel nervous when I'm with you -- that's
my mask. I look confident and powerful but I'm not really.
I'm about to take it off and become serious because I have
important information I want to give you.

Mad in England - A memoir

...It's now off!

Please forgive me for any bad language or lairiness or even badly composed sentences but that is just me! I can't help being in your face.
One important fact to know. Last night when you were all sleeping I was writing this for you. I went to sleep at 5am. I found it easy and I enjoyed thinking about you all. I stayed up late for you.
I will read it to you because I'm too nervous to do it off the top of my head because, it needed composing, tactfully and correctly. If you want a photocopy of this afterwards, you're welcome to one!

I'm taking a big chance by taking off my mask because I'm now powerless, so please don't interrupt me or take the piss because it will hurt me without my powerful mask on!

Here is my heart and I am wearing it on my sleeve for you to see. This is a speech, it is not a lecture, I am trying to touch all your souls. It isn't Victor Kennedy's speech, it's your student rep's speech. It isn't your rep showing off, it's your rep doing his job. And that job is to serve you – I am your slave and I have been for the last three years. If you choose not to support your rep then tell your rep your reasons because your rep cannot serve you correctly if your rep doesn't know something is wrong. I'm not just talking now as a rep, either.

Some people here have judged me and these people have got me all wrong. I am not brilliant, I am certainly not "the best" on the course, I am just a person on the course.

Simple:
Not compound
Consisting of few elements

Victor J Kennedy

All of one kind
Not complicated, elaborate, adorned, involved or highly
finished

If I can use the analogy of football then you could call me a
member of a team and think now. Football teams have
different players with different abilities, who play in
different positions yet they are an entity, a collective, they
are a team. Maybe I am just the Paul Gascoigne of this team
and maybe if I broke my leg then I would not be of use to
anyone who is left on the team.

1. A group is a collection of individuals but...
2. What makes an individual feel part of a group?

They are key sentences, so remember them, forever. What
makes an individual feel part of a group? What makes me
feel part of you lot? The answer could be: just keep being
part of the group you are in. But then join more groups and
meet new people, read new books etc. Try everything!
Put yourselves about and don't try to do everything on your
own because you just can't do it as an isolated individual.

In my RCA moment of terror, I was surprised that I had four
friends helping me to beat the deadline, so in the end we, not
I, beat it. I've tried to think of a time before that day when
I've felt wanted by you lot and I could only think of one. The
day you all voted for me to represent you in the 1st year.
First impressions eh?

I work hard, I enjoy what I do and I love this degree!

My secret's out. What's yours? Why do you want that degree
scroll and what number do you require on that piece of paper
to progress to the next level? Being professional is a state of
mind, not a title, a qualification or a large wage packet! Do
you want a '1st' or would just a '2.1' do? Or are you happy to

aquire the knowledge that is available for free, from just
being accepted on this course?
Get your direction in life now! I've got mine. You lot gave it
to me in the 1st year after only knowing me two weeks.

I've been a servant for three years because everytime I've
gone to step down, I couldn't, because every one of you, said
"I'll do it but only if no one else will volunteer." So I chose, I
made the decision who I thought would do a good job! And
the rest of you at that time could fuck off. In the end I would
still be the mug representing you and caring about you. And
look how badly some of us have been behaving recently and
I'm talking about tutors as well as members of this group!

And if how we've all behaved recently when we were under
pressure is how we will behave under pressure in a future
'professional world' and more importantly at the show, if we
ever get our fucking fingers out and help each other produce
it (never mind decent enough work to show anyone) then
this course and college will always look like 'poor old'
Harrow!

I don't care where you're from or what you look like. All I
know is that behind your skin, the masks we all wear, there
are potentially competent and maybe a few brilliant graphic
information designers trying to get out. So I want you to take
your masks off while you do your major projects. Do the
best piece of work not just for yourself as an 'isolated'
individual but also for the course and your team members!

Now, in a way, I am relieving myself of duty for four
months and I'm throwing you all in at the deep end. I want to
be proved wrong. I want to see you swim and not sink. After
that, I'll jump in and catch you up and we can all ride the
biggest wave of self-satisfaction that GID has ever seen!
Remember Megan told us in the first year 'GID is fun' and
I'll tell you what, I've had the best fun of my life on this

course. I've met and been touched by thirty four people and probably, if I'm lucky, maybe ten of them might be arsed to keep in touch afterwards.

That's it. I'm stepping out of the microscope now and sitting amongst the group and I'll put my mask back on.

We then proceeded to have an all out ruck about who was to blame against what on earth were we going to do for our final degree show. Eventually it settled down and people began drifting off for lunch but a lot of them patted me on the back or said thank you for saying what I said. They all felt the same pressure as me, or did they?

I'd noticed during the speech that Ruth was drawing all the way through so once she had left I went over to her pad to have a look. They were quite 'dark' drawings. There were black crows and sketches of Darth Vader's head next to a stick man on a skateboard with "TWINKLE" written above it. The whole thing intrigued me as much as it worried me. I knew the drawings were about me because they were done while I spoke. I wasn't sure about the TWINKLE reference but maybe it was to do with that bloody gas bill again. I took the drawing but I dared not confront her about it. I respected her and the realisation that someone I respected appeared to be in opposition hurt really bad. I was reading way too much into things.

A couple of pretty first year girls had been standing in the doorway listening to parts of the speech and had already, over the last few months, begun a dialogue between me and Nath. In fact they had created dialogues with lots of boys because that's what you do as a first year.

On the Friday I was at home with Tanya having another one of our domestics at her house. Lewis had been up the bar and got drunk with these two girls. At some point in the evening, late on, I needed to get changed so I was ready to go to Essex in the morning when Tanya's dad came to pick us up. I popped back to my flat to discover Lewis on the sofa with his arms around these girls, Sheryl and Lizette (known as Lisa), while watching my Empire Strikes Back video. I couldn't believe it. He was such a dog. What about Justine? So I went in and broke it up. In the middle of Lewis protesting his innocence, Nath appeared in boxer shorts from his bedroom looking tired. Straight away everyone started flirting and within minutes Sheryl followed Nath back into his room and I pulled Lisa into my room leaving Lewis alone with the film. I did fancy her and after enjoying a cheeky snog I told her that was enough and that she should watch out for Lewis. Then she said she'd only come back for me. That neither of them wanted Lewis. Sheryl fancied Nath and Lisa fancied me. I was flattered and excited but I couldn't do anything because firstly I had just popped in to get changed and secondly, it was complete madness to nip home for a shag when I loved Tanya (even though we were not getting on that well). I told Lisa I had to go back to my missus and she asked if she could sleep in my bed as she wanted to wait for Sheryl, who was currently with Nath. I said, "Fine but keep your mouth shut about that snog or I'll be in trouble." I grabbed some clothes and legged it. Lewis shouted down the stairs, "CHEERS MATE!" I didn't need that complication but I couldn't help myself. When I got back, I had to mention it to Tanya and it only led to another confrontation. I felt I couldn't do right from wrong. I didn't know why she was so impatient with me and agitated by me. When she went to sleep, I switched the bedside lamp back on and started writing down all my frustrations and anger over the past few weeks. It was an uncensored rant that was expanding on the energy of my speech from a few days before. I now had huge issues about Nath and the way he had been manipulating me since the first year and I didn't see him doing any of it. I couldn't see what he was doing until now. Even Shumana didn't know what he was doing right now with another girl. Nath cared for nobody and could not be trusted. He was evil and my writing was explaining why

Victor J Kennedy

he had become evil. Once again, I never slept that night. I just wrote and thought and then wrote some more.

A kid at school can copy over his friend's shoulders and claim to have done the work himself. If he continues to do this he will look very intelligent but it is his friends' intelligence he is riding on, like a wave! If he rides the wave forever he is the most intelligent and powerful looking man on the face of this earth where we all live and have to share with him. Children that are spoiled at school will have inadequacies when they grow up if they continue to copy their friends' answers.

A group is a set of individuals but what makes an individual feel part of a group?
I am not a working class dirty northern bastard, there should be no class system because there are too many 'Nazis' on this planet! That is the lesson I learned at school! I read books, magazines and I watch a lot of television and I pick the best ideas and concepts from these media. You could say I'm still the same kid. I do still look and act like the same sixteen year old but I step over the things I acknowledge before I judge them. Basically, I steal maybe two or more concepts and experiment with them. It is the same as playing with a photocopier, I like to experiment and understand a medium before I use it, before I can value its use. Before I can use it to my advantage. Maybe I am a businessman because businessmen use people and experiment with human minds better than any trained psychologist could ever learn to do.

Do I scare you with my truths! ?
I am not trying to rule the world, I just want to tell you about Victor Kennedy.
Professional surfers can only try to become good enough that they never get thrown from their board. They make mistakes just like 16-year-old kids! There is a saying that, 'Children learn from their mistakes' and the mistakes I made

at school have made me pay for the rest of my life. I am 23 now. This is what I learned from maths, you can already see how bad my English is. This is my equation $23 - 16 = 7$. Maybe I've got the 'seven year itch' and maybe it's come at a bad time? Maybe this is a good time for it? Only time will tell me. I am not brilliant I am very simple! I love simple people because that is my background, that is my psychological make up! And we all know that make up can be defined as cosmetics and humans use cosmetic surgery if they are psychologically affected by their nose. I love my nose, its my father's nose and it's very big and it sticks out really far so everyone can see my father for the rest of my life. Even after he has passed away.

Question yourself now. Have you already made your judgement?

Do you really know who I am?

Do you really know yourself?

Are you too frightened to let my mind loose inside your space?

Let's see!

Definition of Simple:

Not compound

Consisting of one or few elements

All of one kind

Not complicated, adorned or highly finished and over written

A working class farmer who cannot read is knowledgeable. An upper class aristocrat who owns a library but also cannot read appears intelligent.

Knowledge is Power

The internet is empowering

The Bible reads, 'and the meek shall inherit the earth'

It doesn't take a euphoric speech by a copying American leader like Al Gore to understand what the 'Information Superhighway' will do to the human race. Is it fair that an

Victor J Kennedy

American flag was placed on the moon even though it was a human that stood there and struggled to stick it in the dust and rock?

Is it coincidence that Arpanet was invented in 1969, the same year?

Is it also ironic that as the good old US of A took control of Earth's destiny and branding peace then selling freedom back to everyone else. Maybe it is a coincidence that Russia 'cracked' under pressure of the termination of the cold war. Everybody in the west were told by the media that Russia was evil. Someone has to lose.

Isn't it also weird that news reports tell us the Berlin Wall fell over but the Great Wall of China didn't? Isn't it spooky that racism has allegedly ended in South Africa. Look what happened to Nelson Mandela, he is an icon in every sense of the word. The media says that so is Bob Geldof, also referred to as a 'star' or a 'celebrity.' The main message to remember is how Bob Geldof helped the Third World compared to Britain's First World or 'The West' (almost sounds the Best) George Best! Look at what happened to that footballing 'God.' He fell back to earth with a big bang! Just like a nuclear bomb dropping!

Bob Geldof helped the poor starving kids from North Africa By the way, Africa is a continent too! So is North America. World domination, that is all these copying children want! It's how humans develop, by ripping other humans off! And it's got to stop. I want you to know that I've never voted and I never will! Because you'll never find someone who can honestly say, "I'm not greedy. I just love every other human!" A group is a shared set of individuals. What makes an individual feel part of a group?

Vic Kennedy (11.2.95)

PS Blighty won 'World War II' because of propaganda. Whoever controls the media can control the people, sometimes referred to as 'The Meek'!

Mad in England - A memoir

I couldn't show this rant to Tanya because she would freak out. Everything was getting confused and blurred. I was losing track of what was research and what was real. This distortion was leading me to believe I was more than special. That I might just be a reincarnation of Jesus Christ. The Second Coming. No one told me, I just suspected it. I couldn't tell people because it was going to freak them out. They would probably think I was mad and then lock me up in an asylum. I had to be some kind of superhuman because I had not slept for four whole days now and I felt fine. Well, apart from feeling like I had lived about a five months in the last five weeks.

I went into college for a change to see what was going on and to print my almost completed dissertation so I could proof read it. I was sat in the studio at my desk just chatting away with Jah, Anthea, Sharon and a couple of others about the internet. I was preaching basically. These print designers all became interested in the mumbo jumbo I was waffling on about and between us we all joined collectively and intellectually for about an hour's brainstorm on subjects like velocity, volume, electricity, light speed, time, biology, quantum physics, geometry, cosmology, gravity and how all this fits within a computer screen to deliver wishes as soon as they form in the mind of the person in front of the four sided mirror. Everyone scribbled on this A2 sheet of layout pad after reliving their individual experiences of each individual piece of theory from school. Between us we created a theory. A basic set of rules that if applied to a technology which could cope with the amount of data passing through it in both directions would enable human beings to fully experience Teleprescence. Which means to put yourself inside the four-sided mirror (computer screen as we understood it). It would be a projection of yourself into television a la Willy Wonka. You could publish yourself! You be the star! Express yourself. That was it! My Eureka! moment. I immediately stopped the brainstorm and scribbled

Victor J Kennedy

T E L E P R E S S ! in big letters across the whole page. Like a paranoid barrister, I asked everyone present to date and sign that sheet of paper so we all owned intellectual property rights over it. I then ran with the sheet to the student office and asked them to rubber date stamp the sheet as I folded it up into a small compact square in the centre of my hand. Then I signed and dated it, put it in an envelope, walked down to the post office and sent it recorded delivery to myself in Millhead. I phoned my mum up and told her not to post it back to London when it arrived because it was from me. She had to hide it somewhere until I got home at Easter. It was very, very important that she did that.

I went home from the post office and continued to work on my dissertation but my computer kept crashing or locking out and I would have to restart thus losing the work I hadn't saved. I didn't need that right now as the deadline was looming large. Late that evening Tanya came round about 11:15pm. Lewis let her in and she came upstairs to my room where I was deeply engrossed in my work, hunched over the computer keyboard with a single lamp on. She sat on my bed behind me and said, "Alright Treacle."

"Whoa, you startled me there. I didn't even hear you come in. How did you get through the front door?"

"Lewis let me in."

"Oh, he's in is he? I never heard him come in."

"You don't notice much these days do you?"

"What do you mean?" I got off my stool and sat on the bed next to her. One look and instantly I knew.

"You're drunk aren't you?"

"No."

"You are."

"I'm not. I'm just fresh."

"You're more than that. You've got red wine lips and dark gums."

"I've only had a couple."

"Where've you been?"

"At Gideons."

"At Gideons? His house?"

"Yeah. What's wrong with that?"

"You got pissed with him at his house."

"I'm not drunk. He cooked a meal and he bought a bottle of wine."

"Oh, he fucking did, did he?"

"Ah, come on that's not fair. He wanted to talk to me about his film."

"Why couldn't you meet him in a public place. Why do you have to go and enjoy a meal with him?"

"You just don't understand do you?"

"What?"

"It doesn't matter."

"No, it does. Tell me."

"What's happened to you Vic? I've lost you."

"You haven't lost me. I'm right here. I'm always here, in my room. You know where I am."

"But that's where you've gone. It's not you anymore."

"Shut up, it is me."

"It's not. Something has happened to you."

"To be honest, I can't go into that right now. Things will become apparent in time."

"I don't know what you mean?"

"You will. In time."

"But we don't have time. I need you now and you're not there for me. It's all about work."

"You're working too."

"Not as hard as you. I'm still having a life."

"Babe, we've got the rest of our lives to have a life. Right now at this time I need to make sure I do the best I can to get ahead. To make our lives easier later on and then we can enjoy it more. You're thinking short term. I'm thinking long term. The bigger picture."

"You're not. You're just thinking of yourself and I may as well be invisible. I have to find attention elsewhere."

"What, with Gideon?"

"Not just him. You've haven't been up the bar at all this year apart from your birthday and then you were totally out of it and embarrassing."

"I don't remember, what did I do?"

"That's not my point Vic. I'm talking to loads of guys, not just Gideon and I have a good time. I feel like I don't have a boyfriend, you know?"

"No, I don't know what you mean."

"We haven't had sex since we were up at your mum's at Christmas. Do you know how that makes me feel?"

"Hey, hey! That's not fair. We had Thrush for a while and I've been working really hard. My focus is there." I pointed at the computer.

"Ok then, let me climb under the desk and I'll give you a blow job while you're working."

"Look at you. You're out of it. You cannot even sit up straight. You look a mess. Your hair is everywhere. I bet you've already shagged Gideon tonight and now you've come round here for some more."

"I didn't shag him but we snogged on his doorstep when I was leaving." She grinned.

"You are shitting me." I started to feel sick. That feeling you get when you receive bad news in your heart.

"No, I never." Her face dropped to sadness. She went silent and then a tear fell down.

"Why are you doing these things to me?"

"I don't know baby. I'm so confused." She put her arms around me.

"Let's getaway from all this."

"We can't escape it now."

"We can. Let's go on holiday in the semester break. Just like last year, only I'll pay for this one."

"Let's do it at the end."

"In the summer?"

"Yeah."

"Where do you wanna go? Just say it and I'll book it tomorrow."

"But you've got no money babe."

"Don't worry, I'll find some. So where do you wanna go princess?"

"Bodrum."

"Where's that?"

"It's in Turkey. There's this blue lagoon..."

"Don't say any more. Your wish will come true."

"I love you so much."

"I love you too." We hugged on the bed until we fell asleep. Well, until Tanya fell asleep in my arms. I had another night awake only this time thinking about that fucker Gideon and what the bastard was up to. What a fucking great trick to pull someone else's bird. I was gonna break his fingers if he had touched her or even tried to touch her.

The next morning I got showered for the first time in a while, had a shave and then went into Harrow town centre with my cheque book to find a travel agent and grant Tanya her wish. I popped into Lloyds and discovered I was still inside my overdraft limit so I knew the cheque would clear but I had to explain myself after the fact to my bank manager. I would work that bit out later on. I found a Thomas Cook and went straight in, grabbed a brochure on Turkey and within fifteen minutes it was done. I took the receipt home and knocked on the door of Tanya's house to tell her the good news. Cathy answered the door, Tanya wasn't there but I asked a million and one questions about Gideon and what Cathy thought of it all. I didn't hear the answer I wanted to hear, "I think he's really sexy Vic, for what it's worth. A lot of girls do find him attractive. It's that rugged thing. I wouldn't blame her if she had snogged him to be honest Vic. You haven't exactly been a great boyfriend recently." She slammed the door.

I didn't like that exchange at all and alarm bells were now ringing in my head. I was back in that state of anxiety again and I went home to work so I could avoid the feelings and channel my energy into something positive. I hated Cathy for that. That Gideon bloke had some kind of mind control over women that made me feel nervous of him. He appeared to be a very powerful man. Maybe I wouldn't chop his fingers off after all.

The mindset I started to encourage within myself was that Gideon was cleverer than me. In evolutionary stakes he was better adapted to university life in it's third year than I was. Maybe he made a risk assessment throughout the first two years and then decided he would take my bird instead of anyone else's. He'd been reading all that Shakespeare; maybe he had discovered a trick which I never found inside the research books I was digesting. I took my eye off the ball and he slid in and took it away from me, legged it up the other end of the field and stuck it in the onion bag. I was left with nothing. A loser. A dinosaur with no girlfriend. I also thought a lot about how much I invested in Tanya over the last two and a half years, both emotionally, spiritually and affectionately. Was it enough? Yes it fucking was. I was in love with the woman. Deeply in love with her and it felt more real than it had with my first love Faye. I wanted to spend the rest of my life with Tanya. I loved her family too. I was in deeper than ever before. They all loved me. But had I got too complacent? The night before she said I had and then hinted I would pay for any more of that behaviour. I had to put the mouse down and step away from the computer. But not until she came round to mine to discover I booked two weeks in a self-catering apartment in Bodrum during the first two weeks of July. Right on cue, the door bell rang. I went down the stairs to get the door. It was Tanya. I said, "Hi babe, come in and check out the brochure for our holiday in Bodrum. I've booked it!" I smiled but she wasn't smiling at all. In fact she was red around her eyes. "What's up?"

"I can't come in. I've got something to tell you."

"What?"

"I wanted to tell you last night but I couldn't. I'm sorry but I've been seeing Gideon."

"Just bef..Wha..Look, er... Can you explain what seeing Gideon exactly means."

"Well, it's been building up for a bit. Can I come in?"

"No. Carry on."

"But it's a bit cold and the neighbours might hear."

"I don't know my neighbours. Carry on. You were saying."

"It's just the way he's been talking to me over a period of time. Those meetings. We started off talking about his film and as time has gone on we've talked less about it."

"And more about what? You and him?"

"No, just stuff. Normal conversations."

"And then what happened."

"You were right about last night. I never expected him to set up a meal and candles but he had a few extra bottles of wine hidden in a cupboard. I thought there was only the one bottle on the table."

"Ok, so he made the move on you? Not the other way around?"

"Yes."

"But you didn't say no either?"

"I wasn't thinking straight. Before I knew what I was doing it had happened. I came straight to see you."

"So let's get one thing straight. You are not leaving me for him?"

"No."

"You haven't come here to tell me goodbye."

"No. I want to stay with you."

"But last night you were not sure."

"Last night was very draining."

"Ok, while we're confessing. Let me level the playing field."

"Oh no, Vic."

"No, this is not about what's happening now. There are things that have happened in the past."

"Well then I don't need to know about them. It's ok."

"No, you do need to know because it has been on my mind and this is a good opportunity to start a fresh. Remember Julie up north? Her. You know that Scott with the curly hair, his girlfriend. The blonde one? Her. There's another one who you may not know called Lucy. You might have met her dad at Christmas. Her too. All involving alcohol much like yourself last night."

"Vic, this is not gonna help."

"You started it."

"No! You did. All those girls were at the beginning. Last night was my cry for help. And now you tell me this."

"Well, I think we've both got a lot to think about. You'd better go home before you catch a cold."

"So what happens then?"

"I don't know? Maybe we finish, maybe we don't?"

"Oh Vic, I'm sorry I've done this. Please let's talk about it."

"There's nothing left to say. See you around." I slammed the door in her face and then burst into tears as I walked back up the stairs to my bedroom. She rang the bell. I shouted at her to go but she continued. Eventually she left but around an hour later the doorbell rang again, and again, and again. I lifted my heavy body from my bed and pulled the batteries out from the doorbell so it fell silent. Then the letterbox opened and it was Tanya's mum, shouting through the letterbox, "Victor, open the door my love. We just want to talk to you. Tanya is really distraught. She rang me in a right state and I've come straight over to help. She loves you so much Victor, please don't do this to her. We all love you and care about you deeply... Victor!" I was in pieces so I let her in. This was the very last thing I needed to happen at this moment in time. I was under so much pressure with so many other things that I just couldn't cope with the prospect of it all. She gave me a keynote speech on behalf of her daughter by the side of a bed to a shivering wreck under a duvet and then after thirty minutes and many tears, she hugged me before saying goodbye. She left me to wrestle with the decision and all the guilt too.

I stayed in bed for a couple of days and I swear, I never slept a wink. I watched the sun come up twice and go down twice. It was a very, very, strange time where I developed a belief system that Gideon was the devil and I was Jesus. We were both back on earth to fight it out, once and for all. Good versus evil. I knew he was here and he knew who I was and where I lived. He was fornicating with my lover. I was petrified of him and if I left the house for food I would run everywhere so he couldn't get me or shoot me with a sniper rifle. I never once thought about how I had to kill him. My thoughts were all about defence. How can I stop him killing me. It was very very sad and nobody was around to talk to. Not Nath. Not Lewis. Not Tanya. I wasn't coping on my own at all. I was ill. I needed to get some rest but instead I fed myself ProPlus and kept writing the dissertation.

Chapter 7: Breaking Down

In my capacity as Student Representative I'd received a letter from Maggie Tyndall, the Harrow Provost, who had asked me for my presence at a meeting to talk through the experience of life on the new campus from the point of view of all sorts of students and all sorts of staff. She put in her letter of 2nd February:
There in the meeting to listen to you will be an assortment of people involved in planning and preparing the campus. Some of them will say nothing at all but just make notes. Please don't be put off by this; they are going to go away and think about what you have said. I look forward to meeting you on the 10th.
A lot had happened to me in the past eight days, the majority of which I had been awake on Pro Plus tablets washed down with Nescafe Gold Blend. There was the over compassionate letter writing to Sean, Alice and the Access Fund. Sean up in Staffordshire, I had heard, was found by his disturbed housemates hammering an upturned table into the kitchen floor at 3am. Turns out his dad, a carpenter himself, had died and this devastating news had a massive impact on Sean's mental health. I'd spent many drug-crazed nights back in Carlisle 1991 with Sean and I felt for him, especially in the

Victor J Kennedy

strange state I found myself in at the moment. Also from Carlisle was Alice, the hugely talented and gorgeous girl I'd sat next to in Graphics classes. Katie told me Alice's mum had died so I felt in my new found capacity as the saviour of the twentieth century, I had to let her read some kind words of support too. My third letter was an application for the Access Fund, a pot of money the university advertised to financially ruined students. After writing to Sean and Alice this emotionally charged ramble about why I needed more of the university's money probably raised a few unintentional laughs in the office.

In that state of what I now refer to as 'religious mania', I was stretching myself all over the place with belief systems so warped that I knew I couldn't tell anyone but at the same time, I couldn't help myself from acting on them. It was like obsessive-compulsive disorder. I would be in my little bedroom with the door locked, Nath and Lewis totally unaware that I was experiencing and carrying out bizarre rituals, in between knocking out a dissertation and contextual study, something we were not asked to do. It was one or the other and I chose both. Nobody stopped me. Nobody was taking any notice.

One day while in my little room, blasting out The Stone Roses new album The Second Coming, I over analyzed the lyrics and began to get a massive guilt trip about having stolen a Phillipe Starke stool from the college bar, after my Argos stool finally succumbed to my weight. When I stole it Tanya was with me, egging me on and giggling after a drunken night at the bar. It was a brilliant bar stool, ergonomically designed to nurse the backside in all the right places. We brought it back under the cover of darkness but now I had to take it back before God put me into eternal damnation and shame as a thief. I left the music and computer on in the bedroom, picked up the peach coloured stool, ran down the stairs and out of the flat, as fast as I could. My mind placed so much symbolism and social weight behind this stool that it became an icon of evil as I ran through the streets to the Northwick Park roundabout.

Heaven's gates won't hold me
I'll saw those suckers down
Laughing loud at your locks when they hit the ground
Every icon in every town
Hear this, your number's up, I'm coming round

I was scared, petrified even, as I made it to the campus fence
and in one movement, brought it down from my shoulder,
pirouetted and threw it over, only to hear the "Oi!" of a
patrolling security guard. As I ran off, cleansed and angelic,
purified, I thought to myself, why shout "Oi!"? I'm bringing
it back, you prick! My mind wouldn't let me rest, I had to get
back to the confines of my room before something fell out of
the sky on to me, like a giant crucifix.
I'd played games as a kid on my own, walking back to
school from my gran's house after fish fingers, chips and
peas. I would race cars against trees. If I ran past three trees
on the pavement before I got overtaken by a car, then I got
one point. I would end up sprinting all the way to school
sometimes, in a bid to beat my best score. I think when
you're losing your mind it is difficult, near on impossible, to
see the line between recreation and reality. My belief
systems were so distorted by now, there was the inevitable
deterioration of trust and the growth of paranoia just round
the corner.
I got back to my chairless but purified room to find Tanya
on my bed looking sad, confused and a little afraid. She
asked where the chair had gone and I had to pretend I'd
decided it was wrong to steal so I had returned it. I was role
playing. I was telling her things I thought she wanted to hear
because I was convinced she wouldn't like to hear the rest of
the stuff going round in my head right now. To keep her
from suspecting anything I agreed to everything she wanted,
we made peace but she left confused.

Victor J Kennedy

Around this time I was getting affected by the media,
especially stories in the news. A murder had occurred near
Scarborough. A woman was stabbed to death in a country
lane. Her surname was Kennedy and I was convinced her
Christian name was Heather. I rang my mum to check it
wasn't her. She told me not to worry, she was fine. I rang her
again at work one afternoon feeling really insecure and
needing reassurance, she answered while all her colleagues
were around her.
"Do you love me mum?"
"Yes I do."
"But say "I love you Victor""
She said, "I can't say that just now because people are
listening"
"But just say out loud that you love me"
So eventually she did. That was the end of the conversation.
There was also a report on the news a few days later of a
man called Victor who had either jumped (or been pushed!)
from a train near Oxenholme, the station nearest to my
parents' home. This one was scarey because the man who
owned the house in Millhead before my parents had died
after falling from a train. His son was called Victor and his
bedroom was now mine. It all felt too close to me, like a
conspiracy was forming by a government agency who
wanted me stopped and were sending out convoluted and
creepy warnings.
The paranoia finally started to rear it's ugly head when on
deadline day for the dissertation, after another long night
awake putting the final touches to "Internet or Not" I shut
down the Quadra and lay back on my bed, set the alarm for
9am, in about four hours time and dozed off into a light nap.
When the alarm sounded, I was up with a start. I hit the
startup button on the mac, then quickly brushed my teeth, ate
some Bran Flakes and gulped down another coffee. When I
got back to my room, ready to copy the Quark file onto an
Optical Disc ready for printing, there was a 'sad' face icon
and nothing else. I felt sick. Everybody knew that icon was

bad news regarding your hard drive. I tried to restart and got the bomb icon for a crash. My heart rate was increasing and my mind was spinning. Why me? Why now? I waited for the restart, rebuilt the desktop three times and got the same end result. FUCK! FUCK! BOLLOCKS! CUNT! All my hard work since November. All my fucking research. All that time last summer saving up for a fucking computer and for fucking what? This has to be Nath. After all that shit with the RSA applications and his comments to Shumana, which he blatantly made sure I would overhear. He hates me, He's jealous and he's killed my computer. Either when I was asleep or some kind of Trojan horse shareware program that he's found on one of those magazine CD-Roms. He can't stop me. Maybe he's found that Telepress work I've been hiding in the cistern cupboard, behind the tank? That'll be it! He's from the future and he's come back to steal Telepress from me. He's trying to stop me saving the world.

I unplugged the tower, put all the leads in a bag, wrapped it in a blanket and carried it all the way to college and found the IT support guy in the teaching block who saved my hard drive, my life and not to mention my sanity. Well, for a few more days at least. The dissertation deadline was met.

By the time the 10th February had arrived I was becoming suspicious of everyone, especially people I was unfamiliar with. At the discussion of life on the new campus, I took notes on every person around the table. Notes which were inspected, over my shoulder, by the Rector. Not that I knew or cared who he was but I was a little embarrassed when he acknowledged what I was doing. I counted twenty people in this meeting, which starting at the chair, Peter, who was number one and moving clockwise to Maggie, was the last person, number twenty. I was thirteen, the Rector twelve. My tutor Noel, seventeen, was there. Brian the security guard, nine, and Miriam from the refectory, eleven, were there too. The guy in position sixteen disturbed me and as the discussions went on about 'people define their own areas' he always dictated, or at least in my hypomanic state of awareness, seemed to cleverly guide the collective opinion to synchronise with his. I wrote his name down because I thought he might be the devil incarnate. It was Dennis Chorley, History of Media from Riding House Street, so he wasn't even on our campus yet he was shaping it's future. I wrote under his number sixteen, 'A very brilliant, cunning man'. I sat back to make sure the Rector could read it clearly. The meeting was magical for me, in the sense that if I was a professional snooker player or tennis player, this was the final I had trained all my life to win and everything was going to plan. I was at the top of my game, or as close as I was going to get to insanity. I absorbed and recorded all the cross section of insights about moving around within the confines of a university campus. We had just finished the 'Way Finding' module, based on the campus, that Eric had given us so I had research and understanding already. The thing is, great communication and design is all about insights and this meeting was a gold mine. That great feeling you get when you have an idea, that one when you cannot get it down fast enough, everything speeds up and you feel alive so much that your mind expands. You understand the world that little bit better. I had one of those but to the power of ten. In a one hour meeting, I wrote down this: The Eleven Commandments: 1) Security, Personal Safety 2) Attractive Environment 3) Social 4) Eating, Drinking 5) Buying Things and Services 6) Events 7) Information 8) Learning Environment 9) Pride and Belonging 10) Contact 11) Support. It may look like the ramblings of a madman but six years later this list, or a version of it, would eventually be published as part of the Telepress synopsis. Back in February 1995 I left the meeting having experienced a eureka! moment and not being able to transfer the inspiration. Jahan bumped into me in the refectory as I was leaving the meeting. I grabbed him by the shoulders. "Jah, will you do something for me?"

"Yeah man, what it is?"

"Just do that signage project as your major project. OK?"

"Which one?"

"That one we just did! I told you before, if you've got no idea what to do for your major project, you should do that. I'll help you."

"What, we'll do it together?"

"No. I've got something else in mind. Something big."

"Why don't we do that then?"

"Sorry Jah, you're not getting it. You do the signage project. I do mine but I'll help you out on yours."

"I dunno man, I think we exhausted that signage thing before. Anyway are you alright, you seem agitated?"

"Never better mate. Never better."

"Do you wanna hang around while I get a pint of milk and a flap jack?"

"Sorry Jah, gotta shoot. Too much to do. Later."

"Laters. Take it easy Vic."

Thing was, I didn't take it easy at all. I went back to the studio and got everyone else in the vicinity of my desk to sign, date and witness a few equations next to some scribbles of eleven commandments because I was going to be famous for this eureka! moment. It was going to bring great things and it had to be protected. My class mates were a bit confused and probably thought it was a joke but I took their signatures to the front desk and got the whole thing sealed and date stamped. It then got posted to my parents house for safe keeping.

Over the weekend I couldn't settle and Lewis noticed. He popped round to see Tanya and between them decided I needed to see a film so on the Sunday night she turned up looking to make things right and they both convinced me to see Leon. Nath didn't want to participate because his new best friend Rory was coming round to work on their latest project together. So off we set, for a ten past eight performance at the cinema on Station Road. The three of us took our seats near the centre, there were loads available. We sat there chatting, waiting for the previews to begin when in comes a rowdy mob of students from our campus, some of whom I barely knew but one of them was that Lyndsay girl who shagged Lewis at Christmas. Lewis hated her now because she got obsessed, started knocking on our door at all times of the night. She spotted us and nudged the rest of the gang towards our direction. They sat exactly one row behind us. She had balls. She also had popcorn and when the lights went down it was her exacting revenge to begin an assault of popcorn. The other members of her posse followed until I could take no more. I stood up, climbed over the seats towards them and began showering them, not with popcorn but, with double the amount of four letter words. I proper lost it, absolutely enraged and Lewis had to jump back and stop me lynching them. Tanya started apologising, staff came out and I demanded we move seats down towards the front. In angry whispered voices, both Lewis and Tanya started having a go at me as the actual film started. I felt betrayed by them, how could it be my fault? My heart was racing, my mind accelerated and then the guns started. The first sequence of Leon is a huge gun fight with lots of blood and violence. I had no idea what the film was about but I hadn't anticipated this and my eyes couldn't take the images, nor my ears the Dolby surround automatic weapons. I just told them both I was pissed off and going home but the truth was my head was caving in if I stayed in that theatre.

I got back to the flat and sat with Nath and Rory, watching them work, Nath controlling the computer. I told them a pack of lies when they asked why I was back so soon. Shit film, shit acting, shit dialogue. It didn't really matter what I said, they didn't care and they had better things to do. Eventually I got that feeling you get when you're not wanted so I went to bed with feelings of resentment, self-hatred and anger. I couldn't sleep for trying to work out all my relationships with everyone I knew. They all seemed damaged.

Two days later it was Valentine's day and due to my head being in books or facing a computer screen for the last eight weeks, I hadn't got anything for Tanya and I wanted to make

Mad in England - A memoir

it up to her so I decided to go into town on a travelcard and try central London. What happened next I can only describe as a 'trip' to a parallel reality. It was like my mind took a rest for most of the afternoon without the aid of any hallucinogenic substance. It could only be mania. I can't remember where I got off the tube but most of the latter part of the morning and early afternoon I browsed Oxford Street, Charing Cross Road and most of Covent Garden. I felt I was being guided by signs on posters or album sleeves and books. Without consciously trying, I had reached that religious state again where the world revolved around me. That I was controlling space, time and the physics involved to enable me to watch as life unfolded before me. The sad thing about it is nobody could tell I wasn't well and Londoners would do nothing anyway even looking the way I did. At one point of consciousness I found myself in a bookshop on Neal Street because it had Wilbur Smith's book Sun God in the window. I looked at it's vibrant turquoise jacket, an Egyptian sunset over a silhouetted pyramid and it felt like it had been instantly put in that window by a higher source. Wilbur Smith was my dad's favourite author and I'd grown up with those books all over the house, on shelves and bedside tables. It had to be about me. I am the Sun God and this book is the proof. I shall buy it for my dad right now.

After I had it in a plastic bag I felt like I was carrying The Bible around Tottenham Court Road so I decided I had the power to heal and change people's lives. Each beggar I came across, I would withdraw £10 from the cashpoint next to them, put it in their hands and place my other hand on the top of their heads. "Bless you, my friend. You're gonna be ok, I swear. Things will get better. Goodbye, God bless." I know I did this about sixteen times because my bank statement told me later I'd spent nearly £200 that afternoon. At one point I found myself outside the church on Tottenham Court Road and stopped to talk with anyone wearing a red ribbon supporting the Terrence Higgins Trust.

Victor J Kennedy

In my little world of signs and icons, that ribbon meant you were HIV positive so I gave each person a hug and put my hand on the top of their heads and blessed them. They would now be cured.

I popped in to see Isaac and Simon in the Webmedia studios under Cyberia, the cybercafe where I'd done all my research on Goodge Street. They had no idea anything was array. I just looked like I'd been shopping, not saving the world. We had a little chit chat about this and that, Isaac asked me, "If you want a drink you should help yourself." He pointed towards a filter coffee maker on the back wall. As I walked down towards it I saw an old fifties radio on the floor with all it's wires hanging out. Again, my manic brain worked out in four seconds flat that Isaac and Simon were actually astronauts sent back in time to come and get me. They were a threat and I should get out of there NOW! I looked at Isaac, straight faced and asked "Is this your time machine?" "What, the filter machine? Yeah, man. That machine certainly makes me work far too many hours than I really should."

"I think I'll pass on the drink Isaac, I've gotta go. It's Valentine's day and all that." Hopefully they couldn't tell I was on to them.

"No problem Vic, you take care mate. Keep in touch, we might need you when you've graduated."

Keep in touch? With a pair of intergalactic time travelling pirates, coming back in time to steal my invention from me? No chance. I was out of there, on the tube back to Harrow, slightly afraid that there were higher forces at work. That feeling of being chased but not knowing by whom. Like in a dream or a nightmare.

I got back to the flat with nothing for Tanya, not even a card. I picked one up from an off-licence shop with bigger ambitions and then popped round hers to ask her out for a romantic dinner at Pizza Express outside the station. It wasn't romantic at all, it was like peace talks. She also did a lot of worrying and I made sure I didn't mention any of the strange thoughts I'd been having, otherwise it would turn into the Spanish inquisition. I handed over my card and she gave me two back. The first one was a rustic design in reds and oranges and pinks. It read simply, in her handwriting,

Victor. Just to say I love you. Tanya xxxxxxxxxx

The second one was more bizarre and obviously a reference to the amount of time I'd been awake over the last few weeks. It had a black front with a pair of eyes and a thought bubble saying, If I had a penny for every minute I lay awake dreaming about you... On the inside of the card it read,...I'd be the richest insomniac in the World.

Happy Valentine's Day. All my love as always. x

Tanya had a skill, or should I call it a quality, for hitting your heart where it hurts. It's like someone caring for you so much that it takes advantage of you. Over that pizza we tried to solve all our problems, including Gideon as well as my money situation which was now terrible after buying the computer. Tanya always wanted to help, even when we weren't seeing eye to eye and although we didn't work everything out and the meal ended frostily, the following day I found this note left in my bedroom.

Dear Vic,

I seem to have missed you, but had to leave as my dad arrived. I've included my Visa card in case you need any money (4901). Take as much as you need and we can sort it out later, but don't go without.

I love you more than ever, so sorry I missed you. I wanted so much to see you for a cuddle. I'm glad everything's okay between us now – I love you.

Be brave, don't worry and I'll see you soon.

All my love, Tanya. Xxxxxxxxxx

Victor J Kennedy

She'd left it under my keyboard, the only place she could guarantee I would find it because my bedroom was upside down, like my head. The flat was a shit hole too. It had been ruthlessly neglected by all three of us. The systems we had in place in September were gone. It was anarchy and in the scheme of things it felt like I was doing everything, Lewis was doing his best, which was shit and Lord Nath of Foreman was off round Shumana's palace or his mum's mansion to get fed, watered and cleaned. I'd stayed at Tanya's the night before, so when I saw the state of it, I'd had it. With Nath at least. Mauli phoned mid-afternoon and said Alan was watching the Ireland v England friendly at his mum's favorite Irish pub in Wealdstone and would we like to go? I told Mauls to come over at 7 and we would walk down for kick off. By the time he'd turned up I had completely cleaned the whole flat but left every dirty dish piled up outside Nath's bedroom door, ready for him when he finally got his lazy, fat arse back in the flat. Mauli absolutely loved it when he came round. He was giggling in his Malaysian high pitched voice for about ten minutes before I said we had to leave in case we were late for the football. For the next thirty minutes, all the way down to meet Alan, we took Nath to pieces. All the pent up emotion from the last two years of duress came flooding out of Mauli, with full support and agreement from me.

By the time I got to the pub I was wound up so I ordered a pint of Guinness and sat down amongst Alan's family and friends, who appeared to have been drinking all day. This fact didn't help when English hooligans began tearing up Lansdowne Road and fighting the Irish fans after Kelly had scored for the Irish. The game was abandoned 27 minutes into the first half and everybody in the bar went nuts, drunkenly blaming the English nation and scaring me out of the bar. Obviously Malaysians were okay so Mauli stayed. On the walk back I became massively agitated and over sensitive to any pedestrian's body language as they approached and passed me. I convinced myself that I was going to get my head kicked in any minute now. That was my perception after what I'd just witnessed. I felt there was an air of it, some kind of disturbance in the universe due to the fairness of time. There were times of peace and times of war and since Heysel in 1985 I'd lived through a peaceful time but now? Like a superhero I sneaked my way, under the cover of darkness, back to Tanya's and proceeded to tell her, using verbal diarrhoea, every detail of my afternoon and evening. From my passion towards Nath's 'washing up lesson' to how the world is becoming a more violent place again. She ran me a bath, gave me a massage and put me to bed but my mind didn't switch off. She dropped off to sleep beside me but once again I went through my ritual of thinking about everything and anything, three million times over until the sun slowly made it's way around the planet again.

It was now a couple of days since Valentine's day. It could have been five for all I knew. At this point I had lost all rational notions of purpose, there were no college deadlines and I knew it was between semesters. The dead zone. The thing is, it was more than that. I was starting to take a holiday from reality, like that carefree feeling you had in the middle of your six weeks' holiday from school, three weeks in just before the end became closer than the start. It's like zero responsibilities, slightly anaesthetised to any form of structure, especially time. I was whimsical and I still had my over generous head on. After breakfast I decided I wanted to say thanks to Tanya's mum for single handedly saving our relationship a few weeks before with her mother Teresa-like mission from Woodford to my bedside, counselling me back to her daughter's side.

I walked into the flower shop, chest puffed out and said to the girl behind the counter, "You're Interflora, right?"

"Yes we are but it's a minimum of £10 bouquets for delivery."

"That's fine, because I want to send the best bunch of flowers you have."

Victor J Kennedy

"Ok, that would be the Summer Pageant bouquet with Lillies and Roses."
"Look it's fine," I interrupted, "I've got my card."
"It's £45 sir, is that ok?
"I said it's fine so it's fine." She filled out the slip in triplicate before asking, "And what's the card message sir?"
I thought for a second before deciding the nicest thing I could call her was 'mum,' at least that was my megalomaniac projection of how she would receive it. "Just put; Thanks mum from Victor and Tanya." She'd get it! I was sending great thoughts towards her so that when she got the flowers she would see everything and understand what I understand. After I'd done that good deed, I strolled through the town centre shops for what seemed like minutes but was actually hours. This afternoon of quiet contemplation and observation calmed my whole constitution, the input of external stimuli and the idle nature with which I absorbed it left me at peace, like a contented sponge. This stable mood was shattered after I had finally plodded back to the flat.
As I made it back to the top of the stairs I noticed the pots and pans were missing from Nath's bedroom door. I shouted out but no one was home. I turned left down the corridor to my room and was confronted by a note on my door from Nath.

Dear Vic,
I hope you find the washing up and general tidiness of the flat to your satisfaction. I know I've been spending a lot of time at Shumana's but there was no need for this. I don't know what to say? Maybe I just need some time out, move away from things before it gets out of control. I'm going back to Rickmansworth to see my parents now. If you need to talk, ring me: 0923 284 337

Your friend,
Nath

Mad in England - A memoir

I felt terrible and instantly sat down at the top of the stairs and phoned the number which went straight to answering machine. "Hi, this is Joshua and Evette Foreman. We're both away for the next few weeks at the villa so if it's urgent you'll have to ring the office on 0171 686 2040 and they'll get in touch with me. Otherwise, leave a message after the tone."

"Oh fuck" I thought, as I quickly put the phone down before the tone started, he knows they've gone away and he's not answering the phone. But why would he do that? Because he was about to do something drastic which only his parents would find on their return. "Oh fuck, oh fuck." I've really upset him and with all this pressure of the dissertations, RCA applications not to mention how difficult I must have been making his life recently that he's decided to end it! My mind was projecting and assuming.

I read the note again another ten times, each time finding added meaning and subtext, like I was jousting with Nath's intellect, decoding the emotional bombs while looking for a method or a way that I could stop him before he did it. I rang the number again and waited for the tone, "Yeah Nath, er, it's Vic. Look mate, I'm really sorry about those pots and pans. It was a stupid joke and I shouldn't have done it, can you pick up the phone if you can hear my voice?.....er, maybe just ring the flat when you get this message. I'll be here, I'm not going anywhere tonight so if you fancy coming back we could talk and stuff."

I put the phone down and started pacing around the flat as my brain went into overdrive. I walked in the kitchen and it was absolutely spotless apart from three mugs left out on the centre of the empty kitchen top. I carefully leant forward to get a closer look at the arrangement. Tightly sandwiched between the Nescafe cup I used frequently and Lewis's Dairy Milk cup, was Nath's "favorite" floral mug, which he ALWAYS drank out of because it was a gift from someone special. As I stared at the composition, like a piece of art, I translated the meaning into an insecure kid wrestling between mine and Lewis's attention. I felt sorry for him, almost sad for where we had ended up, until I stood up straight and looked around the rest of the environment, the gallery or maybe even the theatre. Call it what you will, I was deteriorating again into the mindset of a Crime Scene Investigator and this flat harboured a psychopath, the clues were everywhere. The actual truth being that the flat harboured someone struggling to hold off a psychosis. With no idea what a psychosis was but imminently about to experience one.

I moved out of the kitchen slowly into the lounge and noticed the ironing board was closed but lying flat on the carpet like a surf board. On top of it was a die-cast model of Pocahontas, from the Disney film which had just come out. I read this display as a warning from Nath to Dean, through me that he needed to back off or suffer violence. I related this back to my experience of Nath and Rory with the replica Reugers last term. I'd also seen how he operated with Mauli last year and the strength he displayed, not to mention his ultra competitive streak when playing football with the Monday night lads in the gym.

There was stuff to interpret everywhere, I was like a small child seeing things for the first time and finding everything slightly magical but at the same time disturbing as I felt they unveiled Nath for who he really was. I looked at his drawing of the three amigos from the year before, bluetacked to the wall like a trophy. However innocent that insignificant scribble was I was overwhelmed by it and had to take it down before it brainwashed me. I hid it under my bed and then went into Nath's room. I rooted through most of his drawers but only found the usual nonsense. I made sure I was extra careful not to disturb anything unless it was mine. I would then reclaim it, taking it back to my room to hide it under my fortress-like bed. I got really freaked on my final return to find his own personal collection of original Star Wars figures. The sight of his own private collection was chilling and I had to leave his room before I had a panic attack. He was stealing my identity!

I put on my Beautiful South Greatest Hits CD to calm down but I couldn't choose a track which would be suitable to calm my mood. I was helpless, unable to even listen to music or settle down in such a claustrophobic space. I reached for the phone and my little black address book to get some answers.

I rang Shumana's house, Ruth answered, "Heeelllo!"

"Ruth, it's Vic. Look, is Nath there?"

"I don't think so but Shumana's not been down from her bedroom all day. Are you alright Vic, you sound funny?"

"I'm not great to be honest but I think something's happening with Nath and need to contact him. Can you check if Shumana's there?"

"Sure, hang on Vic." I heard her footsteps run upstairs and knock on Shumana's bedroom door but I couldn't make out what was said. Two sets of footsteps came back down and Shumana picked the phone up and put on her sweetest voice, "Hi Vic, what's up?"

"Is Nath there?"

"No, I haven't seen him all day."

"When did you see him last?"

"Oh god Vic, what's a matter with you?"

"Why can't you just answer the question?"

"I think it was a couple of nights ago."

"You think? Surely you know when you last saw your boyfriend?"

"Look Vic, why are you getting angry at me? It was two nights ago because I didn't see him at all yesterday ok?"

"I'm not angry, I'm just worried because he left me a note and has gone home to Rickmansworth. I rang the house but it's gone to answering machine and the message says his mum and dad are in the South of France, so he's on his own."

"Mmmmmm, I don't know what to say?"

"If he rings you, please, please tell him to contact me or at least let him now I need to talk to him."

Victor J Kennedy

"Ok, no problem. See you Vic." The phone went dead and once again I felt like she'd got the upper hand in that conversation, all airy and carefree on the execution but ruthless on the delivery. That woman got to me. Full stop. I made phone calls for the rest of the afternoon and early evening, working myself into a real frenzy, playing my favourite dance compilation tapes and drinking coffee until somebody finally rang me. It was Ruth and she asked if I was ok, then invited herself over. Five minutes later, after jogging across the iron bridge, she was ringing the door bell. I let her in, she hugged me and we sat on the stairs talking for what felt like hours about the current fucked up state I'd found myself in. She opened up too, explaining everything about her deteriorating relationship with Shumana, her views on Nath and their maltreatment of the people closest to them. She demonstrated this perfectly by telling me that Nath had emerged from Shumana's bedroom at dinner time to pop out, in his car for some food. That meant they both lied. They both coerced. They both deceived me and that made me rage with anger because I was trying to find out if he was still alive. That observation was the reason Ruth took action and came over, at least I hoped that's why she brought the truth. Maybe she wanted to gossip because at times the conversation contained some cutting vitriol, with real and honest hatred. My mind also wandered into the prospect that Ruth was a spy sent by Nath and Shumana.

As it got towards midnight, I offered to walk Ruth back over the bridge and through the park. We said our goodbyes, I said thanks and then Ruth grabbed my hands, looked me in the eye and said, "Just take care of yourself Vic." When I got back to Manor Road I didn't fancy staying in the flat on my own so I woke up Tanya by throwing stones at her window. She let me in but before I got into bed, I had to tell her everything that Ruth had just told me. I could tell Tanya was exhausted and wasn't listening so I stripped down to my boxer shorts and got into bed next to her. She turned the light off and got into her classic fall asleep position on her side. I didn't cuddle up to her, I just lay on my back and stared at the ceiling till my eyes got used to the darkness. Once again the thoughts and anxieties started to descend from the ceiling where I was transfixed. I began processing the problems without finding answers. There was silence in the room, the house and the street. My ears began to focus into every creak of every floorboard and any drip from the bathroom taps. I was completely tuned into my own universe which only existed in shadow as the earth spun. It was a universe I'd been visiting far too often in the past few weeks. Thoughts began to race through my head, jumping from idea to idea or playing out future scenarios like scripts, where I never fail to come out on top in confrontations with Shumana and Nath.

Hours must have passed without moving physically but my mind had travelled a vast distance. Tanya had moved a few times and I felt very pleased with myself that I was allowing her some sleep, rather than involving her in my trauma which was about to get a whole lot worse.

As I stared at the ceiling I spotted a hole, the diameter of which was similar to that of a drill bit. The edges of the hole were in agreement with the drill exiting on our side, which meant someone from above, from Cathy's room had drilled a hole through the floor to look down on Tanya (and me) in bed. Fucking deviant, like that bloke I'd seen on that Shallow Grave film, drilling fucking holes through the ceiling from the attic and frightening his flat mates. I thought about it and the hole started to scare me but I kept staring and thinking. I was trying to work out who was guilty of peeping. Then I heard Cathy turn over on her antiquated futon. I imagined her being forced into the bed, restrained by a male hand angry at her for moving because that would give the game away. The bloke held her still but was staring down the hole at me, smiling, almost laughing. It's her dad I thought! I'd remembered him from that visit in the first year, to Tring where she grew up and he'd freaked me out then. Cathy had also told us a few stories about her tough upbringing and this was it, unfolding above me. The jealous father turns up at his daughter's university digs, rapes her and then holds her captive before going after the other four girls in the house. It seemed so simple, so obvious the more and more I thought about it. I spent the next few hours as the sun came up, preparing for the breakout, exactly how I was going to set these girls free and get that pervert locked up once and for all. I didn't once think through the realistic consequences before I acted. I just jumped up out of the bed and locked the bedroom door from the inside, then pulled out the key holding it tightly in my fist. I moved towards the window and dragged Tanya's dressing table to one side to get the larger window open. Tanya woke up at this point with a startled question, "Vic, what on earth are you doing?" I jumped on the bed and put one hand over her mouth and the other towards mine, two fingers over my lips to confirm I needed silence and this really was vital. I then gestured her towards the end of the bed to make sure she was away from the drill hole, then it was safe to talk. I whispered, "There's a madman upstairs and he's holding Cathy hostage."

"Have you been taking something?" she frowned.

"No, nothing. Look, I've been listening to him raping her all night. I've not slept a wink, I just couldn't."

Tanya took evasive action. She tried the locked door and started shouting through the walls, "Sam! Cathy! Shelly! Miriam! Can someone please come up with the spare key to my room please?!"

"What are you doing that for? He's just gonna come down with a knife to Cathy's throat." I pleaded.

"You're not well Vic." She shouted.

"I'm fine but you've got to trust me on this one." I moved towards the window again and this time opened it wide. I looked out and saw some school kids going to school and a milkman so I thought I would do some shouting aswell, "Oi! MATE! LOOK! HERE, AT THE WINDOW! CALL THE POLICE, THERE'S A MADMAN IN THE HOUSE!!" The response was not good enough for my liking and now the girls were all outside Tanya's bedroom door. I picked up a pint glass with Tanya's water in and threw it far out on to the road, where it smashed. "Oi, MATE!" I threw another glass, a perfume bottle and a coffee cup, "Oi! CALL THE COPS NOW!!!" Tanya was crying now, screaming at the girls through the door, "Where's the fucking key? You've gotta let me out, he's throwing my stuff out the window!"

"We can't find the key Tanya, who did you give it to?"

"It's in Miriam's room on the window sill." I left the window and calmly walked up to Tanya by the door. She slid down it to her knees in terror. I lent over her and whispered, "It's pointless asking them, he's with them and he's got a knife to Cathy's throat. Don't worry, I'm gonna climb out the window and get help." I moved towards the window and Tanya shouted, "Quick, he's jumping out of the window!" As I looked down I could see Cathy's Land Rover parked right under the window. It was not more than six feet to it's roof. I could make it easily I thought, so I dangled my legs out but Cathy came running out with her car keys. "What are you doing Cathy? Be careful." I warned her.

"I'm moving the Land Rover so you can't get out." I gesticulated towards the front door below my feet, trying to mouth the words, "Is he there? Is he standing in the doorway? Can he see me?" All I got were vacant looks from all three other house mates now gathered at the door. Shelly ran out of the front door as I threw another cup out, followed by a glass ash tray. I saw her go into a neighbours and point back towards me from the doorstep. The whole thing was pandemonium for the next five minutes before the police arrived and threatened to knock the bedroom door down if I didn't open it. This went on for longer than it should have because I couldn't trust them. That part of me was gone. I was psychotic. They had to explain to me that no one was in the house and I would be fine, Tanya would be fine and the girls were all fine, if a little shocked. Eventually I let both Policemen in and they ran towards me, pushed me to the

floor, then one of them held me while the other let Tanya
'escape' from the real madman in the house, me.
They sat on the edge of the bed and interviewed me for ages
about such things as when was the last time I'd taken drugs
and whether I'd been sleeping badly or was stressed. Each
question was like a reality check that I didn't pass. All the
girls gave statements before I was escorted back to my flat,
which was hugely embarrassing, actually it was humiliating
because Shelly had phoned Dean, who was outside with
Diago and Jase. All three were perched on their mountain
bikes outside looking sad as I got frog marched down the
road. It was like a neighbourhood scene from ET. Once I had
changed clothes, washed and had my home inspected I was
paraded back to the squad car and taken to my doctor's
surgery. Once I had answered the same questions to the
doctor he prescribed three Valium tablets for the next three
nights to break the insomnia. I was also told to rest, possibly
have a break from college. The thing is, I had completely
gone by this point. "Off with the fairies" some people call it.
In my head I now believed there was a conspiracy to take me
out, to obstruct my progress towards completion of a
grandiose ambition to make Telepress. I knew but they
couldn't get to me because I was playing a role of someone
who was compliant. I agreed to everything the two
policemen and one doctor advised me to do but underneath I
was convinced they were aliens. Part of the conspiracy
against me. They were evil, whatever they were and I had to
fight it, whatever 'it' was.
The squad car dropped me back at Tanya's who was
magically packed and ready to travel. Her eyes were red and
inflamed, puffy like she hadn't stopped crying for the whole
time I was at the doctor's. "Where are we going?" I joked.
"I've rung your mum and dad, they're really worried about
you. They said they would come down this afternoon but I
said it would be best if you weren't near college. It's not
doing you any good Vic." She started crying again, I could
see how destroyed she was. I'd done a bad thing, I could feel

it in the pit of my stomach. She pulled herself together and said, "I've put some of your stuff in this bag, Lewis let me in. He's going to look after your stuff and Dean has let your tutor's know what's happened. I rang my mum and she said I can borrow the car for a couple of days so I can take you home to your mum's. I think it's best you take some time out because you're not well are you?" She took my arm and we shuffled off towards Northwick Park Tube Station for the journey to Woodford. When we got there her mum was waiting at the tube station in the car. Tanya got in the driver's seat, me with my bag on the back seat and her mum in the passenger seat. Nothing much got said until I pulled out my Valium prescription so we stopped off to get that at a chemist. We dropped her mum off at work and then popped back to Tanya's house so she could bring some extra things. Her dad was trying to convert the front garden to a car port and there was a pile of pebbles ready to lay. While Tanya dashed upstairs, I picked up a big pebble and studied it. It was fantastic, ergonomically perfect for a remote control for Telepress, I surmised. It was cold in my hand, this was February after all. With all this analysis my mind traffic was still going at a hundred miles an hour because I'd decided not to take any Valium before bedtime. I got back in the car and hid the stolen pebble under my passenger seat while she came back. When we made it safely onto the M1 I loosened my seat belt, put my hand between my knees and proudly produced the rock, while announcing I had found the interface for my big idea, the final part of the jigsaw. I also told her to look in her driver's mirror and see the past leaving us behind, look out of the windscreen and see the future. This was the start of a verbal onslaught for the next two hundred and fifty miles for Tanya. I talked a lot. I talked fast. I dominated conversations. I felt like a man of destiny, maybe even destined to change the world. I was suspicious and felt hostile thoughts towards many unmarked lorries and vans, like they were chasing me with people hidden inside, trying to stop me achieving a successful journey. The same paranoia was projected onto factories or refineries that we passed which had no signage or means of identification. In my cinematic psychotic world they were terrorist cells producing horrible chemicals or nuclear bombs, which were then transported around the country in unmarked lorries and vans. What ever happened to England's green and pleasant land? All I could see was an infestation of evil that needed cleaning out. As we reached Birmingham I looked up at the moon and imagined it to be a space station that Nath lived in and controlled the world. That all this was just a software program running which he had designed in a distant future but would come to an end in the past, our present. But why 1995? It must be me, I must be about to invent Telepress and he is trying to stop me.

At Manchester the heavens opened and a huge storm began. Tanya was petrified as the windscreen wipers hardly coped with the battering of water and the wind blowing the car about. I put it all down to Nath controlling the weather and he knew I was about to reach my goal so he pulled out his joker card. I talked her in past Preston, Lancaster, off at junction 35 by Carnforth and then home. We made it! An entirely different kind of journey to the one in the opposite direction three years before with my dad.

My mum came out and hugged us both, she'd helped carry in the luggage and made a cup of tea. Then she started asking the same questions as the police and the doctor. I was fine with it all because I was playing a role again, this time the happy-go-lucky son. I shrugged everything off nonchalantly but my mum could tell by the state of Tanya that something traumatic had occurred overnight down in London. She said, "Why don't you go up to bed love? I've made up your own bed so Tanya can sleep in your sister's room in peace." I complied but I knew she wanted me out of the room to interrogate Tanya for a full version of the truth. As I got upstairs I went to the loo. After I'd finished I put my hand in my pocket and pulled out the pill bottle, looked at it, decided it was poison and flushed all three Valium tablets down the toilet. They couldn't get me now.

Surprisingly I had a good night's sleep, which was probably down to the home comforts and familiar smells. Who knows? But I was up early, downstairs for a bowl of bran flakes and a coffee. I read a week old copy of the Westmorland Gazette, checking out the sports pages for anyone I knew or had played against in the past. Eventually my mum came down in her dressing gown and sat next to me. She gave me a stern look and grabbed my hand with vigour, then looked me in the eye, "What are we going to do with you, eh?" Her eyes were pink and puffy. Tanya walked into the kitchen with a packed bag, her car keys in her hand with an anxious look on her face. I instantly had a bad feeling in my stomach, "Where are you going?" I asked. "I've got assessments on Monday for my patterns to go into the major project. I haven't finished them yet so I need to go back to Harrow." I looked at my mum, who looked guilty and then back at Tanya in silence. Even though my mind was not exactly firing on all cylinders I could tell that wasn't the only reason for leaving me there. She'd delivered the catastrophy two hundred and fifty miles north to unsuspecting parents and now Tanya needed to escape the nightmare. I thought about how, only weeks ago, after she had the keyhole surgery I'd been at Tanya's bedside, sleeping on the floor next to her. I went through it with her. I didn't run away or avoid the situation then, so I couldn't understand why she was not standing by me now? Looking at it from Tanya's point of view, she was probably still freaked out by her boyfriend and just had to get away. The silence was starting to get awkward before my mum stepped in, "Shall we see her out then Vic? I won't look while you two have a kiss and a cuddle." That was it, I had to submit and not cause a fuss, especially as I was still trying to deal with the 'fuss' I made twenty-four hours ago in Manor Road, hanging out of that window.

Victor J Kennedy

She gave me a limp kiss but an enthusiastic and quite caring hug, then she got into the car and drove off without looking back. She was probably still exhaling a sigh of relief by the time she got to the motorway junction. I felt a rush of foolishness run through me like I was simple, sort of child like. My childish thoughts took me to a near future, where all my friends sitting with Tanya chew the fat round a pub table, taking me to pieces. What a train wreck! What a fuck up! I was feeling humiliation and self loathing.

The rest of the Saturday I avoided anyone seeing me from the village. I watched my old club Crusaders play Halton on a very wet and muddy pitch from the window of the lounge while my mum served snacks for convalescents. I wished I was out there on the playing field, just like when I was sixteen and the world was simple and new. My dad came back wet from golf and asked a few more of those difficult questions, we had dinner and while watching Saturday night entertainment I suddenly decided I wanted to go and see my Nan just up in the village in her little flat, so me and my sister, who had arrived from Bradford that night, set off in the pouring rain. My mum hadn't told my nan anything about what had happened, just that I was at home for a few days. She didn't want to worry her but after me and my sister had left the flat, she levelled with my mum, "He's having a nervous breakdown, isn't he."

I took an early night and seemed to sleep ok, just had that weird 'did I or didn't I get much sleep?' feeling in the morning, which went pretty much the same as Saturday.

In the afternoon it was time for a super hyped up Sky Sports extravaganza of Manchester United playing host to the resurgent 'mighty' Leeds United, whose fans and a minority of hooligans were making the journey across the Pennines. The coverage was skewed towards the prospect of Man Utd losing and there being loads of fighting, started by the 'thugs' from Leeds. I had sat down to enjoy the game but in my frail mental state, I couldn't cope with the propaganda being spouted by Sky and I had to leave the house and go for a walk in the park.

Dermont Park is a huge deer park next to the river Kent on the edge of the estuary to Morecambe Bay. It has hills, trees, wildlife and due to it's size, you can often find yourself alone. The perfect antidote to hooligans and hype. I had a magical euphoric experience that afternoon as the winter sunshine streaked across the hills. While I analysed its topography from the shadows cast, comparing it to the shape of the bark on the corresponding trees as if they were mimicking their environment. I checked out snails and leaves, discovering things about nature I had never seen before. It was wonderful, honest and free from anxiety or paranoia. After two hours of peace all those feelings returned as I walked back to my parents house, hoping that the war of the roses had not broken out in Manchester. Luckily it hadn't, Man Utd 3-1 Leeds Utd and tea was on the table.

I spent the rest of the evening with my mum, taking about what happened in a relaxed way with low lighting, a glass of wine for mum and some water for me. She was trying to get to the bottom of why I lost it so I explained how hard I'd been working from right back in the first year. I pulled out my end of year appraisal from 1993 and began reading it out to her:

21/6/93 Victor Kennedy Level One. Tutor: Elena. Marks: The Graphic Experience 60% B, The Graphic Language 85% A, Information Carriers 73% A, Visual Representation 71% A.

Topics Covered: Victor likes the whole idea of exploring and pushing ideas around. Learning skills – really valuable experience from the design studio – Management and organisational skills – useful for working in groups – Had to work hard to get where he is today – flunked school...

All of a sudden I couldn't continue, "What's wrong?" my mum said.

"I don't know but I can't read any more of that. It's making me feel weird. I've got a funny feeling in my chest and I feel a bit hot."

I became very hot and went into the living room. I remember the TV was on, my dad was watching a news programme reporting two murders in Bradford. I marched up to the TV and turned it off. I then opened the patio doors gasping for breath and paced around in the fresh air. I couldn't stand it any longer

"Come on, let's get you up to bed." my mum suggested. She escorted me gently up the stairs, watched me brush my teeth and then tucked me into bed, putting her cool forehand over my brow just like she did when I was a kid. "How are you feeling now? Better?"

"Yeah, a bit better. Just stay here for a while and stroke my head."

"You're a real softie, aren't you?" I knew she was being affectionate but I was no softie, I was battling some sort of internal force. Something unfamiliar was inside my body and my mind which I was struggling to control.

"Mum. I feel better when you're here. Can you stay in here?"

"I can if you want but I'd rather you just give it a go on your own. Be brave!"

"Ok I'll try but I might need to come and get you in the night."

"Don't be disturbing your dad if you do. I'll leave the door open a bit so you don't make a bang when you open it. Try and come round my side of the bed so you don't wake him. Ok?"

"Ok mum." She kissed me on the forehead. I was being compliant again when I should have explained my needs a bit more. I wasn't being assertive. I felt like I was about to have a fit and she was off to bed.

I called her back in and said I was hungry, could she make me something to eat. So back down we went and she mustered up spaghetti on toast from a tin, in next to no time. When I sat down and started eating I felt massively ashamed of my behaviour and went into denial. I said something really irresponsible under the circumstances, "You have passed the test. I wanted to see how far you would go." She was not pleased to say the least and she escorted me back to bed as soon as I had swallowed the last piece.

"Night night love. We're only two doors away." and she was gone. I was in darkness inside a tiny attic room with a low ceiling and light shade to bump your head on. I had to open the curtains to let some of the orange street light in because I felt so claustrophobic. Then I had to let the windows open to let some air in because I couldn't breath. Then I had to close them again because I got too cold. Then I felt I should close the curtains because it was too bright. Then sit on the edge of my bed, lay back down, rollover, turn the pillows over, roll back and then sit up again. I tried lying flat on the carpet, one pillow and half a duvet but I couldn't settle anywhere. This routine went on for three hours of ritualistic obsessive-compulsive behavior until I accelerated myself into a frenzy again and had to find my mum for help.

I crept into their room, heart racing, I tiptoed around the bed and whispered at my mum's face like I used to as a small child, her eyes closed and mouth open.

"Mum............mum........wake up." She woke, startled by the closeness of my face and my warm, rapid breathing.

"Come on." she whispered as she threw the covers back, grabbed my sweaty hand and lead me back to my room. "Get into bed." she was quite stern at this point as I was trying her patience. We assumed the same position as before, her sat on the bed, my head against her leg. She began to stoke my head again in an attempt to soothe me. It didn't work. "I'm really agitated mum, there's stuff all around me. In my head, attacking me like wasps. I can't get it to go away and my heart rate is up like I've been running or something. Can I put my head on your lap for a bit?"

"Ok, if it helps." But I didn't find that stabilizing, I could hear her stomach and bowels but I wanted to hear her heart and her breathing and get in sync with it. As my head moved

up her body towards her chest I was thinking about Freud and that eternal desire to get back into the womb. I could hear her lungs and the air moving in and out. "That's it mum, just keep breathing like that. It will calm me down."
"What's wrong love?"
"Look, just don't talk. Breathe!" I think that demand frightened her because I had feedback as her heart rate picked up. It was like I was wrestling her in slow motion, pinning her to the bed and she was too scared to stop me. I didn't like the dynamic so I jumped up and pulled back the curtains before being blinded by streams of orange from the street lights. I screamed in pain as my retinas received the floods of colour. I thought I was tripping like being on LSD. Now I was frightened! My dad burst in the room and flicked the light switch. "AAAARRRGGGHH! TURN IT OFF YOU CUNT, YOU'RE FUCKING BLINDING ME!"
"Gerald, turn the light off please." my mum had the calmest voice now, she knew she was in a serious situation. My dad didn't.
"What's up? Why all the swear words son?"
"Shut up. Shut up. Don't say a fucking word and don't fucking move either! Mum, you stay on that bed and don't move either. I'm going to the toilet." My metabolic rate had increased and I starting pissing all the water out which I'd drank in the evening. I could hardly see so like a blind man, I used my hands and my memory of the house layout to get to the toilet. After emptying my bladder I then filled up a pint glass with water and scrambled back to my petrified parents, who were like shivering statues in the dark. At this point they had become hostages in their own home and because they cared so much, their compliance and patience allowed me to begin to fight and exhaust the panic attack. I can't remember how long this pattern of behaviour lasted but as soon as the water went down my throat, it seemed to be coming out the other end. By the early hours of the morning things were getting worse and my mum was finding it difficult to calm me. No amount of holding, touching,

stroking or talking seemed to work. I was so desperate now that I wished I hadn't thrown that fucking medication down the toilet.

I was now begging my mum to get help. A doctor. Not an ambulance as I couldn't bear the noise of the siren. Mum persuaded me that if she were to get help then I would have to let my dad stay with me. I agreed. I would've agreed to anything at this point. The GP was reluctant to come out, as there wasn't much that he could do. Casualty at the hospital couldn't give us any help and referred my mum back to our GP. She didn't know who else to turn to at this time in the morning, so she came back upstairs and managed to persuade me that she was exhausted and needed some sleep. She lay down on the other bed praying for me to go to sleep, so that she could sleep also. Her prayers were answered. When I woke, my dad was quietly sitting on a stool next to my bed, keeping his eye on his son. It was by far, the worst night of their lives. Their healthy, youngest child, 'the baby' had developed into this? They'd held hands, cried and prayed to 'him up there' to help us all get through this nightmare. Whatever on earth this nightmare was.

Lashing down with rain, with me covering my over sensitive ears with my hands to stop the deafening traffic noise, my parents escorted me to see Dr Wright, the village GP and he arranged for me to be checked out by a Dr Dawson. After a big chat with her she suggested I stay in hospital and I agreed. She made some calls and everything was set up, mum and dad took me home, we packed and jumped in the car. I made my dad drive at fifteen miles per hour all the way there because my head was still throbbing from the harrowing night before and with the G-Forces of each corner he took. Nobody spoke but every time he changed gear he held my mum's hand.

Walking into the ward was weird but I was not in a good state of mind anyway. There was all the beeping and security doors to go through, like I was gaining entry into the United Nations. We were greeted by different people, all with

Victor J Kennedy

smiley faces and everyone of them said, "You must be Victor. Nice to meet you." which was nice. We had a group chat in what they called a 'quiet' room, which had paintings of chrysanthemums on the wall and a snooker table in the corner. Everything was pastel or mauve. The nurses took down all my particulars, also my parent's phone number and put my wallet, travel card and keys in an old shoe box. That was the bit that freaked me out. I'd been wrongly arrested and put in a cell overnight when I was nineteen so I knew they took your belt and your shoes to stop any suicides. This now felt officious and dogmatic because they started interrogating me again like the police and the doctor had in London. My mum was helping me answer based on what Tanya had told her but the facts were slightly embellished so I decided to have a confessional. I let rip on every question until the nurses asked my mum and dad to leave the room. Once alone with the nurses I told them about all the drugs and the sex ...and the guilt ...and the religion. I felt pretty cleansed when I'd finished. I knew I was in 'trouble' and that this was serious now but I didn't even think about telling them of my constructed reality back in London or my beliefs about my purpose on this planet and the people I thought were trying to stop me from achieving great things.

After I appeared from the quiet room my parents said a sad goodbye but I didn't quite get it. I thought they were popping out for a coffee and they'd be back in a minute. I was shown my bed by someone I thought was a patient because he had a speech impediment and was as tall as Frankenstein's monster. He showed me his badge which was not on his lapel but down on the corner of his cardigan at ninety degrees. I didn't believe him and it made me sad that a patient had stolen a nurse's badge and was parading as a member of staff. But he was legit and I was breaking down. My distressed state continued for the next few hours, as I tried to get used to the other patients and their strange eccentricities. It reminded me of the Mos Eisley Cantina Bar in Star Wars with all the different monsters stopping off for a little break before they go about their business. What sort of a monster was I?

There were times when I was replacing heads on bodies and projecting or at least perceiving that these people were friends of mine or relatives coming to visit, yet they all looked so traumatized that I believed they'd been brought through some kind of worm hole in the space time continuum. So what year was this then? It was all very mad. When my mum and dad came back to visit that night I said, "I want to come home mum, I don't like it in here. This is not me."

"Look love, it's the best place for you right now."

"But I'm fine, I just need some sleep. In my own bed!"

"That didn't work before did it? These people know what they are doing and once they've assessed you, if they think you can come home, then I don't see why not."

"It's not fair." My attitude didn't change after that. My parents went home and I was given a white shiny pill, like a mint with a sugar coating, before I went to bed. I slept. Andre Whittaker NA (Nursing Assistant) in the red team was my key worker. I had to report to him about everything and anything I needed. He was from Leeds and I reckon he hated anyone who supported local rivals Bradford because he was a right twat to me. I disliked the man, I couldn't help it. I overheard him talking about my admission as I walked past the nursing team's office, "It's cruel I know, but I always get allocated the stress heads. I wish Edwin would give me patients on the opposite end, you know? Less fidgety." he said to another NA regarding the fact I was designated to his care. I instantly felt compelled to walk in because the door was wide open and confront him. My mum worked in the x-ray department as a clerk. I knew where it was in relation to the ward I was in so I thought I would go and visit her. At least then I could slag him off to her, get my mum to complain and hopefully move to another, more compatible key worker. I stuck my head round the door, "Andre, I'm just popping down to x-ray to see my mum ok?"

Victor J Kennedy

"You'll need a coat then."
I referenced the Fast Show catch phrase, "Ah, okay I'll get
me coat!" I raced back to my bed and put on my jacket, I got
back to the main entrance to the ward and pushed through
the doors. As soon as I did this, I broke a connection
between the two doors which set off an alarm in the office
like a high pitched electronic beep. Andre came running
after me, I was almost outside the doctor's secretaries
offices. "Victor, stop. Where are you going?"
"I'm going to see my mum?" I was confused now.
"You can't do that mate."
"Why not?"
"Because you can't leave the ward. You're not well."
"But you said I could get me coat?" I referenced the Fast
Show catch phrase again.
"I'm sorry, I was joking. I didn't think you were serious."
"My mum's just down that corridor. Why don't you just let
me go? I've got me coat!" Catch phrase again.
"I can't, I'll get in trouble by my boss. I'm supposed to be
keeping my eye on you Victor and I can't do that if you're
not on the ward. Come on, let's go back." I was so angry I
could've exploded. My liberty was being taken away and I
was imprisoned in a self enclosed unit. This was effectively
prison and I felt I'd committed no crime. When was I going
to get out?
When we got back on the ward he explained to me that I had
been placed under a seventytwo hour detainment order under
Section 4 of the Mental Health Act. I just wanted to go
home. I couldn't deal with all this. At twentythree years old
my reality had just gone wrong. Badly wrong! I walked into
a quiet room, sat down in an upright chair and began staring
at the lightbulb in some kind of silent protest. This turned
out to be the most frightening part of the whole breakdown.
After thirty minutes sat in that position I ended up in what I
can only describe as a semi-paralysed state, where every
muscle in my body relaxed apart from my heart, which
increased it's rate so high the doctor's had to stop me from

arresting. They were outside my world but I could see them in my peripheral vision. They were rushing around me in a blur, pumping drugs into my arm, oxygen into my mouth and checking my blood pressure. In my mind everything seemed very calm and the light bulb was very comforting, like a place I was escaping to but that trance-like rejection of my life was wrapped inside multiple layers of anxiety, confusion and fear that took me to the greatest panic attack I've ever experienced or survived from. It was frightening for my family too, my mum wrote this entry in her diary:

I phoned Edwin (Staff Nurse) and he told me to expect a great change in Vic. My god what a change. He was sitting in a chair holding on to the arms, his face and eyes looking up to the ceiling and no movement whatsoever other than breathing through his mouth which was wide open. Edwin wanted me to go in and talk to him so they could observe Vic's reaction if any... I found the strength and went in, touching his hand and talking to him. He squeezed my hand and as I moved across, his eyes did seem to follow me. I could not stay with him for too long as it was too upsetting. What on earth was happening to him. I sat in the nurses office and Edwin came to talk. I was crying. I had this terrible fear of death. It seemed so close.

There was no neat and tidy end to this. Just the darkness of unconsciousness after the drugs had taken effect. I don't know if they put me on a stretcher or over someone's shoulder but in the morning, rejoice, I woke up in my hospital bed. I had been moved away from the male ward and into my own private room, curtains closed.
There is no right or wrong in this situation. Good or bad doesn't exist here, only opinions. My life was in their hands so was my gentle head.
After I had shuffled around the ward for a cup of tea and some toast the Staff Nurse and two other Nursing Assistants from the red team took me into the infamous quiet room and

sat me down. They explained to me what had happened, 'a Stress Induced Hypomanic episode', the seriousness of it and the implications moving forward. My life was about to change forever. They did it in a kind and compassionate way but it didn't lessen the blow when they served me my Section 2 papers and told me to have a good read. I was being held 'for the interests of his or her own health or safety and for the protection of others'.

Section 1 of the 1983 Mental Health Act explains what the Act is about and who it is intended to deal with. It attempts to provide a legal, rather than a medical definition of the four types of mental health problems the Mental Health Act is intended to cover. Severe Mental Impairment, Mental Impairment, Psychopathic Disorder, and Mental Illness.

Section 2 allows the authorities to keep you detained for assessment for up to twentyeight days, section 3 is for treatment for up to six months, section 4 is for emergency admission for up to seventytwo hours.

So I knew I would be looking at a twentyeight day stretch, with an assessment or 'ward round' once a week before I would be allowed to leave. I was told if I tried to leave before then, the police would come and catch me, then bring me back.

The ward rounds were me, sat in front of a social worker, psychiatrist, occupational therapist, solicitor and various members of the nursing team, who would bring the extensive notes they keep about your progress. I found ward rounds intimidating because, it was like a job interview infront of an audience when you have the biggest hangover of your life.

One of the nurses handed me a blue hardback notebook and advised me to start a diary. She said it would help recovery, especially if I put my thoughts and feelings down. So when I felt well enough I did.

Vic Kennedy's Major Escape: Monday 20th February to Monday 10th April is 49 days.

Mad in England - A memoir

I counted the days in scribbled groups of seven, like on a jailbird's walls.

Thursday March 2nd – I have no solitude. No break. I must spend time with me. Why am I here? Stupid mistakes. So sorry.
It was a bad day. I must have my solitude, I must have my solitude, I must have my solitude, I must have my solitude. I cried with mum today. We both got upset. This diary might help me get back to 'normal.' Bed at 8:30pm.

Friday March 3rd – Awake at 5:50am. Can't get back off. I think I'm turning into my dad. I'm bored as soon as I realise where I am again. Frieda is stuck in the bog and is trying to find the door handle, she's been in there for 10 minutes. I wish I had a camera. This place is so funny/comical sometimes. I think I'll have porridge today as I'm planning a late night, Fantasy Football is on BBC2.

8:10am no date. Fed up of them taking the piss out of me. It's not funny any more. I'm sick to death of being whispered about and helping them with ward round. Meal times are shite! Not funny at all. I want out! ASAP!
I must start to behave. I must start to get better. I don't know why I'm here. I do 'know' know but I'm so dazed and confused. I got rushed in! All I want in life is to help others and to be happy. Being stuck in here and having your independence taken away is like putting a lion in a cage. Or to quote today's news (I have watched it twice) which is all about fox hunting. I feel like the fox and the hunters are trying to dig me out. I'm not even allowed to be responsible enough to make a phone call on my own. I feel like a little kid who has reins strapped to his back, like rubber bands. Or it could be like a dog on a lead that can only be let out so far before being brought back to the kennel and locked tightly inside. I know this is for my safety and for the 'safety of others' but I'm not a violent person. OK, I may have broken

someone's jaw with one punch when I was 19 but I was looking after younger kids than myself at the time. Meal times are really tough!

9:45am no date: All hell has broken loose. Esther's fallen. Frieda's on the bog again. Paul's room is going mental. No sorry, outside the workmen are going mental and now all the patients are going mental including me! This place has become funny again. And I'll forgive the cleaner (June) for patronising me because she didn't know that I'm getting better. I think I'm getting better a bit too quick sometimes. This place isn't too bad!

They're giving me brain relaxant. Paranoid thoughts. Not ready yet. Back to square one. Monitoring.

Questions for ward round
What am I taking? Has it been altered since I started the medication? What about physio? What are your thoughts about my circumstances before and after my episode two weeks ago? I have told the whole truth. What are your plans for me, next two weeks? Have you diagnosed me/my problem i.e. what am I? How am I doing? On a scale of 1-100 how would you assess me? Could I try taking my medication at home? How soon would you estimate it to be? I feel sad (not angry) that I am here for such a chunk of time but I have come to terms with it but I will not ever stop asking questions about me because you've all told me I've got rights. I hate taking pills to look after my moods. Basically this week, if it is okayed, then I would like to set up a '400 meter hurdles' situation where I am getting my independence and private 'own time' back in stages. Like, going to Kendal Leisure Centre for a swim or doing weight training or playing football or running. Maybe even going right into Kendal and getting a haircut from my 'usual' hairdresser up here. All these small things seem to me to be a test of my responsibility to myself and others i.e. How I

conduct my life. Physically I feel 99% but I get panic attacks when I feel under pressure from a face with a badge who visits this ward only on certain days. Basically I feel I'm getting too comfortable in that room on this ward to the point of my head turning off! Life is almost too easy for me in here.

Monday 13th March – Had enough of the pills. My mouth gets salty and dry. I am trying to keep drinking but I keep running out of spring/bottled water. At least I can nip down to Asda. I want my bank account unfrozen. I know I look nervous at meal times and when I ask to go out. It is my nature. It may be hard to believe but I am shy. Could I go home for two nights this week? My mum could bring me in of a morning. Dinner times are still peculiar because I'm not used to living in this environment. I have to deal with it. I know how to relax now. My main aim is the drugs. I want to keep cutting them down as I am slightly running my day by them and I don't want to get hooked. If I didn't feel like taking a pill in the future could I ask not to do so? I keep tidying up for something to do.

The ward had a collection of old books along with Cluedo, Scrabble and Monopoly donated by caring pensioners for lost people like me to find some salvation. I found this poem in a dusty old book, probably circa 1950 but it resonated in my mind like it had been written just for me. Waiting to be uncovered in 1995.

Exhaustion
I'm tired from inside out. My spirit craves for crumbs of comfort anywhere!
A body lost at sea, I sink in hopeless search for your attention.
I'm almost proud of my exhaustion, I wear it like a medal to prove "he tried!"
But now's the time to say "I quit" and let the pain begin.

Victor J Kennedy

Fatigue and pain must fade away through ticking minutes of my alarm.
And only then will I become more than I was before all this happened.

There was a programme of things to do and events designed to aid recovery, while they also had a cupboard full of traditional family games and I became fixated with Scrabble and the formation of words. HOspiTEL, HOSPEL, HOSTEL, HOTEL, HOSPITAL. I would analyse patterns of the twentysix characters until I found one which allowed the maximum meaning with minimum means. I also worked on Telepress but without a computer. I was limited to sketches of the pebble from Tanya's driveway which now would become a remote control. I would also think deeply about the TV in the lounge and look at it's interface for any insights. I played alot of cards with myself, usually clock patience because Telepress was all about circles. The nurses offered assertiveness training and educated me about the five stages of problem solving, the anxiety spiral, common thinking distortions, emotional sequencing and how to challenge negative thoughts – ten common irrational beliefs. I also went to a presentation on body language. I couldn't understand how it would help but entertained me all the same. There was also relaxation every morning next door in Garburn House, the outpatients unit, where we would lie down on huge pillows and be taken off on a journey through the sky, where we can breath clearly, to be coached gently back down to earth, all in the space of thirty minutes.
The get well cards started coming in from all the different parts of my life, past and present. That's when you know something has gone really wrong with you because of their effort to say 'Get well soon' in their own individual ways. Some people even travelled long distances to visit unannounced but I didn't really want anyone seeing me in there like this.

Mad in England - A memoir

I think in life, whenever a human being experiences great
trauma directly, there is an initial shock and reaction but the
real struggle comes later. The indirect trauma suffered by the
human beings around the individual and their reaction will
form the new landscape in all your relationships. We all
understand what love at first sight means. Well, other
people's initial reaction to learning of my diagnosis whether,
positive, negative or indifferent have become a long-term
effect of this traumatic event. It's a scar nobody can see and
it's very difficult to understand and therefore empathise with.
If someone finds it difficult to be around me, the hypomanic,
I can smell it a mile off. You cannot hide it, in fact you
amplify it through your face, your body language and your
words. You give yourself away. It's a fact of post-diagnosis
life.

Dear Vic – Take Care of yourself and never forget how
much everyone cares about you Vic – hope to see you real
soon honey! Lots of love from your chum Ruth xxx ----------
----STOP--------------Vic, sorry to hear about the way things
are at the minute, but me, Billy and Craig are coming up
there to sort things out. Dale R --------------STOP--------------
To Victor, Best Wishes from Bob (University Security
Guard) Terry Venables has been looking for you. Get Well
Soon. --------------STOP--------------How you doin' nutter?
Call in and see us. Stan --------------STOP--------------
Sending thoughts to cheer you and hoping you'll soon feel
better. Mrs Crinkley Bottom "The Granary" With all my luv'
Nan xxx--------------STOP--------------You soft northern
bastard, I thought you lot were made of stronger stuff! Get
better soon Robbo. --------------STOP--------------Hope alls
well – Cathy. --------------STOP--------------At least I'll get a
pass and end up top scorer now! Gazza. Look forward to
seeing you after easter. Mark. Gazza said "can he lend your
predator boots?" See you when you get back – Paul (2nd top
scorer!) Hope everything's fine and you're feeling better now
Superman! We've only played one game since January (we

Victor J Kennedy

won 2-1 in the cup) – yeah! It would have been 8-1 if you were playing! So hurry back! All the best Bobby. ------------- -STOP--------------Just thought I'd send you a bit of a card to make you chuckle for a while. Take care of yourself, love from your Big Sis. xxx --------------STOP--------------To Victor, nippet, cheese toastie, nip, nipping, brussel sprout, mini action man, nipped, twinkle etching: "Virtual cross Hatching" all make a little twinkle, see you soon. Carl-------- ------STOP--------------Vic, I hope you're having a good time relaxing. We all miss you. See you soon. Shumana x ps. Enjoy the apple flavoured chewing gum--------------STOP---- ----------Dearest Vic, Hello, it's Katie here, just thought I'd write and tell you how much I'm thinking of you! Well, not much is happening in sunny Harrow – the gruelling task of final collections is upon us, so no time for partying! I'm having a tough time at the minute, my dad's walked out on my mum for someone else and has completely left us all, me, my mum and sister and he's not interested in us at all. My head is confused by it all and I nearly left college but I'm staying on now for my mum. Nothing else matters to me. I'm lucky I've got such good friends down here and you are too, as everyone is always thinking about you and wishing you well. Alice is about to arrive today for a couple of weeks and she's feeling alright within herself, she has her ups and downs but she's keeping her chin up. She was really touched by your letter and felt really glad you had written.

Well my darling, I must go and do something like eat or I'll have no energy to do my work.

Thinking of you always. All my love, Katie x p.s. If you need a chat, don't hesitate to call me anytime!-------------- STOP--------------Dear Victor, How you doing mate. I was very sorry to hear you have been unwell. I really hope you are feeling better, and shall be back soon. Harrow remains the same, but with the worry of leaving etc. Football continued to deteriorate after you went home, and we missed your silky skills on the left wing. Bobby continued to be the backbone of the team until he was injured last Sunday after a

Mad in England - A memoir

'delicate' tussle with a member of the opposition. We have missed your unbelievable pre-match tales of daring-do aswell. But rest assured my man, while Harrow has missed you, you have certainly had very little reason to miss Harrow. I spoke to Tanya a couple of times to get your address, and she said you were improving rapidly, and I was pleased to hear that. I would love to hear from you, so if you fancy writing me a letter, I would be most grateful, but only if you get the time. Anyway you Northern Bastard, better go and watch the telly or something equally interesting. Cheers mate, All the best Daz Brooke. ps- Write Soon--------------STOP--------------Vic, Hope things are seeming a little better and brighter. Don't forget I love you and that my thoughts are with you. Take care. Missing you more than ever. Tanya xxxx--------------STOP--------------Dear Vic, Hello love, how are you? For some reason I'm missing you more than ever tonight. I keep thinking of you there in hospital and so wished things were different and you were here with me. Anyway chin up hopefully you will be soon, so I'll stop moaning! I've included a copy of the album for you, I bought the CD today but taped it for you so you can listen to it in the mean time. I've also put in another write up on Gumbet that I thought you may be interested in. Anyway my love I won't keep you – just remember I'm thinking of you and can't wait for the weekend. All my love + thoughts as always. Tanya xxxx

These kind words of support meant nothing to me in 1995. Not because I didn't appreciate them but because I was not well, in fact I was very ill. Tanya continued to visit every weekend on the west coast train, with the the financial backing of my dad, who felt it would help my progression if she was by my side. Sometimes she couldn't cope with the sight of me. She told me later that it was like looking at a different person, sitting on my bed stroking my head while I was unconscious or on other occasions she might be unlucky enough to witness me having a manic rant. Seeing your boyfriend in that state can be pretty alarming, like you don't know them anymore. It's difficult to see how her visits helped either of us individually or as a couple. It's an exposure to trauma for the relationship. So the visits would often be Tanya sat with my parents in their house, crying their eyes out over me. Her relationship with them deepened at this time and it must have been very difficult for her. I had no idea what was happening to her.

Nath also felt compelled to help by managing my affairs down in London while I was away and got in touch with the RSA to make sure I still had a chance of winning, even though I obviously couldn't make my finalist interview. It was a great gesture but I always question the motivation of it. Is it hypocritical to perform a 360° reversal of behaviour after all Nath and Shumana's campaign of aggression towards me running up to my breakdown. Was it purely selfless or did he feel obliged to do it because of our fall out before I got ill? Either way, does it matter who's signature is on the letter. Someone tried to help me, I guess.

My old boss Reggie also made an impromptu visit, which I found massively embarrassing. All visits were difficult because it was my first experience of stigmatism. I mean, I didn't have anything as serious as cancer but all things considered it was probably thought of as fairly serious and therefore well worth a visit. The thing that got me was the conversations always ended up with the same subtext "you've done this to yourself" and I didn't think I had. My views back then were as equally stigmatic as my visitors because I was diametrically opposed to what I considered to be a 'substandard' or 'weaker' person. I didn't belong here with these people and this was just a blip, a hiccup. Your friends and ex-colleagues walk onto the ward at visiting time and that is what freaks them out. Seeing a lot of people unwell in the confines of a Psychiatric Ward is not a pretty sight but each person visiting me would open on the following statement, "Christ Vic, what on earth are you doing in here!?" They would probably leave with a picture etched on their brain to keep them in check whenever they thought they might be cracking up. There are all the undesirable visual cliches from films like "One Flew Over the Cuckoo's Nest" and putting a friend or a loved one into that scenario makes it difficult to deal with and affects your perception of that person's mind forever. They become a 'substandard' or 'weaker' person in your eyes.

By the time April came round I had put on weight and made enough progress to be allowed out for a few days to go to my interview at the Royal College of Art. I'd already been informed by the RSA (Royal Society of Arts) that due to missing my finalist interview my work was unsuccessful. I didn't want that to happen with the Royal College of Art interview so I had nagged everyone at my last three ward rounds to let me do it. I'd wanted to do the Computer Related Design Masters for over twelve months and I wasn't going to let it slip away from me now.

The ward gave me enough medication to last the visit and we were off. My dad drove and my mum came along for a break in London. They stayed in a bed and breakfast about two streets from my flat and I slept in my own bed at the flat. While I'd been away Lewis had decided to apply last minute as well but had been sent his portfolio back, which meant bad news. Nath was preparing his outfit because he got through. I hid in my room, still too embarrassed to deal with seeing people. It was a bit shitty being back in Harrow, where life had continued fine without me. Things were moving on, I could tell. The chlorpromazine medication I was taking didn't help either, I spent most of my three days in bed with the curtains closed feeling really down. Tanya was acting weird too. She had no patience for me at all. On the morning of the interview I got ready with Nath, we left the flat together and walked towards the tube station until I stopped outside the bed and breakfast to wait for mum and dad. He leant towards me and held out his hand. Slightly confused, I leaned forward and grabbed it. He shook my hand, "May the best man win." He winked and walked off.

Victor J Kennedy

All of a sudden it had become a competition. I thought back to the applications in January and remembered him filling in a form completely last minute. This was not a positive omen as far as I was concerned.

I thought my interview went fine apart from my mouth being dry from the drugs. I noticed self consciously that I'd slurred a few words but I hoped they wouldn't notice, until about a week later I got this handwritten letter:

Royal College of Art Kensington Gore, London SW7 2EU
Telephone: 071-584 5020 Fax: 071-584 8217
11/4/95
Dear Victor,
I am sorry we weren't able to offer you a place this year. Raymond explained to us that you had been ill and, indeed, we felt you weren't able to do yourself justice at the interview, given the high quality of your portfolio. I hope you will consider applying again next year; clearly we cannot predict what the competition will be like next year but we do think it worth trying again.
Yours sincerely,

Geraldine Copthorne-Scott
PROFESSOR Copthorne-Scott

I was absolutely devastated for about thirty seconds after reading it before my thoughts turned to anger and revenge. I wrote a vicious, stinging attack on Nath, blaming him for the triggering of my breakdown when Ruth had discovered he and Shumana had lied to me over the phone and the subsequent heartache it had caused me including the rejection from the Royal College. It was a huge setback in my life and my career because the 'best' man won. Yes, Nath got in. He made it and I didn't. The course I'd worked half my degree towards, the reason I worked my arse off in the summer of 1994 to get the computer, the only person on the GID course to write a dissertation and produce a contextual study about the immediate relevance of the internet. How ironic. I'd just missed the cruise liner. The extra effort counted for nothing.

I'd only just been discharged from hospital, which should have been a celebration, yet I found myself sinking, almost drowning in a chlorpromazine soaked despair. Back up north, I watched the whole of the World Snooker Championships with my Nan but I just wasn't there. All I could think of was losing my degree, the MA I wanted so badly, all my friends and of course my girlfriend. It was all two hundred and fifty miles away and it was going further away from me.

My mum and sister took me to Salts Mill in Bradford to see the David Hockney exhibition. It was like they wanted to get me out there looking at art and being inspired. I think they knew I was depressed and they were trying to help me bounce back. My mum bought me a Keats notebook and told me to start writing a new diary 'on the outside.'

Nath and Lewis drove up to visit one weekend and said stuff like, "You look fine" and "You look like you can come back!" I had to apologise to Nath for the letter and he brushed it off like it was nothing but you guess that's the etiquette protocol in action.

May arrived and I was really down, totally missing Tanya. I had a constant sick feeling in my belly, a nauseating nagging about Harrow in general. Everything was up in the air. Was I leaving or was I coming back? I was feeling strong mentally so I asked my mum if I could go down for a week but we ended up in a huge discussion about my belongings being stuck in the flat. My parents were still paying my rent and wanted to end it, get my stuff back home and prepare for taking a year off. Eventually we agreed that if I went down then I had to pack everything up ready for both of them (in two cars) driving to London to pick it all up and take it back on the Sunday. The deal was done and I got on the train. Just like the RCA interview I spent the whole week in bed, hiding from the overwhelming feeling of being left behind

Victor J Kennedy

by everything and everyone. I guess that is what a ghost feels like because I sort of felt like I had died in February and now eveyone was over it. No one more so than Tanya. Through the week I'd tried to see her but her major project demands were too much, at least that's what she told me. She couldn't even let me sit in her room while she was working on the sewing machine. I don't think she ever really wanted me in that room ever again. The thing was, she was distant. It was like I didn't know her any more because she spoke to me like any other person from college. The other girls in the house were obviously nervous about having me around again but soon warmed to me. They had a barbeque on the Saturday and quite a lot of people from college turned up and got drunk. This was quite an intense experience for me because I had to explain myself to everyone and then tell them what my plans were one after another. The awful thing was, a few of them leant forward and whispered things like, "It's rumored Tanya is seeing Gideon behind your back" or "I saw them come out of Trinity together" or "Ahhh Vic, you're so lovely. Tanya doesn't deserve you, after everything that has gone on."

It all got too much so I went inside to find her. Nobody could find her or knew where she'd gone but she had sneaked off all the same. I went up to her room and got into the bed to wait for her to get back. As the party progressed, more and more people would come up, sit on the bed to see if I was alright. It was embarrassing and made me feel like I was unable to cope, in my eyes all I was doing was waiting. I guess to everyone else I was sick, sad and a potential problem waiting to happen. A head case who needed help. When Tanya got back we talked for about an hour on that bed about a lot of things. I asked a lot of difficult questions and she answered as honestly as she could. She didn't once hint at finishing with me but then it may have been the cruelest, unbearable thing she could have done but she didn't.

287

Mad in England - A memoir

I went home in a packed car thinking me and Tanya were
fine and I'd work something out later in the year when we
were in Turkey. Come June, all that was blown right out of
the water when I received this letter in the post:

Dear Victor,
I have been meaning to write for a while now but as usual
have had trouble putting my feelings into words. A lot has
changed in recent weeks and I have learnt a great deal about
not only others but myself. I understand how much you must
have been through, it must all seem like a horrible
nightmare.
The thing is Vic, it hasn't been cosy for me either and it's
changed me so much – it had to, as otherwise I couldn't have
coped with the situation. I was so weak that I could never
have survived if my outlook on things hadn't changed. I
simply would have been crushed and not been able to cope
myself.
The last thing in the world I want would be to cause you
anymore pain or suffering but I have to be aware you
understand how I feel. The only way I learned to cope with
the situation that was thrown upon us was to harden up to a
lot of things. I do care for you so much Victor but in a
different way to how it once was. I'm sure you understand
this from what I said last time you came down. You
probably even feel the same, so much has happened we had
to change and this means our relationship had to change
also. Victor I feel so awful about this and I'm so very sorry
but we have to be realistic and look at the situation – for a
start we live at opposite ends of the country and until you
move back to London it will be hard to see one another.
I'm so very sorry for all of this I was just so scared of telling
you. I hope you understand and can forgive me – ? With all
this in mind I'm not sure how you still feel about coming to
the show, I have sent your sister's cheque in case you decide
to no longer come.

Victor J Kennedy

If there is any chance you still want to – just call Cathy or my mum and they'll get a message to me.
I'm so sorry Victor – I do miss you so much.
Love and thoughts,
Tanya xx

I showed my mum the letter and we cried. After I had composed myself we decided that I should ring Tanya to see if she would change her mind. I played it like I hadn't received the letter yet and this call was only an enquiry about the tickets for her course's end of year fashion show,
"Hi Tanya, it's me. What's happening about tickets for the show?"
"Look Vic, I don't know how to say this but I'm seeing Gideon and he's having your ticket. I'm sorry. I'm really sorry, I've been trying to tell you for ages but you've not been well. Did you get the letter explaining everything?"
"No, I haven't. Does your mum know you've been having an affair behind my back?"
"My mum's met Gideon loads of times. In fact, he's been over and met the whole family for Sunday lunch."
"And what does your mum think of him?"
"She likes him. She's sitting next to him at the show."
"But why did she come through to Harrow after our fall out in February to get us back together? Talking to me about looking after you in the future? Did she know you were seeing him then? I can't believe this Tanya."
"It's difficult to talk about all this now and I don't think it's going to do you any good."
"Don't worry about me. You were seeing him then, weren't you?"
"Yes but it wasn't serious then."
"I knew it! That night you came back with those red wine lips. You'd been with him then, hadn't you! People were telling me before Christmas that it was going on. I didn't believe them!"
"It doesn't matter now."

"But you loved me. Two and a half years. We were gonna get a flat together. What about the holiday in Turkey? I've done nothing wrong. Nothing!"

"Vic, you're no Angel yourself and you've been stupid enough to tell me about them."

"Yeah but I've never extorted money from your dad."

"What? Neither have I?"

"So why come up and visit me on a train every weekend for two months when you're living a double life down there with Gideon?"

"You don't know how difficult this has been for me. Look Vic, I'm sorry but it's over now. I'm with Gideon and I'm happy."

"Well, as long as you are. I guess this is goodbye then?"

"I'll see you." She put the phone down. I couldn't even cry I was so shocked. My mum was angry and sympathetic but was also pleased another loose end was tied up. I wasn't, and I spiralled into a deep depression for weeks. Some days I would lie on my bed not moving all day until five minutes before my parents got home from work. I would jump up, go downstairs and eat dinner with them both, then sit silent infront of the TV until nine o'clock and make my way back to the sanctuary of sleep. It got so bad that I slept way too much. When my parents were due to go on holiday they organised for my sister and her boyfriend to come up from Bradford and keep an eye on me. The summer of '95 was a summer of darkness for me. I thought I had nothing. But then on the 10th August I got a letter from Shirley Armstead at The University of Westminster informing me I could take a year out and return for the final semester in February 1996. I still had the chance to salvage my degree and my life. The brightest dawn follows the darkest night.

Victor J Kennedy

Chapter 8: Fighting Back

I spent a lot of the summer of 1995 in bed, alone in my parents house inside that bedroom where everything happened. I felt paralysed with despair, which after a few panic attacks and follow-up appointments with the team at Garburn House, had turned into a clinical depression. The doctors prescribed more drugs to give me support, which I resented. It was like I'd survived a spectacular plane crash and now I didn't feel brave enough to leave the wreck. My mum would invent tasks to go see my Nan in her flat to watch the afternoon sessions at the Embassy World Snooker Championships on BBC2 with a cup of tea, chocolate biscuit and a fag. This would give my Nan enough time to counsel me and report her assessment back to my mum, who would then probably have a chat with one of the nurses from ward 4 while she took a break from the x-ray department at work. Through June and July I became progressively worse. I actually looked forward to going to bed at night time because it meant I would get a few pills that knocked me out and I would sleep. When I slept all my worries were gone. That's why I stayed in bed. To try and always be asleep. I think, deep down, I just wanted to die. I just hadn't worked it out consciously how desperately lost I actually was. Everyone had graduated. They had all left Harrow and grouped up to live together in new and different parts of central London to begin their professional lives. I'd been told how many of my classmates had got First Class Honours and I could in no way be happy for them. I could only despise them for it because they had what I wanted all along. Even worse, three of them were off to the Royal College to do the CRD course I wanted to do, one of which was Nathan. All I had were the letters informing me about the suspension of my award from Cumbria County Council and a deferment letter from Raymond Beattie and Shirley Armstead in the main office telling me I had to decide whether I was taking out more than a year or not. All these types of decisions were huge for someone in my weakened state of mind and they just got on top of me and made me want to go to sleep. To escape. I tried to motivate myself by going out for walks in the Lakeland countryside with the Kendal Mind and Garburn House outpatients but it was really tough trying to be sociable. The exercise got me fitter but the loss of Tanya was getting to me as much as my imposed isolation from my education. The frustration made me jump on a train to London and I caught a central line train to South Woodford where I walked up the high street after buying a bunch of flowers. Now, in my mind it seemed like a really straightforward thing to do but as I walked through the front door of Carolyn's letting agency I could see her face drop and fear flood through every blood vessel in her body. As I walked to her desk, I could see a wall mounted colour photo of Tanya wearing her mortar board. She was obviously a very proud mum. I had bought the flowers for Tanya's mum to butter her up and allow me to find Tanya to win her back from Gideon but I changed my story last minute, due to the colour draining out of her face. Her look made me feel like I was holding a gun instead of a bunch of flowers. I offered them to her and I said, "Carol, I'm really sorry about how all this has turned out but I want you to know I still care about Tanya and wondered if you could give her these flowers from me and say that I'd love to speak with her. Only if she wants to. I mean, she can ring me up in Millhead on my mum's phone anytime and I'd be glad to speak."

"Ok Victor, I'll pass that message on to her. If it's ok, could we get on with our work now as things are really busy around here at the moment?"

"Oh yes, no problem. Are you ok?"

"Yes, I'm fine. Just very busy. I'll speak to you soon. Take care."

"Bye bye."

I turned around and frog marched myself out the door and sheepishly made my way back to Millhead and my bed. I needed a very deep sleep after that hammer blow.

Victor J Kennedy

My sister and her boyfriend Alvin had come up from
Bradford for a holiday. They proceeded to get me out of bed
everyday and visiting things or doing errands. I hated them
for it but eventually I came round a bit. One day they took
me to IKEA in Warrington and we sat in a traffic jam on the
M6 for an hour but it all seemed to be thawing me out. At
night time we all sat down with my parents after a good
meal and talked through my problems. All attention was
focused on me and sorting out my life. They had me writing
lists of my problems and fears, then each person would take
two or three off me from the list and next day they would
sort them out or help me to get on top of things. For
instance, Lewis had sent a letter demanding my share of
joint bills for the summer term amounting to £116 which I
didn't have and therefore stressed me out. My dad sorted that
one and told me he had given him and Nath money already
so was slightly annoyed. My family were brilliant at this
time. It was like boot camp for the disaffected soul. They got
me so motivated I decided to ask Reggie if he had any work
for a junior and if I could take up my old job again. He said
yes. We got the formalities over and I informed the
Occupational Therapist at Garburn House that I would no
longer be using the day centre. They posted a really nice
letter to me, congratulating me on finding a new job. Holly,
the Occupational Therapist even asked me if I'd like to be
discharged. Of course, I said yes. This time it felt final. This
time I felt ready to quit the support and go on my own. By
now I knew I had to wait until February before I would get
back to London and at least knowing that was formalised
gave me something to work towards. To get ready for. I
planned from this point forward to go back and complete the
degree. I was getting back my mojo. My ambition. The
embers were breaking out in flames inside and I could feel
the drive slowly coming back. It was pre-season too, so I
went down to the Crusaders and started training. Before long
I felt like it was 1989 again and my life was as it was. The
friends I'd made in the village were still there for me.

Mad in England - A memoir

Everything picked up where I had left off in 1992. Like putting the needle back down on a record.

Getting up early and being driven into Kendal by my dad at 7:30am was difficult to get used to again. He was an early riser my old man, liked to open the post in the office and get his troops up to speed as they entered the front door. He would drop me off by the Cock and Dolphin then I'd walk to work along the riverside, looking around at ducks, trees and architecture while my mind wandered towards Tanya. I would spend a few minutes tripping around different scenarios and wondering all about the 'what ifs'. The 'what ifs' would lead me towards 'the whys' and then they would push me over into darker territory and more negative thought processes with regards to Gideon. He had won. He had the girl but he had stolen her. That should be punished. Not just the theft but the subsequent cause and effect it had on my mental health. He deserved some karma. In fact, as my head spun downwards into the helter-skelter I decided he should suffer some physical pain at my hands to even up the score. Sometimes I would wish terrible things to happen to him 250 miles away. There was no way I could seek him out and attack him but I had to plan for the day our paths might cross. I would cut him down with a comment constructed over years of pondering. Each time I created the scenario and the line I would deliver, I would always end up at the front door of work and once inside forget completely where my mind was at. I never recorded any of it, I just thought about these things every morning without fail. I believe that this is part of the healing process. Working these things out from inside. Tidying your head up. Then moving on.

Those journeys in the car with my dad could be quite annoying with him being an Insurance Broker. One day he got in the car and told me I had to inform the DVLA that I had a nervous breakdown. When I asked why I had to do that, he said if I ever had an accident driving then I wouldn't be fully covered if they had not been made aware. I felt the indignity of doing something like that. It made me feel ashamed of what had happened to me. I felt stigma. But it also showed how much the media had influenced my perception of mental illness because I felt shamed by having had a nervous breakdown. It's not something people are necessarily proud of. I mean, if I'd been in hospital with cancer and then told to inform the DVLA, would I have felt the same way? Would people feel shame towards me for having suffered cancer and then recovering? Would my capacity to drive be monitored?

After a few weeks with my driving licence in Swansea, I got a letter informing me to go to see a doctor in Kendal for a mental assessment. They wanted find out my suitability as regards me sitting behind the wheel of a one tonne lump of metal and rubber. I can see the DVLA's point of view because I'd just grassed myself up for having been ill and they needed to find out just how ill I was. The doctor explained to me that older people who may be susceptible to Alzheimer's would have to go through the same thing as me. It was too dangerous for other road users if the DVLA didn't keep risks off the road. I was now considered to be in that risk category and I personally didn't agree because I know myself. I was in a bad way back in February and March but it was now September and I honestly felt back to my old self. I really did think I was over it all, the trauma I mean. It was a blip and the blip was now behind me. But no, it was going to stay with me for as long as I could drive a car. The doctor told me that should I pass his tests, my driving licence will be reissued for a short-term period of between eighteen months and two years. Then the same assessment would have to occur before another driving licence would be issued. I told him I'd passed my test at 17 years old and never had an accident and that my licence was not due to expire until 2039 and I liked that long-term licence, could I ever get permission from the DVLA to have that long-term licence back? He told me I would be reassessed for the rest of my life. His words were a massive blow to my confidence and I felt policed by the state and reliant on a doctor's opinion of me on the day I visited him. What if I'm having a bad day in 2014 and I get banned from driving? It could be at a time of my life when I needed a car the most. When we actually got down to the assessment, his first question was, "Who is the Prime Minister?"

"John Major!" Easy! This pub quiz was going to be like taking candy from a baby.

"Who is the leader of the opposition?"

"Ermmm..." I started to panic because I knew the answer, it was that smug twat from the Labour party but his name just wasn't coming to the front of my mind and I didn't really watch the news that much so I hadn't heard it that often. I was starting to get worried because the doctor would think I was unwell because the question was so fucking easy. Jesus, what's his name? Brown hair, always smiling. He was new. Just made leader and was pretty young for a politician. "Tony Blair!" Phew.

The rest of the questions were not general knowledge but did actually get into the relevance of what they needed to know and luckily for me, a few weeks later I passed! My new driving licence arrived in the post. I got to use it for the first time on the way to my cousin Dylan's wedding in Copmanthorpe near Scarborough. It was the first real event and family outing for me since the breakdown so it was quite tough and another test for everyone. On the way we passed York and my dad asked me if I wanted to drive for a little bit because the roads were straight and mostly dual carriageway. It was a great gesture but as soon as I got in and buckled my seat belt. Myself, mum and dad all went tense. I did okay and never went over sixty miles an hour but the atmoshphere or should I say, atmos-fear, was too intense for me to continue all the way to the hotel in Copmanthorpe so I pulled over after five minutes. The point was proved and I was grateful to my dad for again forcing me to be brave and get in the saddle. A bit like when he taught me to ride a bike when I was little.

Victor J Kennedy

The wedding ceremony and evening do went without a hitch for me. All eyes were on the bride and groom from the wider family so nobody really took much notice of me. They all asked how I was because they obviously knew and some had even visited me in hospital. Again, the feeling of aloofness and taboo that a breakdown brings to a family is amplified only to the person who actually experienced the symptoms. The other people are concerned only about politeness and empathy. Maybe it's the British stiff upper lip thing but I wouldn't have minded talking about it to clear the air, rather than ignoring it. If I could be interrogated by a DVLA nominated doctor to get my license, surely I could talk to my cousin's about it? But again, I could not impose myself on them, it was Dylan's wedding and big day. I'm a bit part player and I'm also going to do the British thing and smile for all his photographs, like absolutely nothing has happened.

I didn't drink alcohol at the wedding. In fact, I hadn't drunk alcohol since that Republic of Ireland v England game which got abandonned just before my breakdown. That was nine months ago and due to my training with the football club and all the larking about with Smudge and the lads, I was starting to feel pressure to go out. I kind of felt like this was the next step for my rehabilitation, to get back on the booze, but I was apprehensive I might regress if I started to drink again. It was a drug after all. But then again, my breakdown was a 'stress induced hypomanic episode' not a 'drug induced' one. And alcohol is not exactly a class A drug is it? I talked to my parents at length before I accepted to have a drink after one of the pre-season games at home. The clubhouse was right behind my parents house so they could run across the field if anything went wrong. What was I on about? What could go wrong with an innocent pint after a good run around on a football pitch? I was nervous but as me and Smudge walked out of the changing rooms towards the clubhouse, he asked me what I was having. He always asked first. He was very generous like that. I told him I'd have a pint of lager and his face changed to a look of surprise and delight, "What's a matter with you?" he said. "Oh, I reckon it's about time I got back on the drink." "And is all this cleared with your mam 'n' dad? I don't want to get in trouble for turning you to the dark side." "It's cleared by half of Westmorland General's doctors. Just get 'em in." "Good to have you back Vic." This was quite a watershed because I was telling him I was fit enough to play football and now I was fit enough to start socialising too. That meant going through to Kendal, which was seven miles away, in his dad's car and meeting up at 7.30pm on the dot, in the Shakespeare or the Cask. Basically any pub that started after Kirkland but before Highgate in the first 500 metres of the one way system. Kendal has a massive amount of pubs and on any given Friday or Saturday people do 'the circuit', which is a pint in every pub around Highgate and Stramongate before ending up at the George & Dragon in the market place for last orders and a fight. Or maybe if you don't get caught in a fight, then jump in a taxi to Netherfield football club. They had made a nighclub under one of their stands for some extra revenue. It had turned out to be a gold mine because everyone wanted to be seen there. It was called The Park and it was a proper northern night out. They had Athena posters in glass frames all down one wall. Loads of boobs and beaches, there was even that one for the ladies of the bloke holding the baby in black and white. Proper classy. I didn't care though because by the time my drink intolerance had dissappeared, which was about a month later, I could hardly ever remember what had gone on in that club. I was just there to have a laugh with my mates, Smudge, Gibbo, Mitch, Ernie and the remnants of the football team dotted around. Unlike the George & Dragon, The Park had bouncers and if there was a fight, it was over before you could turn around. Then all you could see were two blokes being carried out by a couple of contestants from the world's strongest man. The Park DJ was

Victor J Kennedy

a legend. A legend of cheese. He played all your Take That
tunes, bit of Celine Dion and healthy amounts of Robson &
Jerome. In between all those guilty pleasures he stuck on
some floor fillers you might find in a decent club and a bit of
Rock 'n' Roll in the shape of Roll With It from the up and
coming band Oasis, which all the lads just stood there and
sang. They don't do dancing unless it's to pull a bird. That
time of night was when Back for Good came on and you
dived in and grabbed the girl you'd been staring at all night
through a drunken haze. One night I'd been on the
dancefloor to take the piss out of Shaggy's Boombastic and
started girating my hips whilst generally making a twat out
of myself as three other blokes started doing the same thing.
I think it was to do with losing confidence in dancing, after
all my clubbing on drugs in London, bouncing around for
seven hours sipping water. I couldn't see the point in dancing
if I wasn't taking chemicals. It just didn't have the same buzz
any more so I just took the piss. As I was doing my Shaggy
impersonation I could see this brunette watching me and
smiling. She was absolutely my type exactly. She was
beautiful. Dark skin. Sultry eyes and a bright smile, perfect
teeth. She was wearing a silver sequinned mini dress and
was gleeming right at me. Unbelievable figure too. Perfect
breasts, ample but not too big. Slim waist but wide hips,
athletic looking legs. She looked a lot of fun and if after
eight pints of lager and a few bottles of Hooch, that's what
love at first sight felt like, then it's fair to say I was in love.
At the end of my Shaggy routine, Ernie grabbed me and
dragged me to the bar. It was my round. After I'd bought
sixteen bottles of Hooch for the gang of lads, I turned around
to find her but she was nowhere to be seen. I walked, sorry
staggered around the club hoping that I wouldn't find her
snogging another bloke but she was nowhere. I even stood at
the bar next to the girls toilets for twenty minutes, watching
like a hawk but it was no good. Then, Back For Good came
on. It was five to two and if I didn't find her now, it was
never going to happen. I walked onto the dancefloor

between each couple smooching, staring through each gap to try and find the girl in the glitter dress. The floor was packed and it was almost hitting the chorus, I spun around and she was there, amazingly alone. So I darted across with excitement and grabbed her. "Can I have this dance?"
"What?" She shouted into my ear over the Take That boys. "I said, can I have this dance? I think you're completely gorgeous!"
"Yes! I think you're fit too."
We smooched for the rest of the song. I could feel her breasts touching my chest and as I moved my arms around her waist and her bum I was getting aroused and then embarrased that she might noticed and think I'm a dirty letch. I must've disguised it because I got a kiss right at the end of the song but as the lights went up she let go of me and said, "Wait there, I've just got to find my friend."
So I waited and waited, like a twat, until Smudge came over and slurred, "Come on, Ernie's got a taxi waiting." It was chucking out time and the bouncers were coming acros to have a word for the fifth time to get out. I asked one, "Have you checked the girls toilets mate?"
"Yes sir, I've told you already there's no one in there. She's left you sir. Try the burger van, she might be there." I told Smudge to sit tight in the cab and I ran down to the burger van but she wasn't there either. I was gutted. My heart actually sank because it felt right. I think deep down I'd been looking for someone to replace Tanya for nearly six months now and I felt like this was it. And now she was gone. I didn't even know her name.
Over the next three weeks I made a consolidated effort to go to The Park every Saturday night to try and find her again. I hoped she was not a tourist in the Lake District and had gone back to wherever she was from. But alas, it never happened. I never saw her and I gave up hope.
As luck would have it, I'd found another girl in the mean time and started dating. It was a bit of a weird one because first of all I played football with her cousin Dominic. It was

Victor J Kennedy

him who introduced me after the second team had lost away to Keswick in the Westmorland Cup. On the way back in the mini bus Dominick mentioned his cousin and that he was going to her parents 25th wedding anniversary party that night. My mum was going to that party because she worked at the Hospital with the girl's mother Laura, who I knew very well and got on with. I thought I may as well give it a go as my dad would probably turn up to give my mum a lift home and I could hop in with them. When I got to the party there was a lot of Netherfield players there and Kendal lads because her brother Liam, was a good player and played for Netherfield. He was also a bit of a loose cannon after he had had a drink and was a reknowned fighter. I personally didn't like him or his reputation. That was the only minus of dating his sister.

I met Dawn Bailey in her mum's lounge for the first time. She was the spitting image of her mum. She even had the same laugh and was very friendly. I liked her instantly as a person but being the superficial bloke I was at the time, I wasn't blown away by her looks. Don't get me wrong, she was an attractive girl and she definitely looked after herself but I think she was just too blonde for me. The conversation was great and I sat with her and her friend in the lounge all night, telling stories and hearing stories. We had a good giggle and got to know each other quite well. She worked at the TSB on Stramongate, not more than four hundred paces from where I worked at Reggies. We could easily do a lunch. By the end of the night we were pretty drunk and her friend wanted to go to The Park. We discussed this to the enth degree. All the permutations and the logistics of taxis or walking etc. This was small talk in my opinion because Dawn had already told me she had her own house and mortgage somewhere near the train station at Oxenholme. I could tell she was stalling and wanted to dump her mate and get me back to her place so we had all played the game for long enough. The catalyst was my mum coming into the lounge and asking if I wanted a lift home because my dad was outside. Dawn jumped in, "He's staying here. We're getting on too well." She winked at my mum and gave her one of those beaming cheeky smiles.

"Is this true?" asked my mum.

"Yeah, I think we're going to The Park."

"Have you got a key?"

"Yeah, but don't expect me back in the middle of the night. Dawn lives round the corner from The Park so I might get my head down on her couch and come back in the morning on the 555."

"We might even miss out on The Park and stay here with all my parent's free booze, eh Victor?" Dawn gave my mum another wink and another big smile.

"Ok, you three have a good time, don't drink too much and I'll see you tomorrow." and off went my mum.

As soon as she had gone, Dawn called a cab and the three of us headed for The Park, which I thought was going to be our destination until we parked up and her friend jumped out saying, "Tarra, you two be good!" She slammed the door and the Taxi turned around and went back to Dawn's place. I got quite excited at that point, I was on a promise and we had just ditched the mate to go back alone. When we got there we had a fumble and a snog on the couch but she stopped me getting serious by standing up and throwing a blanket on me. "That's enough young man, I'm not that kind of girl. Not on the first night anyway. You'll have to sleep there, I'm going to bed. And don't try to sneak in my bed in the middle of the night because I've got a lock on my bedroom door."

"Aw, come off it Dawn. You can trust me. I'll hardly sleep on this sofa."

"I've slept there many a time and it's really comfy. Just make sure you're there in the morning and I'll make a breakfast. We can go for a walk or something? Get to know each other when we're sober."

"Have you locked the front door then, so I can't escape?"

Victor J Kennedy

"It's a deadlock. So if you feel the need to run, make sure you close the door behind you. I'll understand. But it would be nice if you stayed."

"Ok, I'll see you in the morning. Can I have my eggs unfertilised?"

"Very funny. See you in the morning."

"Night sexy."

In the morning she came down in her dressing gown and no make-up, I was sober and I wasn't quite sure what the fuck I was thinking of twelve hours before. We had a breakfast and a difficult post fumble chat. I hadn't had sex with her yet and I had that feeling you get as a bloke the morning after an alcohol induced decision made the night before. I just had to leave. We exchanged numbers, I didn't really want to but I was now coming to realise she would get my number from her mum, who no doubt had called my mum in the past. I'd done myself up like a kipper and I was going to have to find a way out. Hopefully with a clean set of heels.

I was coerced into a few dates, which seemed harmless. I took her to see Goldeneye at Windermere Odeon. We also spent time round her house watching videos designed for couples. Eventually we were an item and it was realised by her parents, my parents and especially her brother Liam. He kept speaking to me if he saw me out on the town. He was always pissed and slurring his words like an English hooligan who wanted to welcome you into his family. This was not what I wanted for my future. However, it was making me think less and less about Tanya. I was ridding her from my system by exorcism through another woman. A woman I didn't really care for but was getting me back into the scheme of dating again. I'd been deeply in love with Tanya and I thought I would always be in love with her till the day I died. To fall out of love with someone who left you for someone else means altering your mindset and letting your opinions occupy a different part of your psyche. I should have been in a single bedroom flat in London, with a blossoming career in Online Advertising, with the woman I was going to make my wife, who I'd met at university. But now I was back working as a junior at Reggie's doing the Cumbria Tourist Board Guide and dating a bank teller who's mum is good mates with my mum. Everybody would have loved it if me and Dawn would have made a go of it. Proper happy families but that was not what I wanted at all. I think I needed to sleep around and treat women like shit. It was an infantile way of dealing with the chronic rejection I felt, now the shock of Tanya leaving me for Gideon had sunk in and was becoming a manageable proposition. These women from Kendal were gonna have to pay for what Tanya did to me. They would have good sex, maybe not great sex but they would never control my heart.

The following Saturday I was out with the lads again after we'd beaten Pheonix 3-2 at home. I was celebrating after setting Geordie up for the winner. We all did the pub crawl thing and ended up in The Park as usual. I was fairly blathered and doing my usual dancing mickey-take to Simply Red when I got a tap on the shoulder. I turned around and it was that stunning brunette. I couldn't believe it. I leant forward to hear her over the music. She shouted in my ear, "I didn't know you were a fan of Mick Hucknall?"

"I'm not. He's a red head and I love brunettes!" I gave her a wink and she smiled.

"Sorry about the other week. My friend was really drunk and I had to take her home. She puked up everywhere."

"Don't worry about it. That's a shame about your mate. Is she okay?"

"She was fine in the morning, just a sore head."

"Is she here tonight?"

"No. I'm with my sister tonight. She's over there with her mates. Do you want a drink?"

"Are you offering?"

"Well, I'd rather sit and chat with you than stand over there with my sister. We'd cramp her style."

"Okay, I'll get 'em. What do you fancy?"

"You." She winked at me.

Victor J Kennedy

I couldn't believe what I was hearing. We got the drinks and sat on some leather sofas then talked the rest of the night away. She was called Sonia and she worked in Pain De Paris, a sandwich shop I often bought a ham and brie stick from. The thing was I never noticed her at work, when I was sure I would never miss anyone who looked as stunning as she did. Oasis came on and she was up there with all the lads, singing all the lyrics to Roll With It, like she wrote them herself. By the time the last dance came on, we knew each other really well. It was Take That again and we snogged all the way through it. She stopped at one point to whisper in my ear, "Will you come back to mine, we can walk it from here?"

"I'd love to. Grab your jacket and let's get out of here."

She said goodbye to her sister and I gave Smudge a nod and pointed at her, then winked. He put his thumbs up and I left with Sonia on my arm. We walked past the burger van chatting all the way over the river and up past the college towards the Underwood estate. It was quite a walk but we had time to really get to know each other and I had managed to sober up a little bit. As we got to the house I realised she still lived at home. She confirmed it by asking me to stay as quiet as I could until we got inside the house. She ushered me into a low lit lounge and got me a Baileys. When she came back in the room from the kitchen she was already changed into sweat pants and a baggy t-shirt. She looked fabulous. We sat on the floor practically in darkness and began kissing. This inevitably led to a lot more touching and caressing. Eventually, things were getting out of control and we were both down to our underwear, so she asked me to come up to her bedroom in case her parents came down and witnessed something they didn't expect or approve of. Once installed in the bedroom she put on the Oasis album, What's The Story Morning Glory and flicked off the light so we could continue where we'd left off. As I lent over her and began kissing her neck the bedroom door flew back and the light switched back on. It was an angry looking bloke with

brown hair and he stank of booze. He was shouting, "I hope your fucking pleased with yourself, you fucking bitch!"
"Give me those keys. You've got no right to let yourself into my parents house like this." Sonia stood up to him to grab the door keys. I stood up and by now realised this was the boyfriend and I was in the middle of a serious situation. I assumed a queensbury rules stance, in my underpants, to try to defend myself should the boyfriend lunge at me. He looked at me with a pathetic stare.
"There's no need to worry about any fighting mate. I'm not gonna smack you. It's her I've got the problem with, not you."
"Just get out Woody. Give me the keys and leave. It's over." She held out her hand and he dangled them in front of her.
"DAD!" She shouted. "WILL'S BROKEN IN!" A couple of seconds lapsed and then the whole fucking family came to the door. Including her younger sister! And I'm standing there with a semi on wearing only a pair of Marks & Spencer black briefs on.
"Who's this?" Her dad said.
"Er, it's Victor sir." I replied.
"I wasn't asking you son. Sonia, why is this lad standing in front of William in his underwear in your bedroom?"
"Me and Will have split up."
"No we haven't. And you're shaggin' around. Look at yer. Shaming your parents." Will interjected.
"Bollocks Will, I've told you numerous times it's over. I've had enough of your drinking. Now give me the keys and get out. Dad tell him to give me the keys."
"William, give her the keys. You're going to have to leave. I'm sorry son."
Will handed over the keys and the crowd dispersed but before he turned to leave he said to me, "Please don't shag on that bed. I bought that bed from Argos for me and her for our flat. If you have to shag her, do it on the floor and have some respect." And then he left. I was agog.

Victor J Kennedy

She went down stairs with him and locked the door once he was outside. By the time she returned I was totally turned off and completely bemused by what I'd just experienced. What a way to get introduced to mum, dad and her sister. Not to mention the ex-boyfriend. We lay in the bed talking about it in the darkness, listening quietly to Oasis on repeat. By the time the album was on it's third rotation we were having full passionate sex. On the bed, not on the floor. We didn't stop there. I lost count of how many times the album repeated because this girl was insatiable. She was also a bit of a nutter who liked to stick her nails into my back and then brand me, as she dragged them down. It was a mad night and in the morning after having had almost no sleep I got up. I had to sit and have breakfast with the family who saw me the night before I slept with their daughter/sister. It was bizarre but they all treated me very well. It was the start of a very bizarre and highly charged sexual encounter, which was based on passion and a shared love of Oasis. It was a relationship very much of it's time and I did not have a clue how it would end up and I didn't care. The main thing for me was that this relationship was what I wanted, not the one I had already started with Dawn. I was in a stupid situation now and I had to try and rectify it. I had to find a way to end it with Dawn and get away without Sonia finding out.
The opportunity arrived soon enough after a catalogue of schoolboy errors on my part and the effect of living in a close community such as the one involving 18-25 year olds from The South Lakeland area that gather in Kendal pubs and clubs on a regular basis. I told, or should I say bragged, to too many lads at the football club. These conversations often took place in the showers with soap in your eyes after someone asks, "Vic, are you still shagging them two birds from Kendal?" and I would have to explain myself while keeping face at the same time. These guys would often tell their partners, who in turn would tell someone from work. A lot of the players were golfers so they would chat about the football gossip to their golfing buddies, who in turn would

307

tell their partners about these characters and their despicable behaviour. It would all get embellished. Before long maybe, say, six, or seven weeks of grace, it will come back to haunt you. Phrases come to mind like "what goes around, comes around." and all that. These lessons are valuable lessons and help focus the mind when you understand exactly what the words describe. Sometimes you have to live through the experience to learn that it is wrong to live that way. Learning by experience resonates and focuses the mind. I'd just learned that from experiencing a nervous breakdown and I felt stronger for it. Thing is, my behaviour had slipped backwards again since reintroducing myself to alcohol and my so-called mates who in turn had bought their round of lagers before snogging someone elses' disillusioned girlfriend in the corner of a sticky-carpeted nightclub. I met my fate in the form of a fist and then a headbutt from Liam, the honour defending brother of Dawn Bailey. I was on the dancefloor with Sonia, enjoying the vibe and oblivious to being watched by Dawn's drunken brother, my other squeeze, who had been conspicious by her absence in my life over the last couple of weeks. I'd been hoping she had dumped me in a fit of desperation at the fact I was aloof and generally a crap boyfriend. If that had happened I would have been happy at the outcome. That was my clean pair of heels without upsetting my mum's working relationship with her mum. It was more honourable and respectable to get the push for being a useless sap than for being a womanising cad. What on earth had my mother brought up to do such a callous act on such an innocent girl? I had to be punished and the family's anger recoiled, through Liam. He told me after he struck me, "Leave my sister alone. Stay away from her." before he stumbled and fell flat on his face, only to be pounced on and carried off the premises by the bouncers. Sonia took me to one side afterwards and asked me what was going on. "Do you know Liam Bailey?"
"No, not really. I know he plays for Netherfield but that's about it."

Victor J Kennedy

"Are you sure?"

"Yeah, course I'm sure."

"So why was he swinging for you?"

"I dunno? Maybe he thought I was someone else? He was very drunk. Did you see him fall over straight away? Totally off balance, which to my mind says 'blathered'. Totally out of his tree."

"But you're okay though? Nothing hurts?"

"No. No blood or anything. My cheek is a bit sore but I'm ok."

"Shall we go back to mine and I'll make it feel better?"

"Sure, let's go."

I was concerned it was all going to come out there in an interrogation but I got away with it and I got a night of hot passion as a reward. In the morning we woke around 11:30am and Sonia got me a cup of tea in bed. She told me her mum had asked if I wanted to stay for Sunday lunch. I accepted and then showered. I got dressed into the fancy shirt and trousers I was wearing the night before. The rest of the family wore casual clothes. I looked an idiot sitting there but they all chatted away to me openly. By now, in late November, I was getting on really well with her dad. Her younger sister was a tougher nut to crack but overall it was going really well after the difficult start after her ex-boyfriend pounced when I was only in boxer shorts. Her mum brought out the Yorkshire puddings and the phone started ringing. Sonia jumped up to answer it and then everything changed. "Hi Jerry. You alright? What's up?....yes he is........we were......yeah.......he did......off his trolley......yeah.......when?......who told you that?......for how long?.......really?......no......he's never said anything to me.......that's interesting.........well it's nice the truth has finally come out........I will........thanks for ringing Jerry, I really appreciate it.......no, no babes........let's meet up soon, we haven't been out for ages.......ok...cheers....love you, bye!"

309

Mad in England - A memoir

She put the phone down and turned towards me with a really
stern face. I knew that phone call had just confirmed my
worst fears. Her father asked, "Are you ok, Sonia? Was that
bad news?"

"No dad, it was entirely good news. I've just found out that
Victor here, has been seeing Dawn Bailey at the same time
as seeing me. Basically, behind my back!"

"Is this true Victor?", her dad looking slightly displeased.

"Not entirely sir. There was some overlap but I've not seen
Dawn for almost three weeks now. I presumed she had
ended it so I guess that's where the confusion is coming
from. I apologise for that." I was dying inside. It's bad
enough explaining yourself to your girlfriend but to her mum
and dad, plus her younger sister at the dinner table. This was
something I never wanted to go through ever again. It was
infinitely more painful than the headbutt the night before.
Her dad empathised with me, maybe he'd had this lesson
once, "Well, let's say that evens up the score between you
two, after that episode with Woody the first night you
brought Victor home. Potato anyone?"

After that, the only time I ever spoke to Sonia about what
happened was on a walk along a crag near Lythe Valley, one
Sunday afternoon just before Christmas. We'd got quite
serious by then and the prospect of my return to Harrow was
making us take stock of our relationship. It was a make or
break conversation in front of a fantastic view. She told me
she'd had enough of the small town attitude of people in
Kendal but that did not mean she wanted to join me in
London. She had plans to teach children English and see
some of the world. She was driving the relationship and I
was being agreeable just so we could stay together. It was
basically just great sex. Looking at it from afar, that was all
we had. At the time I didn't want to split up. I suggested we
stay together and write. I'd done it before and I knew the
letters would help me get through the last term. Then we
could both leave England together and travel. She could
teach English and I could be a designer. I could almost speak

310

Victor J Kennedy

Italian. Well, almost is not quite the right word but I would pick it up. I would pick up any language if she said yes to us staying together but obviously in a long-distance capacity. After a couple of hours up there in the wind on top of that crag, we decided to stay together. It felt solid and real after that. More than just sex.

One midweek night after enjoying a fix of passion with her, I set off home in torrential rain in my mum's red Rover Metro. It was a typical Lakeland shower. One of those where the windscreen wipers have to be on full blast and then you can only just see out. It was about 2am and I'd got a Terence Higgins Trust Comedy tape in the car, sent to me from Alan down in London, who I'd kept in touch with since my breakdown. He was staying on at university to complete his MA I just think he didn't want to go to work yet and this was a great way of delaying it. The tape itself had Paul Calf and his alter ego sister, Paulene Calf live on stage at somewhere like the Hammersmith Apollo. It was cracking me up while driving the seven miles through darkness back to Millhead. As I drove up the A6 passing Hale, towards a chicane tree-lined section of the road, I was laughing so hard that tears were rolling down my face. The car was travelling around 50 miles per hour but I had applied the brake before the first bend because I knew from experience that it was tight and the rain was intimidating.

What happened next I can only explain as wet leaves on the road and human instinct. In a split second the car was spinning. When I say spinning, I mean the vehicle had hit something slippery on the surface and was trying to do a 180 degree spin towards the bank at the far side, which was a steep hill into an old disused railway line. When I realised I was out of control, my instinct snapped into action. I turned the wheel into the skid and the car regained it's grip. Once that happened, the momentum of the car took it straight forwards into the dry stone wall on the opposite side of the road. I braked just before impact but it was too late. I mounted the pavement and bang, in an instant the car was still. It was 2:30am on a Wednesday morning and there was no traffic whatsoever. I sat there in shock for a second and then started up the engine without getting out of the car to check the damage. It started straight away and I reversed back on to the A6, put it in first gear, then drove off. I was home in less than three minutes. I put the car into my mum's garage and then had a look at the front end. There was bright green brake fluid coming out from somewhere inside the engine. The outside of the car didn't have a scratch so I sat and watched the green liquid dripping for five minutes to see if it would stop. In that time I decided it was best to tell my mum what I'd done. It was too dangerous to say nothing and let her drive it. I went upstairs and pushed her bedroom door open, much like I had as a little boy, only this time it was her nightmare. My dad was snoring and didn't wake up but I whispered loud enough to wake her up. She came out on to the landing and I explained what had just happened. I expected a rollocking but she just said, "I'm not bothered love. I'm just glad you're safe. You're more precious to me than a stupid car." It was nice of her to say that but the next day she changed her tune when the mechanics told her I'd moved every one of the engine mounts in that collision. That crash would cost my mum's insurance company £2,000 and her no claims bonus was gone. It was the first time she started to warn me that I was doing too much. It was a turn of phrase that politely told you that you're out of control or at least you're heading that way. More haste less speed and all that.

I tried to take it easier over Christmas but in fact things went the other way. Everyone up there drinks too much and it's inescapable because whenever you and your friends go out, everybody buys a round. Otherwise you're stigmatised for being tight-fisted. The whole thing is designed to make everyone involved an alcoholic. You have to drink as fast as the fastest drinker. You also have to drink as much as the biggest drinkers and in a rounds scenario that means drink as much as you can until you become unconscious. It was good

Victor J Kennedy

in a way because I didn't think too much about myself and my recovery. Especially on New Years Eve, when most people experience melancholy about change or the past or even the future. I was so blotto that I couldn't even tell you to this day what happened at midnight. I was with all the lads in a pub in Kendal and Sonia was there with me. I've seen the photos to prove it. Thing is, I just look wrecked and I'm smoking in those photos which is always a bad sign for me. By the time I'd sobered up it was nearly my birthday in mid-January. I'd been thinking about Tanya and I wanted, once and for all, to put it to bed and finally get some closure so I started writing a letter to her. It was all going to be civil and would sort out the money situation still unresolved since she got a refund from the Bodrum holiday deposit. I needed the money now, as I was about to go back to university.

Dear Tanya,

      I don't know whether I've gone soft or what but I'm doing or about to do something I always told you I didn't believe in. I told you I'd never write as it leaves a document of how fucked up we can sound and reflect badly on the person sending the letter (I remember how you felt about Mike - your ex and I don't want you to think I'm doing the same thing). If I'm honest with myself I've been meaning to write since June but I think I was right not to do it.

Amazingly by coincidence, at this point my parents' phone started ringing and I jumped up to answer it.
"Hello Kennedy."
"Er, Hi. Is that Victor?"
"Yes it is. Who's this?"
"It's Tanya."
"Wow! That's unbelievable!! I was just writing a letter to you."
"Oh really?"
"Yeah, amazing. That's fate, that is."
"Why are you writing me a letter?"

"I could ask you the same thing about ringing me up."

"Well, do you remember that blue Levis shirt that I bought for Lewis?"

"Yeah."

"Do you have it?"

"Why?"

"I want to find out where it is?"

"But it's not yours."

"It's not yours either. It's Lewis's."

"So if it's a gift for him then why do you want it?"

"Look Vic, to cut a long story short. Lewis and Justine came round to ours for dinner last week and Lewis was asking where his shirt was."

"So you took it upon yourself to get it for him?"

"I know you have it because I brought it up for you when you were in hospital."

"In between your trysts with Gideon, you mean?"

"I haven't called for an argument Vic. The shirt cost nearly fifty quid. It was a gift for someone else and you have it."

"I don't know how you can talk like this after taking the deposit for the holiday in Bodrum. That was £250 of my student loan and it went into your back pocket."

"Is that what your letter was gonna be all about?"

"No. It was about closure."

"Closure? We've been split up for over seven months Vic. I'm living with Gideon now. I've got a totally different life."

"That's your closure. Not mine. Anyway, I've found a girlfriend and been steady for three months nearly now. I want you to know I'm back on my feet."

"Good for you. I'm glad for you. Now can I have my shirt back."

"It's Lewis's shirt and you can have it back when you give me my £250 back."

"Ok forget about the shirt then. I'll see you around."

"Hang on a minute! Two and a half years together and then you ring me up about a shirt that doesn't belong to you? Are you sure that's why you rang?"

Victor J Kennedy

"Vic, our relationship died when you bought that computer. Gideon paid me more attention than you did during that last six months. I hardly even remember the two years before that. I mean, you were shagging around during the first summer holidays so what chance did we have? Gideon loves me. I don't think you ever really did."

"I did. You have no idea what effect you've had on my life. This last year has been the worst in my entire life. I nearly died in the hospital. I'm only just back to my old self."

"Your old self? Watch out girls."

"I'm back in Harrow in three weeks. Gonna finish that degree I should've finished last year with you."

"And on that note I'm going to hang up."

"No, not yet. I'll bring that shirt down with me. It's too big for me anyway."

"I'm not paying £250 for it, ok?"

"We could meet up somewhere and have a chat? Bring the shirt."

"You've got a girlfriend, remember?"

"I want that money Tanya."

"Well I'm sorry. Best of luck back at uni. Bye."

"Don't hang up..." The phone went dead. I was livid. Thoughts were racing around my head again in a fit of paranoia. Dinner with Lewis? Was she having an affair with him too? No, don't be stupid. But if he was there with her and Gideon all cosy with their girlfriends then they must be friends and my demise must have been a set up. No one liked me. It was not just Nath. He was telling the truth. Oh my god, I deserved this. I'm a horrible person and I don't even realise it. I need to sort my act out. My act? I shouldn't be acting, I should be myself. It's her fault. What was she ringing for anyway? Should Lewis fight his own battles if he wants his own shirt back? What if Lewis doesn't know? But why would she act on her own volition? Ah... she has decided that shirt would look good on Gideon and she's discussed it with him before ringing me. The twisted little bitch. I fucking hate Gideon. It wouldn't suit him anyway.

Mad in England - A memoir

It's not black and it doesn't have ACDC written across it's chest. Maybe she's trying to 'change' him and smarten him up? Maybe deep down she's not into black. What am I on about? I know her! I know her like the back of my hand and she wouldn't like someone like Gideon. She liked me. Someone like me. Someone who hadn't had a nervous breakdown.

I went downstairs and straight to my mum, of course. I don't care what anyone thinks, there are people who love you and care for you, who sometimes after a car accident or a diagnosis of cancer, actually become your carer. They literally have to care for you. Imagine if I had married Tanya and all this had happened later in life, perhaps after our first born child. Would she have reacted the same way? My mum has always been there for me. It's unconditional love and it's proved how strong that is because the last year was no fucking picnic for her. I cannot imagine what it must feel like to watch a healthy boy that you've created and raised, deteriorate into something a shadow of his former self. I nearly fucking died for god's sake! What would I have died for? Tanya wouldn't have got her Levi's shirt back then, would she?

I took all this anger to my mum so she made a cup of tea, sat me down and counselled me. She distributed some wisdom and empathy, whilst making me see Tanya's side of the story. What would I have done had the shoe been on the other foot? Would I have left her in the same circumstances? People should not be blamed for not being able to cope. I didn't quite understand that at the time because there was so much anger inside me but as I listened, I began to thaw. My mum gently made me believe and understand that I had bigger fish to fry. I was about to go to London and get the degree. It was going to be really difficult and I would need to prepare for unexpected obstacles. This whole Tanya thing needed to be less of an obstacle and I had to let her go. I did afterall have a new girlfriend in Sonia, even though it felt temporary. My mum's persuasive tone convinced me I had to set myself free from all the emotions surrounding Tanya and move on to the next part of my life. A clean slate. A brand new start. Don't ignore this has all happened but become focused on 'next' that it occupies more of your brain and the scar of 1995 is pushed right to the back in a small dark recess. I was over it. My mum was amazing. In one cup of tea she had rearranged the whole universe.

My driving licence had finally returned from the DVLA after about three months of interrogation and checks to make sure I wasn't an axe murderer who shouldn't be behind the wheel of a car. Their letter of 31st January 1996 expained that I only had a two year licence because due to the mental health problems I would need a regular review of my fitness to drive. I had to take it on the chin and with my new outlook on life think glass half full. At least I could drive. Some people with fifty year licences can't even do that. The week before I'd been to Harrow to see the housing officer and managed to find a place on Station Road above a chinese restaurant. I would be living with two girls, Hannah and Ilisha, from first year Contemporary Media Practice (Gideon's course). I'd persuaded my dad to do the long journey south for the penultimate time, although he didn't really need convincing because, like my mum, he was there to help me finish my degree. He would have done anything to help get me on my feet again. So he was happy to go through another seven hour tortuous motorway journey before collapsing in the Cross Keys. This time we only took my dad's car because the onset of my studies being focused on computers rather than drawing boards meant we could fit it all in a saloon. I was only going to be there for five months anyway, plus the nice girls I was moving in with had drawn me the short straw which meant I had the tiny bedroom, at the front of the flat, overlooking the kebab shops and traffic. I didn't care because I was focussed. I had a job to do. Go down there, get the degree and get out. Like a Ninja. I'd had a final heart to heart with Sonia before I left and she told me she was going to pursue her dream of teaching English abroad. She had found a school in Corfu town and was finalising her details before going out there for six months. We discussed me going out there after I graduated. Silly plans like me starting a little agency on the island and us having a new life together abroad. She said that if we were still together in July, then why not go over for two weeks sunshine and a rest after working so hard to finish university. It sounded like a plan to me. I needed a rest from the last two years. I hadn't had a holiday since Lanzarote with Ray and Julie in September 1993. And I couldn't exactly call laying in bed with depression all last summer a holiday.

Ilisha and Hannah were really good to me when I moved in. They helped me unpack and flirted with my dad. They cooked food and helped me set up the computer in the back room, which they said should be my study room because I was a third year student and they were first year students who would mostly be smoking dope, watching Eastenders and having their boyfriend's Darryl and Donovan round in the lounge at the front. This split was perfect because I had a quiet room and they didn't have an old man encroaching in their frolics. I empathised because when I was in the first year I didn't really want to hang out with third years. Thing is, maybe they'd heard on the grapevine what had happened to me because they let me into their social circle up at the bar and at home. It was like having a little family back at the flat. Totally different from the competitive and fake-gun ridden terror cell I'd been living in twelve months before.

Vic is our man...
We love Vic

Dear Husband
Just to let you know that your 2 lovely wives have gone to stay with Darryl's granny in Bedford (I can't remember if I told you) in case you're wondering where your dinner is! See you tomorrow evening darling - lots of love, Isha + Hannah xxx

Victor J Kennedy

ps - Please do the rubbish
pps - Practice your dance moves I want to dance with you
tomorrow...

We love Viccy xxxx
Vic is cool

The contrast was amazing and made me feel confident that
the atmosphere which had built up over two years living
with Nath was very, very unhealthy. I wasn't a threat to these
people so I was allowed in. They certainly didn't make me
feel I was putting them in pigeonholes. They didn't want to
control me or steal my identity either. They even invited me
to watch the infamous Brits round at Donovan's house when
Jarvis Cocker jumped on the stage with Michael Jackson.
The story was a little bit different up at the college bar. I was
quite fearful of people's reactions who were in the year
below me and were still there on my return but I hadn't
anticipated the wide range of their reactions. Mental health
stigma boils down to a very simple split: 51% of people treat
you the same as they did before they found out you had a
nervous breakdown. Those are the sorts of people you need
to seek out and be around. They are called friends. 39% of
people treat you like a victim and over-sympathise. They
always ask you if everything is okay and come across as
condescending. Then there's the 10% that are left. They are
your enemies. They're the ones who fear you and fail to even
try and understand what has happened. They are absorbed
with distorted media messages and apply archetype
prejorative labels from historical periods where 'witches'
were burned and 'freaks' were expelled to the circus. There
were more than 10% of these people before the world
civilised. Forever, there always will be this 10%. You can
see it in their faces, that's if they give you eye contact. It's
like they have just felt something damp in their pants or
tasted something slightly odd from between their teeth. Their
face twists in slow motion. It's not like I'm insane on a day-

to-day basis but the thought that I could be is enough to put 10% of people off me. They're too polite and 'British' to ask me to my face about what happened but they are cheeky enough to have joke about it between themselves, often within earshot. You know it's about you, that's why they do it. They speak in code and 'in' jokes to expel the heretic. 'Nervous Breakdown' implies you are weak. You are not. In fact you are stronger for having gone through it. Like a broken bone. I know that now but back in February 1996 I didn't realise I had to curb my enthusiasm for behaving the same as everyone else ever again. This is a huge lesson in the road to recovery and for me it came in the form of Lyndsay from the year below us in Ceramics, that tall leggy blonde girl who had slept with Lewis a few times just before I went in hospital. She remembered me alright. That night she caught me slagging her off to my GID mates for being a cheap slut who was desperate to bed Lewis at that party in Twinkle and Ruth's house. This was pure karma in action and is another thing to watch out for. There's pre-breakdown down life and post-breakdown life. Now I'm not saying you gain more forgiveness post breakdown, after all I'm just talking about behaviour. In fact this whole story is about human nature and how we treat each other but Lyndsay was out for revenge and she unleashed both barrels with similar fury to Nathan Foreman and his pigeonholes speech that put the final nail in my coffin twelve painful months ago. A week into my return I'd got drunk at the bar with Ilisha's boyfriend Darryl and I ended up taking one of the girls there outside and across Watford Road to the pitch and putt for casual sex. I had no idea why it happened, I never saw the girl ever again. She wasn't even a student. And not to mention Sonia back in Kendal, preparing to fly to Corfu. I felt like shit about it but at the same time I felt good that I was back here in Harrow having fun without Tanya. I was allowed to get on with my life and I should not feel guilty about it. Thing is, gossip from Darryl to his mates had spread to Ceramics and Lyndsay had got word of my indiscretion and it had stirred up the feelings of revenge. After a few drinks during the second Friday night back she came over to the bar with a wry smile on her face. "Hi Vic, how's things?"

"Er, good yeah. And you?"

"Oh, I'm not quite myself at the moment."

"What's up?"

"Oh, I don't know whether you've heard or not but I've had loads of problems over the last year since you left."

"What's gone on?"

"Well, first of all I had a secret drug habit that nobody knew about. Then my boyfriend ran off with a girl from CMP while I started to believe my housemates were trying to kill me just when the dissertation had to handed in. Then I couldn't take the fact that nobody was bothered about their work as much as me so I did a little speech and then my head caved in one night at my boyfriends. I locked the door and terrorised his housemates by shouting out the window until the police came and battered the door down, locked me up and sent me to the nut house. I've been in rehab for about a year and now I've just come back to college to try and pick my sorry life up and last week I shagged someone I've never met before on the 9th green over there at the pitch and putt. I'm such a sad worthless piece of shit. Anyway, enough about my problems, what's happening with you?"

"Er,......not much really. Just out for a few drinks with my new college mates."

"What because all your old ones have all graduated?"

"Yeah. I guess I've just got to get on with it."

"Ok then, nice talking to you Vic. See you around."

"Yeah, see you later." She walked off grinning with a confident strut. Like a hyena after it's just eaten a gazelle that something else had already killed. I was screaming inside. It hurt so much because of the way she did it, lured me in to be compassionate about her life and then as her sentences expelled I realised it was a piss take. Massive, massive humiliation. To make it worse another girl from

Mad in England - A memoir

Ceramics overhead and tried to put her arm round me, that 39% of sympathisers which I hated nearly as much as the 10% who attack like Lyndsay had done. I hope she felt better and pre-breakdown I guess I deserved it but if she ever has a breakdown that's the only way she'll know that being on the end of such a hammering is unfair. Especially to tease someone about implications of why it occurred. After that, I knew I had to watch my behaviour because I would not be allowed the same forgiveness as everyone else anymore. In fact, I couldn't make any mistakes on any putting greens. I was a witch and a freak as soon as that information got out. Imagine that you have to be bland and unobtrusive to everyone to get away with this. They kill you if you're loud because that means you're mad. No opinions allowed. That's all there is to the 10% of people. I can spot them a mile off. If I watch my behaviour they'll never spot me. Unless they find out through idle gossip. Then they look at me like I'm not a rounded individual. This type of thing doesn't happen to people with 'sense'. It forces you to be rounded and balanced. You wouldn't survive otherwise. Like a rock star, dead in a swimming pool.

I decided after that episode that I had to educate myself with coping mechanisms. I wasn't looking for quips or put downs that I could drop into conversations like the one with Lyndsay. I was looking for answers. Big answers. Life's big questions answered. So I hit the University library for some extra curricular activity on top of the two modules I had left to do during the next four months; Major Project and Launch Pad. I wanted to find out if I was mad or whether what happened was actually just a glitch so I looked at psychology books and modern approaches to modern problems like the insightful book, Significant Ingredients of Burn Out. Everything that hit home I carefully wrote down in the notebook my mum bought me to use as a diary after I came out of hospital.

Victor J Kennedy

Dedication & Commitment
How many 'musts,' 'shoulds' and 'oughts.'
To friends – was charismatic, dynamic, inexhaustible, super competent.
Couldn't allow himself to ask for help, but had to deny his needs.
Like nail-biting, role playing becomes so much a part of the person that he doesn't even know he's doing it.
They have so much energy, it spills over to the people around them. They are the spark of every project, the centre of every group. They have that special attractiveness for others that we call charisma.
People bore you. Causes seem trivial. Whereas you used to participate at every meeting, coming up with plans and solid suggestions, you now sit silent, wishing you could get away.
"I love you" all the time – the voices belie the words.
Flare ups occur that seem totally out of character.
His speech patterns will falter as he finds himself forgetting what he started to say. Names and dates will elude him. His concentration span will be much more limited.

This stuff was pure gold and although I last summer I'd had support from the hospital and Garburn House, I had never found such strength in self-discovery. They say, a life unexplored is a life not worth living and as the months passed I made it my own personal project to make myself more than what I was before. I'm not talking about a complete moral overhaul but only by getting to the route causes of how I ended up experiencing a Stress Induced Hypomanic Episode would I be able to avoid doing it again. I would be able to recognise the patterns of behaviour – the triggers. I knew I would never take Pro-Plus ever again in my life. That one was easy to cut out. Other things, like alcohol, are more tricky due to how they have been sewn into the fabric of modern life. I'm not just talking about a pump on a bar in a pub. I mean, how we celebrate everything, no matter how insignificant, with a drink. I cannot stop drinking because I give myself away as being 'different' when in the presence of others. So I drink when I'm in company. But my strategy is just to avoid physically being in pubs or on stag do's or Friday lunchtime drinks etc. I try to save myself for certain things I feel are more important to celebrate than others. That way, people just think I'm boring rather than insane. Boring is less threatening. The thing is, all these strategies and the ones in the books follow one simple rule; Do anything in moderation. That advice was also given to me by my mum. Obviously, I didn't take her advice till it was too late but now, after everything I put myself and my family through, I'm an advocate.

The 23rd and penultimate module, Major Project, was worth 45 credits. That's three times greater than a normal module and therefore three times as much pressure not to mess up your degree right at the final hurdle. It was briefed in by Raymond and Sofia Gretchen from Apple Computers in California. She was an ex GID student who had been lucky enough to get into an MA course at The Royal College of Art called Computer Related Design. When she graduated she went straight to Cupertino to work in the Advanced Technology Group set up by Steve Jobs before he left. She was helping develop Operating System 10, which four years later became known as OSX. Apple had a history of innovation and to keep up the advantage, they had created The Apple Design Project. A competition open to all universities of the world, where a brief is set to solve a particular problem using technology. The entries from each university are monitored during the Major Project period and the best ones are selected to be presented at the Apple headquarters 1 Infinite Loop in Cupertino, Sillicon Valley. A week on campus would then be spent refining the solutions into a pitch presentation and each student team would stand up in a theatre full of Apple employees and present on a podium, next to the big screen. After that, commendations are presented and a winner is announced with a bursory or

Victor J Kennedy

the chance to make the project real and join Apple. I guess they were pretty shrewd coming up with such a conveyor belt of ideas and talent, not to mention for very little investment. We were all blown away that Sofia had got Westminster invited to contribute and she was really cool and down to earth about everything. The brief was as follows:

A universal characteristic of humanity is the natural desire for forming communities. Traditional communities have generally been focused on a particular location, and have aided their members in obtaining such basic necessities as food, clothing and shelter. This is not to say that community is merely a mechanism for enhancing our chances of survival in an uncertain world. Much of what makes life rich – story telling, song, art, gossip, friendship, games – is intimately entwined within community.

In this age of rapid transit and mass communication we find other sorts of communities, what might be called communities of interest. In these communities – which may or may not be centred around a particular place – people come together because of shared interests, values or goals, rather than because they are concerned about enhancing their day-to-day survival. Nevertheless, like traditional place-based communities, the conviviality and social richness communities of interest exhibit goes far beyond what would seem to be needed to simply accomplish their stated ends. Community, even though it is a powerful mechanism for collective activity, is also something of an end in itself.

In the 1996 Design Project we invite you to reflect on the possibilities and problems of community, and the ways in which computational and communication technologies might support community. Our definition of community is deliberately broad: a group of people, large enough to prohibit everyone from knowing everyone else well, who share some common interests which leads them to communicate and perhaps act in concert. Over time true communities develop common traits such as histories, traditions, values, and methods for recruiting new members, establishing norms of behaviour, and other aspects of self-regulation.

How might computational and communication technology support the community? There are two avenues to explore. One direction is to focus on the question of how a place-based community might be supported with computational technology – how might technology be integrated in to a place so as to better support the formation, maintenance, and functioning of the community within it? The other direction is to focus on the concept of virtual community, the idea that a network of interest can grow.

Great brief! The one sticking point for me was this had to be a group project. I knew the year below me, the one I had now joined, did not have the same verve and ambition as the year I dropped out of. First of all who would take up the challenge because this was not a mandatory brief for this module. Then out of those that showed interest, who would I want to team up together with. Who would team up with me? I wanted to win it from the outset but I didn't know who could match my drive or my talent. One person who did was Cameron. Cameron was about seven feet tall and loved the Nine Inch Nails. He had long brown scruffy hair which changed red, pink or jet black every so often. He wore army fatigues or black swat outfits with three hundred lace up Dr. Martin Boots or standard issue Marines' footwear. The thing is, he was a really gentle guy and massively intelligent. People looked up to him metaphorically as well as literally. He had matched me pretty much grade for grade up to this point so I approached him and asked how he felt about teaming up. He thought it was cool as long as his housemate Brian could join in. Brian was a Hertfordshire rich kid who came to college in a white Jeep. He was blonde and had grown his hair long which was naturally frizzy, so along with his surfing fatigues and pastel colours, not to mention

Victor J Kennedy

his heavy spliff habit, he was the perfect hanger-on. A stoner who was getting grades by living with the more talented ones and hoping it brushed off. Even worse, for the past year he'd been going out with that gorgeous black girl Siobhan who I snogged in the bar behind Tanya's back. I talked with Cameron about this for a while to gage how close he was to Brian but there was no budging him so I decided I needed Cameron more and I would have to help carry the Stoner through the last part of his degree. While we were talking Peter Farrell came over to do the same thing. Peter was a local Pinner lad and he was a really good footballer. He was a man's man and had a very strong cockney accent. He didn't sound too bright but then neither did I. What he did have was a great eye for design. The work I'd seen of his since my return was very impressive but the deep thinking was not as astute or in evidence. Maybe he hadn't had the right project yet. The three of us chatted and came to an agreement that the four of us would enter the competition with the prior knowledge that if we won, only me and Peter would travel to California as Cameron was getting married after graduating and Brian was flying to Venezuela to pick fruit on a gap year before deciding what to do next. Picking fruit indeed.

After I left the briefing and was walking home, I thought about it and decided we didn't have much conceptual mental strength and also if two would never receive the prize then their motivation could waiver. I knew Alan was doing an MA at Harrow so he would be around all summer. I'd already seen him briefly going into his lectures. I wondered if he had the time to join in and whether that would be allowed due to him not being on our course any more. So when I got home I gave him a ring and we chatted about it. Turns out that Raymond took some of his lectures and had mentioned it to him already. Raymond knew how good Alan was and he obviously wanted his University to do well so he had already drafted him in. All I had to do was speak to the rest of the group and convince them to let Alan join the team.

Mad in England - A memoir

After I put the phone down I practiced my guitar skills using
Donovan's guitar. Donovan, Hannah's boyfriend was a really
talented guitar player. He would play for us, taking requests
and even picking up songs that were played to him on CD
which he had never heard before. His skills fascinated me
and after my love affair with Sonia to the soundtrack of
Oasis, I wanted to be able to play them all myself so he
began teaching me. I found learning to play music very
therapeutic and I would add that to any recovery programme
or coping strategy in the future. The concentration gives
your mind a rest from all the other stuff flying around in
there. It's the same thing when playing football for me. I lose
myself on a football pitch. I leave everything in the changing
rooms and once I cross the lime I feel ten years old again,
only for ninety minutes but that's enough. After I'd finished
murdering Wonderwall, I walked up to Cameron's house and
he agreed to let Alan join the team. Brian was in bed but was
cool about it. I got Peter's number from Cameron and he
thought it was a great idea.

The following weeks we tried to scope out the problem and
create an angle. Early discussions lent towards the
exploration of existing physical community and we debated
whether technology could have a detrimental effect upon
social interaction. Would it be too easy to say that in the
future we will, by the aid of technology, never need to leave
the house; work, leisure, social interaction could be achieved
from home via the screen? Could this situation lead to the
deconstruction of the community till it no longer exists for
large proportions of the population. It would be interesting
to see how technology can be integrated into existing place
based physical communities, instead of replacing them. How
can technology be integrated as to better support the
formation, maintenance and functioning of community? Is
one of the main elements of a community the fact that some
people are let in and others are excluded, communities such
as golf clubs for example remain strongly defined because
they strive to exclude others from joining. Does technology,

Victor J Kennedy

however, give everybody the power to set up their own community? Can new technology significantly alter community and social relationships, has lifestyle become introverted? Has the connection to the world community been gradually replaced with electronics that span great distances (telephones, radio, television, computers), is there a greater incentive to not leave the house, a greater incentive to not seek out physical community? Does an ability to communicate with a much larger wide spread community threaten to isolate us from our immediate community, our friends and family? Will virtual communities become a problem when they displace similar discourse in real communities? We must not neglect our place based communities for new virtual ones.

Before long I'd got immersed in my London study lifestyle and once again the girlfriend had taken a back seat. This time it was easier for me because Sonia was 250 miles north in Kendal (soon to be 2050 in Corfu) and most of our dialogue was over the phone or in letters. I really quite enjoyed some of the rubbish and kinky filth she would send down for me to experience. It really cheered me up each week and I reciprocated with various creative letter writing techniques. Having her on the end of the phone was really supportive too. If I felt down I could call her and tell her how I felt but at the end of the day, it was a long distance relationship and it was about to get longer when she went out to Corfu. Like they say, out of sight out of mind. With all my focus on the Apple project I forgot Valentine's Day. Well, I actually remembered it on the day but effectively missed the post. I wrote in the card;

"Roses are red, Violets are blue, sorry it's late, I am shit! xxx"

I also called Interflora in Kendal and paid twenty quid for a bunch of roses to be delivered to her at Pain de Paris, which would have embarrassed her good and proper in front of her work mates. She wasn't mushy or sentimental like Tanya and I liked that. I obviously felt pressure to get Sonia something but that is pressure from the marketing genius who invented Valentine's Day. The pressure I felt from Tanya was a claustrophobic feeling of letting her heart down. It was the claustrophobia that had slowly squeezed us both together so intensely one of us ended up on Ward 4 doing a twentyeight day stretch, ironically just days after 14th February 1995. These memories or touch points, as I prefer to think of them, when calendar dates or physical places start to remind you as much as smells do sometimes. These touchpoints are where I confront my demons. When I say a demons, I mean in terms of post traumatic stress, there are things that can set off a spiral of negative thoughts and these processes can lead to trouble again. They need to be interrupted. They need to be confronted and not avoided. This is another coping mechanism I knew would build up strength. I thought for a long time about what I would do if I ever came face to face with Tanya again. Or Tanya and Gideon together for that matter. There is a saying that luck is preparation meeting opportunity. I hate laying in bed at night after a confrontation with another human being and running it all back in my head, then realising I should have said something at an appropriate time and it would have fixed everything. I found my thought processes, combined with my studies of psychology, led me to so much personal enlightenment that I began to explore why I blamed Nath, Shumana, Tanya and Gideon specifically for the events that occurred during February 1995 when my head turned inside out and my heart nearly stopped beating. If I could hold Edwin the staff nurse responsible for saving my life with that injection of Haloperidol, how could I blame those four individuals for my hypomanic episode? Surely I had to take responsibility myself. It is my body and they did not infiltrate my body unless they poisoned me? Now there's a stupid paranoid thought that needs interrupting. Of course they played their parts in my deterioration and I would add Lewis to that list too for not telling my parents or any medical staff or tutors at the university about my change of behaviour. They just didn't notice. It was neglect. Neglect and being ignored by the people who were supposed to be my friends and the people looking out for me. That was what I would blame. People who succeed in life are those who have learned how to take any challenge that life gives them and communicate that experience to themselves in a way that causes them to successfully change things. People who fail, take the adversities of life and accept them as limitations.

I took the unforgiving view, that people who think in limits are limited people, into the scoping phase of the Apple Project, which we were now doing in Cameron's living room with This Morning blaring out of the TV and Brian sat in his pyjamas with his eyes wide shut from too much resin abuse the night before. We seemed to be getting nowhere fast because each brainstorm would result into a giggling schoolboy gossip about people from college. Peter had surprised me because he had the worst attention span of all. After one session me and Alan left to go home together and we started talking about how bad it was all going. By the time we got to my flat at Station Road we decided to break away and hold an unofficial brainstorm ourselves to get things back on track. I asked him to come upstairs and offered him dinner so we could work into the night. He agreed and we discussed what this project could possibly become. We had seen that the ability or desire to create relationships and social grouping was a basic human need and developing technology would potentially make it easier for us to create our own communities; technology was giving us the power of creation and community management. Interesting issues were being raised by research into the work of Howard Rheingold and his writings on the virtual community. He spoke of there being three places in life, where you live, where you work and where you go for fun or leisure. He saw places of 'idle chat' (pubs, cafes, parks) as being places where communities can arise and hold together, he proposed that the Internet and the virtual community idea could be classed as being one of these 'third' places.

'The idea that logging on to a community is like peeking your head into a pub for a moment to see who is there'. Where community has been restricted by location and resources, via technology we can now have communities based instead on interest and goals. What role has communication within a virtual community?

Communication is the very core of any social relationship and a community's ability to survive depends on its members' ability to talk to each other, exchanging both views and opinions. But does the culture and methods of communication in the virtual world raise important issues when compared to face-to-face communication. At present, communication via e-mail and chat facilities represents faceless communication. No one really knows who they are speaking to and therefore a communication culture has arisen where there is a lack of responsibility or security in what is being said or read by the users. No one is guaranteed of authenticity or level of interest in a conversation. Is the communication then flawed if both parties in an exchange don't know or completely trust the person they are talking to? If no one can trust each other then nothing significant will ever happen with this medium. Could technology therefore be used to develop safer or new ways of responsible communication in an environment with no responsibility?

Of all the issues raised, the most interesting and potentially strongest, was the idea of technology actually working with the real community, to enhance instead of replacing it. Technology increases the individuals power to create their own communities, giving them an organisational ability that they may not have in 'real' life. It became obvious that for the project to move on, the research must focus now on one example of a community and see how technology could benefit that group of people. With this in mind we concentrated our research on to the physically impaired community, more significantly, the Multiple Sclerosis community. An individual's ability to create or participate in a community is severely restricted by issues such as access, resources and more significantly, the symptoms of the disability. It was clear from this early stage that the virtual community could offer a new opportunity for such individuals.

We put it to Cameron and the team who agreed it was a good angle to go on so we did some extensive research with Laura Hunter of the Harrow MS Therapy Centre and Derek Pryor, IT Manager with the MS Society.

Raymond and Sofia Gretchen accepted our project submission brief. It was then emailed to Cupertino to be approved. Eventually we were told by Raymond that we had been accepted but that the pressure was now on to produce something special as another group from Alan's course also had their project submission approved and only one team could go to the states to present. That meant we had a competition on our hands. I relished it. I had a goal now. Even more focus. We started looking at ways in which a product could be prototyped either on screen or as an actual model.

On the same day we got approval for that project, I had to sit down with Raymond and Noel and review my contextual study from last year. When I got in Raymond's office they told me instantly that I had passed the module because I had written a dissertation and the mark was 70% which put a massive smile on my face. At least all that effort had paid off, even though it helped put me in hospital. This was Raymond and Noel's whole point of reviewing that Director projector I'd spent numerous hours producing above and beyond the call of duty. Raymond spoke up after the presentation on his monitor had ended, "Well Victor, that was all well and good but I don't know why it exists?" "Sorry?" I questioned.

Mad in England - A memoir

"Well it's quite clear you did two pieces of work when you only needed to choose one. This work is superfluous."

"Will none of this go towards my degree?"

"No Victor. Your mark for a single module of 15 credits is 77% and that was based on your writing for a dissertation. I don't quite understand why this piece of work exists. Well, I do understand but I need you to undertand why doing more than necessary is unnecessary and can actually affect your health."

"Oh yes, I totally agree now but it's twelve months later and a lot has happened to me."

"Indeed."

"I've learned a lot about myself. About life."

"There's still a lot to learn. Even at my age. Do you take medication?"

"No. What for? All the medication stopped when I came out of hospital in May last year. I'm fine now."

"I take Prozac Victor. My wife thinks I need it at my age and doing such a demanding job can sneak up on you, you know?"

"Does that mean you're depressed?"

"Not if I keep taking the tablets." he smiled.

"Does it affect how you think? Your clarity, I mean."

"No. I'm doing better than ever. In fact, I've just been offered the Professor's job on the Computer Related Design course at The Royal College of Art. Not bad for a 72 year old?"

"That's brilliant! When do you start?"

"Oh no, I won't be starting there. I'm happy where I am. I don't want to over stretch myself too much now do I?" he smiled again.

"Like a rubber band, you mean?"

"Aye, that's a possible representation. Flexible, strong. Good."

Noel interjected, "I think what happened to you last year was yourself. You pushed way too hard when you really didn't need to. You have the talent. You've proved that in the three years or more that you've now been here. What Raymond is trying to explain is that from now on you must keep an eye on yourself and take regular breaks. Balance work and life. There'll be times when you're a professional when you'll have to put the effort in but being exceptional all the time is not a guarantee of satisfaction. You'll find happiness in a more balanced lifestyle. With your talent you will find it easier than most people to rise up the ladder without nearly killing yourself doing it."

"I understand and I just want to say thank you for allowing me back to finish off the degree. It means so much to graduate."

"Well you haven't done it yet. You better get back to work then!" quipped Noel.

"Aye, go placidly young man." added Raymond.

"Honestly, I'll not be going back in a psychiatric ward again in a hurry."

"Don't be so dismissive Victor, some people do their best work in there. Speaking of which, I hope you will be re-submitting to the CRD course at The Royal College again this year." Raymond smiled his biggest smile as I walked out of his office with a massive smile on my face too.

"I've already filled the forms in. I just need to put the stickers on my work again and that's it." This kind of positive exchange was the antidote to Lyndsay and the 10% of people who chewed away at my confidence. That old saying, divide and conquer rings so true. Raymond had just done the opposite, he just gave me an insight into his private life and that he has problems too. When that happens, when people open up and engage with you without interrogating you about what happened, it is great. They give you energy when they give you information first. It's finding that common ground. All human relationships follow the same formula: rapport equals trust plus comfort. I don't know whether I would advise seeking that kind of information out of other people because the majority of us are still influenced by the media to be ashamed or feel weak about mental illness. Who aspires to be in the mass anyway? To be an outsider can be a great privilege, almost an honorary distinction. Saying that, the so called 'normal' ones are the minority these days.

I knew I was alright but I had to take it easy on the booze in between the studying. I think my tolerance had gone down because of having pretty much six months off drink while I recovered. Mind you the amount I drank with Smudge and the lads running up to Christmas was pretty phenomenal. Maybe it was because I had calmed down since returning to London. Either way I was pretty disappointed with myself when I woke up one morning in my single bed next to a naked girl and I was naked too. I was really angry laying there running the last few hours of the night before through my head. I couldn't see this girl's face because she was asleep on my chest but I knew that Sonia would not be best pleased if she could see me now. I also couldn't undertand myself either. I wasn't in London to sleep around and now this was the second girl in less than three months away from my girlfriend. Drink is the devils work. And look at me, I can't even practice what I preach – everything in moderation! You what?

I racked my brains until I remembered who this girl was. It was Liona Sullivan for god's sake. She was in a bar in Harrow with some mates when I bumped into her. She was Stella Clarke's best mate. Stella was Rory's sexy little sister who had a crush on Lewis and would bring Liona round for Sunday dinners last year. Eventually we would all get drunk and Stella would hook up with Lewis in his bedroom and poor Liona would be left with me and Nath to do the dishes. She was a great girl, a really kind person and very pretty too but she was really, really young. I wasn't sure of her age but I would bet she was not even 19 yet. I started getting flash backs of the filthy stuff we did when we got back to Station Road. We'd even been in the shower together doing all sorts of crazy things. I hoped Ilisha and Hannah didn't see anything. They just thought I was a boring book worm and this would shatter their expectations of me. They also knew about Sonia and would force me to tell her what I'd done. I'd been unfaithful. How terrible. I think maybe with Sonia being in Kendal, I just needed some physical touch and comfort. Liona's naked body laying on mine was certainly feeling good. Maybe I shouldn't feel so bad. If you can't be with the one you love, love the one you're with and all that? When Liona woke up she was fairly loved up and called me "Benny" which was her pet name for me. Oh dear. She told me again how much she cared and was so glad to see me doing so well again. She said she'd been worried about me while I was ill and didn't know what to do. She was so glad to have bumped into me in that bar and that she always fancied me but never wanted to upset Tanya but if she'd known about Gideon she would have gone for me much earlier. It was all very flattering but what about what I wanted? I'd never even thought of Liona in that way until I came round naked next to her after an alcoholic binge.

I went home at Easter on the train for a little rest and relaxation. I wanted to see Sonia and maybe tell her what had gone on but I knew that if I did, it would be over. She was just about to fly off to Corfu in three weeks so I ended up bottling it and just having a great time. She didn't need the stress. We saw Chubby Brown on stage in Manchester and went to Preston to see Trainspotting at the cinema on the night Liverpool drew 4-4 at home to unlucky Keegan's Newcastle. Afterwards I was feeling inspired after seeing someone getting off the drugs and choosing life. For me, this was a positive media message and I found strength from it. Once back in London and having said goodbye (almost for good) to Sonia, I found out that my application to The Royal College of Art was unsuccessful for the second year running. What an utter load of bollocks! I sent them exactly the same portfolio of twelve months ago when I received that wonderful hand written letter from Professor Geraldine Copthorne-Scott. If they said they would take me if I applied again then why not now? It's total nonsense and they've wasted my time. It's the end of a dream for me because I cannot be arsed to keep applying every year then get knocked back again and again. But maybe Professor Copthorne-Scott was pissed off because Raymond had been offered her job? Maybe she'd already quit and someone else took the job because Raymond turned it down? It can't be my fault again. The portfolio is exactly the same. It's down to opinion. Or maybe they don't want a potential 'lunatic' running around the hallowed halls when the project deadline arrives along with the stress. People with mental health 'issues' don't rise to the top like people without those kinds of undesirable issues. I needed to stop and interrupt these thought processes because I was projecting a lot onto this outcome instead of dealing with it and shouting at the top of my voice "NEXT!"

I dived into the Apple Project and tried to sort it out because after all working together on research we decided in May that we would divide the group up for the actual design and production. It was at this point that we agreed a verbal contract to each other that each sub group would not have to worry about the other sub group's work. i.e. 'You would only have to produce what you have said you would produce'. This was put into two parts. Introduction to ideas/concepts and realisation of proposal. I worked mainly with Alan on the first section Introduction to ideas/concepts, although Peter did contribute in two areas of it. I designed and produced early screen layouts of how the introduction would run but as a group we decided not to use them. I then worked up the final screen designs using the circular model. I personally collected all images used on the first section and scanned them all myself. In production I also resized them and built the grid for images and information to fall into. I worked on the script and storyboards with Alan for this section and personally recorded and edited an initial voiceover which acted as a marker for the final voiceover to be used in. I liaised with the Media Degree course leader and set up a meeting with the head of radio production. I then had to organise the whole voiceover and meet with a second

Victor J Kennedy

year Media student, Spencer Hayes. I then recorded and
edited the whole voiceover with Spencer. I also worked on
music/sound selection for the first section, recording and
editing those. I also spent alot of time organising, recording
and editing three of the four interviews with MS individuals.
This involved meetings with subjects, organisation of
messages being put across and actual recording of their
voices. I spent alot of time on the telephone organising
meetings with the MS Therapy Centre and the MS Society. I
also spent time to organise and neatly present all research
gathered along with other group research, personal roughs
and development of ideas. For the record as well, I
contributed a large amount to group communication, morale,
administration and organisation. To be blunt, the other group
of Cameron and Brian did absolutely fuck all. They put the
whole project in jeopardy but then they didn't give a shit
anyway because we discovered the group mark for this
project was divided four equal ways (not including Alan)
and in any case they were either getting married or off to get
stoned in Venezuela under an orange tree in about three
weeks' time.

In the end, what we actually ended up making for the Apple
Project 1996 was not even a product at all. Me, Alan and
Peter made a linear multimedia presentation about the
concept of adapting a television screen into a touch-screen
virtual community centre for people who have keyboard
accessibility problems due to symptoms of Multiple
Sclerosis such as shaking hands. The linear presentation
would run alongside a live verbal presentation made by me,
Alan and Peter:

Apple Design Project '96 Final Presentation Speech

When we started looking at the brief from the beginning we
looked at ourselves and how we are hindered by the
technologies we use to produce our work. The key word here
is 'Hindered'. This led us on to the physically challenged

community and then focusing on the Multiple Sclerosis Community, who, by the very nature of the disease can benefit most from technologies that could adapt to their individual requirements.

Another huge important fact we found is not only do MS individuals have multiple symptoms physically but they can also be faced with multiple problems financially. This could be adapting a car or their home involving rails, bath lifts or ramps. Sometimes they may even have to relocate.

Ideally a way of utilising existing communication technologies they already own, such as a telephone or television would benefit them a lot more than spending x amount of time and money on a new product that they have to learn and understand how to use.

We met with the MS Society in London. Now, through literally cold calling we came across an interesting and massive point that illustrates what an MS community is all about.

We dealt with Derek Pryor, IT Manager at the MS Society over email and the telephone for three weeks before meeting him in person. When we did he turned out to be a wheelchair bound MS individual. Aside from the fact that we didn't need to know he was wheelchair bound, the technology had masked that point from us.

And so we realised a facilitator was paramount. What is needed is technology that lets humans take part fully within any community in whichever way they choose.

MS is a very private and personal affliction and we didn't want to make assumptions about it when researching.

(Videos played of each Case Study here)

So here we are with four individuals isolated from a central point who all have needs and personal requirements. They are unconnected.

Victor J Kennedy

Another message we got through research was; often a person who has just been diagnosed is almost left to their own devices by their GP. They then start, as we did by going to a library or looking for a phone number in the Yellow Pages. Other MS Individuals have mentioned safety and security in the fact that they would only tell someone how they were really feeling when they were inside a therapy centre or amongst people they could 'trust'. Which happens to be a fundamental requirement for communities to form.

We can now see the four individuals connected to a virtual MS Centre and through common interests can now function as a whole.

In the end, all the heartache paid off because Raymond gave us 66% which meant I was still on for First Class Honours with one module left to complete:

Module 24: Launch Pad.
Design an interactive presentation that STRICTLY engages the user. The user was actually a potential employer and the briefing for this 'Interactive CV' was done by Kaitlin Mackenzie, a moderator on our course and also a director of Mackenzie Keane, one of the BBC's main suppliers of interactive content for their CD-Rom titles. Seen as how this was my final hurdle and with my knowledge of my failure to gain a place at The Royal College of Art, I decided to really push the boat out and do my finest piece of work since I began the course. I would not be relying on anyone else as part of a team, I was working solo and I only had to rely on myself. Just the way I liked it. If I wasn't going to do an MA then I may as well launch myself into professional life making a statement. That's if I didn't go to Corfu and set up my own humble studio making flyers for DJ's and fisherman's business cards.
My Launch Pad was going to be an interactive self-portrait designed to present to a prospective employer my range of

skills, my interests, details of my background but mainly to project my opinions and thoughts about work through an extension of my personality. It wanted it to work like this: Part one: Potential employer receives a cover letter, an enclosed CV and a disk formatted for an Apple Macintosh. Part two: Employer opens the disk and the file inside. She/he is then introduced to a looping sequence of images and invited to explore and interact further to receive more information. Part three: Once the person has accessed the information within they will have a good idea of what my personality is like and whether I am competent enough to be given an interview.

Launch Pad - Victor Kennedy

Background
When I read the brief I was very excited and I knew what I wanted to do, I just wasn't sure of how exactly to go about producing it.
I wanted to work in the area of multimedia involving screen design so straight away I decided that my final product for Launch Pad would be produced in Director, on-screen and would be interactive. I wanted to be able to show that I could actually bring an entire contained piece of work from design right through to production. This piece of communication would act as an ice-breaker or introduction prior to me actually meeting the person who receives it. It would be in the form of a disc that could be sent through the post and then viewed on a computer at its destination. I started by dissecting the brief and found that as a 'self-portrait' I could stretch the brief as long as I tried to describe myself in relation to my work and the technologies I used to produce my work. Straight away I knew I could produce a parody about using technology, namely the Apple Macintosh computer by trying to relate my ideas and experiences to the prospective employer. I wanted to strike a chord with

whoever was exposed to the information, something they find amusing.

I split the presentation into 4 sections: Background, Experience, Skills and Interests. These sections do not necessarily come in any order as the presentation is non linear. They all appear as options in a home screen and are represented as alternating photographs. There are no labels or directions just a looping sequence. The reason for this is to invite the spectator to be curious and explore what is hidden behind each set of images by clicking on them.

The section 'Background' is designed to show basic and relevant information about my upbringing that an employer needs to know. Where I'm from and where my home is.

The section 'Experience' demonstrates my ability to communicate by visual means. This section again attracts the person by the very nature of its image (Lottery balls), what it represents and what it might imply.

The section 'Skills' clearly identifies a signified subject matter (Apple Computers) but through the employer's understanding of the technology, it conveys a meaning. The aim of this section is to represent my knowledge of the technology by showing fundamental problems incurred when using a computer.

The section 'Interests' is where I wanted to enjoy myself but also where I wanted the user to be challenged by what they were seeing. There are two simple games for the person to play, based on football. The first is a spot the ball competition, the second game is a more challenging exercise. 'The Net' as it is called, uses fonts as teams that pass the ball to each other in complex patterns that the person must remember and follow to progress.

It did the trick alright, because Kaitlin Mackenzie offered me a job there and then when she was marking it. She probably offered every student a job that afternoon on those one to ones. That said, I was glad of the feedback because I knew if it impressed her it would impress other people. People in bigger agencies than Mackenzie Keane. The great thing about it was that if she liked it so much and offerred me a job then she had to give me a good enough mark to get the First Class Degree I'd spent four years desperately striving to collect. It was within my grasp, I could feel it. I just had to wait three weeks in June doing nothing but watching EURO 96 and playing five-a-side at the Sports Day in Chiswick under scorching sunshine. All I could think about was the marks coming out in the following weeks. Thursday 11th July 1996 was my day of reckoning. The day it was all over. My nightmare would end and my dreams could begin.

I got two tickets for me and Alan to go to the quarter final at Wembley against Spain on Saturday 22nd the weekend before the semi-final. I was really excited. I'd also given my months notice to the landlord of 172a Station Road and my mum and dad were informed that I needed them to come down for my big exit from London. Smudge, Gibbo, Mitch and Ernie were coming down on the Friday for a night out in Chelmsford in Essex, which was where Ernie went to do his Landscape Gardening degree. They had a black tie summer ball with Beatles and Abbamania tribute bands. We all had to wear tuxedos and I got so drunk I woke up in someone's common room kitchen. I thought I was back in Marylebone halls in London. Then the lads came to Harrow to drop me off and have another night out, stopping over and then driving back north the next day. It was pure punishment but a great laugh until I found them all drunk and asleep in Hannah and Ilisha's beds (the girls were away).

During this bizarre period in the degree results deadzone, I was relaxing at home watching morning TV doing nothing but preparing for summer and the rest of my life. The phone went so I answered it. "Vic speaking."

"Hello Victor, it's Raymond here."

"Hi Raymond, how's things? You haven't got my final degree marks, have you?"

Victor J Kennedy

"Ah regrettably no, but at talented lad like you needn't be worried about minor details like that."

"It's driving me mad waiting for them though. Well, not literally mad. Metaphorically mad. You know what I mean."

"Look, I wondered if you have Alan's and Peter Farrell's numbers with you there?"

"Yes I do, do you want them?"

"No, I would like you to ring them and tell them that your work for The Apple Project has been shortlisted for presentation in Cupertino."

"SHIT!"

"I need to know who's going because the University will be paying for your flights and there's a few logistics to get sorted out. We're travelling on the 18th of July. Returning on the 25th."

"No worries. Leave it with me and I'll get you everything you need."

"It's passport numbers and who wants to travel with whom because there's a few connecting flights at JFK and LAX. The University likes to save as much money as possible."

"I understand. I'll bring it all into college tomorrow. Thanks Raymond. Great news eh?"

"Very good news indeed. It is the culmination of all the hard work but you still need to do more but we'll shape it more in the five days you have on site with the Advanced Technology Group. See you tomorrow. And well done Victor."

"Thank you Raymond. You taught us everything. See you tomorrow." I put the phone down and started jumping around the room and yelling to myself. I was going to Silicon Valley, where it all happens. I would not have had this opportunity had I not dropped out last year. It's another positive thing to hold on to for strength, the fact that life sometimes seems to have put you at a disadvantage but then along comes an unexpected benefit out of all the pain and striving. One door closes, another one opens.

Mad in England - A memoir

I called Alan and Peter, who were equally delighted. They confirmed receiving an email from Sofia which I was apparently Cc'd on. Next day, England's semi-final vs the Germans, I got the info to Raymond and checked my in-box at University.

Date: Mon, 24 Jun 1996 10:29:47 -0700
To: Raymond Beattie
From: Sofia Gretchen
Subject: Apple Project 1996 Submission Date and Travel needs
Cc: Victor Kennedy, Alan Kirkby, Peter Farrell
MIME-Version: 1.0
Status:

Deadline
The deadline for submission is 1st July. Apple needs to have your video and documentation by then. So perhaps you should make your actual deadline 28th to allow for getting the stuff to America safely – I strongly suggest you use a courier like Federal Express to guarantee arrival.

Flights
Emily is about to book the flights – she can make arrangements for extending people's stay and may be able to make stopover arrangements in New York. But you must send her the details of who will be going, and the exact dates you want to leave, arrive and return for all flights.

Please try and send the information on who is flying and when, today or tomorrow.

Thanks a lot.

Sofia

Victor J Kennedy

All preparations for travelling to California were practically complete. Now I shifted the focus of my attention to my degree results. The day had finally arrived. My alarm went off at 8:30 to give me a good hour to get to college without rushing. I put on the radio and 'Lifted' by The Lighthouse Family was playing. I took a shower, ate some bran flakes and headed out into the morning sunshine.

The final semester results were due to be posted on the outside of Shirley Armstead's office, which was tightly knitted together with the housing office, next to the new lift shaft that had been erected during the campus improvements. That was another thing I was glad to see come to an end, having lived on the building site that turned my 'shit-hole' second choice Tech college into "the largest Media Lab in Europe." The Queen had opened it during the first semester before I returned to London. This open space really felt like it was going to be something. Somewhere that inspires young people. Mind you, whoever had the decision to put everybody's final results on that office wall was an idiot. When I arrived there was a queue bigger than outside the Wembley toilets at half time during the England v Spain game. People's faces looked just as anxious as well! There was a lot of jostling at the front while people got out a pen and pad to quickly jot down their success or failures. Once this occurred it would start a delayed chain reaction. The failure's made a sharp exit before they burst into tears in front of the inconsiderate twats who jumped up and down next to them with a massive grin on their faces, hugging other twats next to them. I hated all that back slapping American shite. It makes me sick when people have to explode like that. It's bad manners and embarrassing. Try and be humble, it's not like you just scored the winning goal in the World Cup final! Mind you, I shouldn't blame them. I should blame the decision maker who chose such a narrow corridor and foyer. This was the first year that they had posted results in the new building and I thought maybe next year someone would change it to make it easier on everyone.

Mad in England - A memoir

At twenty minutes past ten I found myself at the front. I didn't know the people in front of me and I was ashamed of the idiots behind me, who I didn't know either but I'd had to endure nearly an hour of shrieks and giggles of excitement and anticipation. I could hardly hear myself think as my retina scanned the courses and found course 2902 BA Graphic Information Design. As my eye moved down the sheet of pristine bleached white melotex paper, I read 'BA Graphic Information Design With First Class Honours' in jet black toner. My eye dropped a line to read 03138555F HAMILTON CAMERON DELANEY and then I read the next line under the same column.

09060732F KENNEDY VICTOR JAMES

I calmly went out the doors of the entrance with a smile, into the sunshine and walked at pace to the shopping parade in Harrow town centre. I made my way into HMV and splashed out on various CDs to celebrate my achievement with myself. Some were football related titles because of EURO 96 and Three Lions, others were things I'd wanted for ages. I got the Simply Red latest album and another was The Lighthouse Family album. I took them home and stood in my bedroom next to the double glazed window staring out at the Station Road traffic while Ocean Drive played full blast and on repeat from my old faithful Panasonic XBS. I have to say that being there in that window, above that Chinese Restaurant, looking out onto a sunny afternoon high street, opposite Spud-U-Like, while hearing that tune was the happiest moment of my life so far. Hopefully when my children are born or during my wedding day I'll be as equally happy but for me, having gone through what I'd put in front of myself, that single thirty minutes was the top of the mountain. Then I shared my news with the one special person who endured my pain with me and helped me back on my feet over the last eighteen months. I rang my mum.

Victor J Kennedy

All the cards and emails started flooding in over the next few days.

What a great achievement Victor, Well done!
Now I'll have to buy cakes all round for this greedy lot at work.
Look forward to seeing you soon.
Love mum & Crinkly Bottom

Date: Fri, 12 Jul 1996 17:12:23 -0000
To: Victor Kennedy
From: Noel Palmer
Subject: Well done you First Class Student!!!
Cc:

You should be proud of yourself Vic!
Noel

After my hangover had cleared I tried to find motivation to present my portfolio at the degree show. The GID show was in Regent Street again this year and from the 1st July it was five days of utter chaos and a total shambles. I went down there once during the set up and it looked worse than a bric 'a' brac art fair in the local church fete. I totally withdrew after witnessing that. I know I wasn't being a 'team player' and all that bollocks but I didn't want to put my work up next to this bunch of amateurs with they're fucking sugar paper and Macintosh Performa's from 1986. It was laughable how shit it all looked. They should have spent their money on cans of White Lightening and gone for a drink in Cavendish Square instead of all those colour print outs of Monopoly boards and children's ABC books. Embarrassing.
Once that was out of the way it was full steam ahead for The Apple Project. I'd bought some new trainers and jeans, plus a bright blue shirt for presenting in. I looked really colourful and interesting. Everybody would notice me in that shirt. I got a sharp haircut too and picked up my dollars from

Mad in England - A memoir

Lloyds Bank with a student discount. This was gonna be a great holiday as well as really hard work. Alan was taking his video recorder to capture everything and stick it on a VHS for me and Peter when we got back. Peter was going to travel with me and Alan was going on an earlier flight with Raymond. We would meet at Los Angeles airport because the stopover was about nine hours and they would be sat waiting for us to arrive. Accommodation would be at the Cupertino Inn, directly across the road from Apple. It was $110 per night including corporate discount rate but who cares if the University was paying. The journey was not that great as the morning we flew into JFK was the morning after TWA Flight 800 had exploded on takeoff and everyone suspected a missile had been launched at it from Long Island. On the flight both me and Peter were scared to death that another missile might be launched at our plane because we caught the back end of the story on GMTV before we caught the Piccadilly line to Heathrow. When we made our connection after safely landing we got mobbed by American news crews about how we felt on our flight. I doubt they understood a Cockney or Yorkshire accent so we probably never made the news. The rest of the journey was pretty tiring not just because we did sixteen hours of flying in total but because Peter was reading the horrible book American Psycho and describing despicable act in detail while I couldn't escape on an aircraft. When we finally arrived at the hotel we all stripped off and went down to the pool for a relaxing swim but got sunburnt on the first day. The hotel was amazing and Alan did a full sweep of his 'King size room' and the ten million channels available on the TV set, which was also massive. They had a video library in reception that was free so we could watch films all day instead of doing any work. It was also the opening ceremony of the Atlanta Olympics so we enjoyed a few beers in front of that but it was not quite EURO 96 to be honest. Raymond was really chilled out too. I'd never seen him so relaxed, until of course we had to go over the road to 1 Infinite Loop and start getting serious about the work. When I say 'over the road', what I actually mean is over eight lanes of speeding traffic with no zebra crossing.

Apple Design Project 1996 Schedule

Friday, July 19 3–5pm
Student, faculty and Apple 'social' students, faculty, and Apple staff get together for drinks and get to know one another.

5–7pm Workstation setup
Students configure their workstations and load their files.

7pm Free time
Students and faculty have the evening off!

Saturday, July 20 Free time
Students and faculty have the day off. Students will not have access to Apple facilities.

Sunday, July 21 9am–12pm
Design critiques and presentation reviews, each team gets a one-hour session. The first half-hour is a critique / feedback session with the evaluation 'panel of experts', who will have already reviewed the team's submissions (paper, videotape, and slides). In the second half hour, the team will preview their presentation for an Apple reviewer, who will give comments and advice on refining the presentation.

12–1pm, Lunch

1–4pm, Design critiques and presentation reviews
Continuation of the morning's critiques and reviews.

4pm Free time
Students can use this time to refine their presentations, fix things, and meet other teams for dinner and/or partying.

Monday, July 22 9am–12pm,
Presentation dry run, teams give their presentations in the hall where the final presentation will be held, for final comments, suggestions, equipment checks, etc.

12–1pm, Lunch

1–4pm, Presentation dry run
Continuation of the morning's dry run.

4.30–6pm, Apple tour
Students and faculty visit one or more Apple design groups.

6–8pm, Apple technology dinner theatre
Demonstrations of new Apple technologies and upcoming products, and a chance to talk to their designers
over a casual dinner and drinks.

Tuesday, July 23, 9am–12pm, Public presentations
Teams present their work to Apple, the public, and the press.

12–1pm, Lunch

1–2.30pm, Open house
An open house or 'poster session', where students show and discuss their work with Apple staff, the public, and the press.

2.30–4pm, Press interviews
Individual interviews with selected design publications.

4–5.30pm, Faculty roundtable
A review of the 1996 Design Project. Faculty and Apple staff only.

Victor J Kennedy

6.30–9pm, Awards dinner
Dinner, awards, and well-deserved revelry.

I have to say that I was and still am very lucky to have been
fortunate enough to be there at that moment in history just
before Steve Jobs returned to Apple. I would have loved to
have met him but at least I met people like Gill Amilio,
Jonathan Ive and drank Monterey Riesling with Donald
Norman in a Silicon Valley vineyard. I even bumped into
Geraldine Copthorne-Scott in the Apple Shop and had a
polite chat but she seemed to remember Peter more than she
could recollect me. I never mentioned her kind hand-written
letter to me from eighteen months before. Maybe she
couldn't connect the gesture to my face. Maybe they are two
separate people now? That's why she didn't recognise me or
my work.
Throughout our week at Apple the work was battered with
severe criticism and we even had to rewrite our presentation
on the night before the Public Presentations. We did,
however, win a commendation for best graphic design at the
Awards Dinner, for whatever that's worth. We never really
cut it in the end and I just think that's life. I'm sure there'll be
other chances to change the world. For me I was just grateful
to be alive and on the flight back to London across the
Atlantic my thoughts again drifted to Tanya and my love for
her. I wanted to get past that stage so I opened my filofax
and just began writing my thoughts down while Peter slept
next to me. I wrote for hours and hours occasionally looking
out of the window as we chased the rising sun in front of us.
I felt on top of the world so I decided to collect the thoughts
into a letter for Tanya but actually send it to her mum
Carolyn, which I would post from Heathrow airport after a
safe landing and purchasing a stamp.

Mad in England - A memoir

Dear Carolyn,

I'm really sorry to be bothering you again but I've done my best to try and contact Tanya but obviously I know she doesn't want to speak to me. I know she doesn't want you to give me any details of where she is and I don't want to put you under any pressure but I haven't got any other choice. I'm only doing this because I know you'll at least read/listen and give me a chance. I haven't got a clue what or how much you and Tanya have spoken about what happened but you were there, involved towards the end, towards the breakdown. You and I spoke, very frankly in my bedroom about how I felt towards your daughter and I can safely say I have never been more honest!

Not only did I love and respect Tanya but I felt very strongly towards you and the rest of your family. I hope it showed. I'm trying not to start going into any further detail because I could write for days about the subject.

I wouldn't wish on my worst enemy what happened to me last year. Imagine losing control of your thoughts and not being able to grasp the concept of what is real and what's not. Then imagine while you are the most disoriented, confused and scared that you have ever been in your life, you get institutionalised and have your freedom violated then taken away completely! Try to imagine not committing any crime but being locked up and then think about trying to comprehend why this has happened to you! Now think about all that just being the beginning of a nightmare that gets worse before it gets any better.

Chemicals, drugs, counselling, rehabilitation, realisation, humiliation, contemplation of suicide, loss of confidence not only in every aspect of your life from holding a basic and structured conversation with your close family to the paranoid belief that your heart and lungs might fail at any time. These beliefs result in panic attacks, uncontrollable hyperventilating and fevers. AND, this is not some two-week illness, it's an immeasurable yardstick and for some people can go on for years, like a long, dark, cold and very unquiet corridor. Everything I've just put down is about loss, now here's what you gain!

I've gained a strange sense of respect and silence from my close friends. It's almost an uncomfortable silence sometimes. They have never treated me the same since, and I don't know if ever they will? I no longer feel 100% pure in their eyes, I am lowered in their agendas and hierarchies, like I've been bent, torn or scorched. Never as good as before! Everything that happened last year has altered our relationships. They seem crooked, even askew and sometimes false-hearted to the point where it becomes a sham.

As for friends that are not so close, the situation is amplified and I find I have to break the ice again. People take a step back from you when they've heard you had a 'nervous breakdown'. As for people on the periphery who were around college last year and still there now, well I've gained courage to be able to deal with comments, cruel jokes and careless gossip that I've been unlucky enough to experience. You find you have to live your life as a dilemma: Do I tell the truth or do I lie? Am I ashamed or unconcerned? (Even though you are never a liar, nor are you guilty of anything.)

It is such a huge learning process and builds a lot of character and strength (mental self-defence and fitness). Going back to Harrow College has been the second hardest and most horrible experience of my life and at times I didn't think I'd get back to my old self. Now I find myself writing this on a plane back from San Francisco wondering if my life has finally got back on the rails again and has some direction (tread water).

I'm sure you understand when I say that I've scrutinised every detail, reason and option for answers to what happened to me (cause and effect). I've conducted so many post mortems in my head that I've got enough material to write a book. I've also been doing a lot of reading into the subjects of breakdown and burn out to try to understand it all so I can finally wrap up this chapter of my life and move on. That was the main reason I've been wanting to see Tanya, to get her side of the story as she was an eye witness and also a key player in the final decline of my personality and mental health. In hindsight I need to try and understand more, have a laugh about it and maybe become friends again. There is no other hidden agenda behind this. I have a girlfriend of nearly a year now and I'm very happy in that relationship.

The reason I feel compelled to write rather than phone is because when I have rung up (on the odd occasion) I've ended up coming away feeling like I'm a psychopathic ex-boyfriend who must be avoided at all costs. That's not what this is about or what I'm writing for. It's about being fair and having the guts to see your responsibilities and recent affairs through.

Last year I was in no fit state to try and fight for the things I was losing, including Tanya. I've told her before that I hate writing letters because words on a page can be misconstrued and interpreted differently by the person receiving it, especially if you are writing it in an incoherent state and full of prescription drugs. I just felt that now the time was right for me to talk to her but obviously Tanya does not feel the same way.

Tanya told me once that no matter what happens, however bad it is, it will always turn out for the best and she was right! I wish her and Gideon all the best for the future and honestly hope everything works out for them, the same goes to you and your family Carol.

All my love,
Victor x

---THE END---

Lightning Source UK Ltd.
Milton Keynes UK
07 September 2009
143434UK00001B/18/A